PRACTICAL
Skin Cancer
Surgery

PRACTICAL
Skin Cancer
Surgery

Mileham Hayes
OAM, MB, BS (Qld), FRCP (Edin), FRCP (Lon).

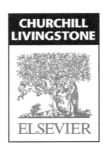

CHURCHILL
LIVINGSTONE

ELSEVIER

Sydney   Edinburgh   London   New York   Philadelphia   St Louis   Toronto

ELSEVIER

Churchill Livingstone
is an imprint of Elsevier

Elsevier Australia. ACN 001 002 357
(a division of Reed International Books Australia Pty Ltd)
Tower 1, 475 Victoria Avenue, Chatswood, NSW 2067

This edition © 2014 Elsevier Australia

eISBN: 9780729579322

National Library of Australia Cataloguing-in-Publication Data

Author:	Hayes, Mileham, – author.
Title:	Practical skin cancer surgery / Mileham Hayes.
ISBN:	9780729539326 (paperback)
Notes:	Includes index.
Subjects:	Skin–Cancer–Surgery.
	Skin–Cancer–Treatment.
	Cancer–Surgery.
Dewey Number:	616.99477059

Content Strategist: Larissa Norrie
Senior Content Development Specialist: Neli Bryant
Project Managers: Karthikeyan Murthy and Rochelle Deighton
Edited by Linda Littlemore
Proofread by Tim Learner
Cover and internal design by Lisa Petroff
Index by Robert Swanson
Typeset by Toppan Best-set Premedia Limited

Contents

Preface

The intent of this text is to detail and teach operations that can be done in a doctor's clinic under local anaesthetic but that can account for most of all skin cancer cases.

Skin cancer surgery is unique in that a hole remains where the cancer has been excised and, somehow, this defect then has to be closed and the wound sutured together without tension. This text details not only how to do so but how to do it best.

The operations described in this book are well within the capabilities of any medical practitioner given the progressive training systematised in this text.

Skin cancer is the fastest growing medical epidemic of Caucasians. Once melanoma or keratinocytic (basal and squamous cell) cancers have invaded by penetrating through the basement membrane, surgery is the definitive treatment. All else is blind, questionable or palliative.

The text moves in a logical advancement from basic, simple, straight-line excisions to more complex flaps in step-by-step, methodical, teaching sequences. Absolute surgical basics, too often glossed over, are documented to provide the basis for progressive improvement, upgrading and advances as well as best possible cosmetic results. No one likes or deserves an ugly scar.

Researched world's best evidence is provided as to margins along with slow Mohs technique, which affords the best results.

Mileham Hayes is a Registered GP and Specialist Physician, having studied in teaching hospitals in Brisbane, Sydney, London and Edinburgh. He was Medical and Skin Registrar at Greenslopes Hospital and then went to Edinburgh and London with further specialist studies in skin. He is a member of the Australasian Skin Cancer College. He is the author of *Skin cancer, melanoma and mimics – practical diagnosis and non-surgical treatments, Surviving the business of medicine, The diet that works* (Penguin) and the HELP series of preventive medicine. He is the Medical Director of MoleChex, Brisbane.

Dedication

This book is dedicated to an increasingly threatened species –
the proceduralist – who makes the diagnosis, accepts
responsibility, makes decisions and does something which,
in this context, is often life saving.

And

to my father G.S. Hayes, a very wise and ethical medical practitioner,
and Sir Fred Schonell, vice-chancellor of the University of Queensland
from 1960 to 1969 who guided and helped me.

Acknowledgements

My thanks to Rosemary Duffy who suggested I write these books, Sophie Kaliniecki who first commissioned this work and the expertise of Rob Kolkman. Dr Ian Thompson for finding and sending me a valuable reference. Alan Laver was able to immediately turn my primitive sketches into, not only works of art, but art that works … and we had fun doing it. I may be wrong but I feel these are unique in the relevant drawings where they show the undermined or bisected fat layer, which is essential in skin flap surgery, whereas most books just show the fat layer intact. Finally, my wife Margo who not only endured the seven years of this book's gestation but prevented my developing trichotillomania or having to resort to diazepam or SSRIs.

I did all the operations, except the split thickness skin graft with compression mould, for which I thank Dr Bill Ansiline. I also took all the photos and typed every word – a number of times.

The evolvement of the Australasian Skin College has seen excellent surgical courses, but also those of the Universities of Queensland and Monash as well as those of individual doctors in various states can be highly recommended. Most countries do not have a cancer registry for keratinocytic (non-melanoma) skin cancers, let alone those proven by histology, but the establishment of the Skin Cancer Audit and Research Database (SCARD) – as developed by Drs Cliff Rosendahl and Tobias Wilson here in Queensland – now does so and provides arguably the biggest database in the world.

Reviewers

Richard Abbott MBBS FRACGP FACRRM DRCOG DA Master Of Med(Skin cancer medicine) Dip ACSCM
General Practitioner at Scone Medical Practice

Steve Margolis MBBS MFM MD DRANZCOG FRACGP FACRRM
Associate Professor of Primary Health Care, School of Medicine and Dentistry, James Cook University, Queensland; Medical Officer, Royal Flying Doctor Service; until recently, the inaugural Chief Examiner for the Australian College of Rural and Remote Medicine

Neil Wearne MBBS BSc (Hons) MSc (Sydney) MFM (Monash)
Rural Generalist Locum, Hunter New England Health

Introduction

Well over 90% of skin cancers and melanomas can be diagnosed and completely excised in the medical practitioner's clinic, office or rooms, under local anaesthetic, to world's best standards and technical proficiency and at an enormous cost saving to both the patient and the nation.

Queensland and Australia have the world's highest rates of all skin cancers and credit must be given to the practitioners who realised this and did something about it. Initially, this saw the establishment of 'skin clinics' but then the establishment of the Skin Cancer College of Australasia and university and private courses with an ever-increasing standard that is second to none.

An overnight 'stay' in a hospital costs well over $1,000 without anything being done. Patients frequently have to see over a dozen staff, from admissions clerks to escorts, to nurses, before they ever see a hospital doctor when they are prioritised and 'listed'. Delays compound. The cost in patients' downtime in waiting and repeat attendances is incalculable and the cost of the hospital bureaucracy incredible. However, for skin cancer, Australian diagnostic and mortality figures are the best, and probably the most cost-effective, in the world and the key, of course, is early diagnosis and correct treatment – usually by GPs.

Diagnosis and non-surgical treatments are covered in the companion volume *Skin Cancers, Melanoma and Mimics* (skincancerbooks.com.au), but this volume details the surgical methods that provide the best evidenced surgical clearance rates as well as the techniques and tricks that provide optimum cosmetic results.

Mileham Hayes, Brisbane 2014

Equipment, sutures and design

It's better to start at the end – that way you know where you are going.

With apologies to Alice in Wonderland

Setting up a skin clinic: essential equipment

Knowing the 'wish list' of equipment that may eventually be installed in the clinic will at least allow for some basic dimensions, a flow chart and better-to-optimum design as and when needed.

Whoever performs the operations, procedures or consultations knows best what is practically needed. It is essential that those clinicians be responsible for any and all basic design and insist that their wishes, based on experience and needs, be expedited and not compromised. Unfortunately, too often medical clinics are forced into shopping centres where limitations of space constrict design and few doctors have the luxury or time to design their own centres. Even in good clinics the operating theatre (OT) is often an afterthought so that lack of space enforces compromises. This then reduces the scope of operations and, hence, the service the clinic can offer its patients.

EXAMINATION ROOM EQUIPMENT

To examine the skin and take biopsies the minimum requirements are an examining couch with a very good light and enough room for the doctor to get to both ends (scalp and feet) plus enough room for an assistant and a trolley. A hydraulic examination couch is a most desirable bonus or objective. Computerised dermoscopy, while not necessary, certainly reassures the patient (the 'wow' factor) and, if wanted, space and location must be planned.

Suggested examination room equipment

It is obviously most efficient to arrange the following items in a logical, systematic way that enhances work flow:

1. Couch + steps
2. Pillow, pillow slips, fresh covers ('blueys')
3. Light (LED preferable)
4. Loupe
5. Dermatoscope
6. Computerised dermatoscope
7. Trolley
8. Insulin syringes/needles or equivalent
9. Local anaesthetic (with adrenaline)
10. Biopsy punches, biopsy blades
11. Adson non-toothed forceps, Adson toothed forceps, jeweller's forceps
12. Stitch cutters
13. Disposable scalpels, 11 blades
14. Gauze swabs, alcohol swabs
15. Dressings
16. Liquid nitrogen (and secure mount)
17. Hyfrecator
18. Curettes
19. Surgical pen/Sharpie
20. Waterproof medium pen
21. Disposable gowns
22. Camera

Most clinics have a combined consultation/examination room where biopsies, cryosurgery or procedures not requiring suturing are done. This, however, traps the medical practitioner into having to wait while the patient undresses which, especially with the elderly, can be a considerable time. (The author's own survey of over 300 patients found the average time to undress and dress was approximately 3 minutes, which translates to 90 minutes per day if 30 patients are seen.) This time could be better used examining patients and finding their melanomas. Thus, having a separate room where staff can initially prepare the next patient is far more efficient.

In some clinics, consultations, examinations, specimen-taking and operations are all conducted in the same room, and these clinics would also include sutures and operation packs in all-purpose rooms.

SCRUB ROOM EQUIPMENT

(*Note*: this equipment may be placed in the OT if it can be located far enough away from the table.)

- Elbow taps or taps with electronic sensors
- Sinks, surgical scrub wall dispenser
- Trolley or shelving for gowns, gloves, masks, caps
- Adequate clearance when gowning and gloving
- Mirror for checking cap and mask (if used)
- Rubbish bins

OPERATING THEATRE/ ROOM EQUIPMENT

Preplanning can obviate the need for later compromises. Not every clinic has the space for a dedicated OT/OR but, for any practice performing surgery, a dedicated OT that provides a private and quiet environment should be instituted as soon as possible. The space should be large enough for the surgeon on a castor chair and assistant to move right around the table (360°). This facilitates surgical access and best approach as well as room for the assistant to be on the opposite side of the patient and not crowd the surgeon. There should also be enough room for trolleys and waste disposal. Getting as much equipment as possible off the floor, especially bulky lights, provides more room and better access.

Dedicated operating tables are a luxury but a hydraulic lift table, which is essentially the same, is a necessity. Most operations can be performed with the surgeon sitting, and a good chair is not a luxury but a fundamental essential. As will be seen in Chapter 7, 'Operating', there are long-term musculoskeletal sequelae for surgeons who adopt incorrect posture/access.

Lapped linoleum or impervious floors are necessary so that any spillages or blood can be appropriately cleaned.

The benefit of a dedicated LED ceiling-mounted theatre light cannot be over-emphasised. Substitutes can be modified from cheaper floor lights. A second light provides a shadow-less field.

A basic list of OT essentials
1 Hydraulic 3-break table
2 Chairs for surgeons, assistants, nurses
3 Computer terminal
4 Room for trolleys, diathermy, smoke evacuation
5 General, special lighting (theatre light); emergency rechargeable LED and spot lights
6 Emergency call bell/intercom
7 Clock – wall-mounted behind the patient

RECOVERY AREA EQUIPMENT

All operations should be done under local anaesthetic and after a full preoperative assessment. This should minimise any recovery problems, but a room where the patient can sit and recover is recommended, with:

- portable oxygen, suction, monitoring equipment
- emergency trolley with defibrillator.

Equipment required for skin surgery

The Elephant in the room
Journal of Education *1915;37:288*

Equipment becomes larger and larger, more and more expensive and more and more 'necessary' and, unless medical practitioners dictate where it is to go, it will be sited where the installer feels it is best or easiest for them. This may not be medically efficient nor the best site had there been some pre-planning. Unfortunately, most clinics are pressed for space and, even if it is the doctor's own clinic, often it is the doctor who ends up compromising or accepting this 'elephant in the room'. The message is: don't order anything before you have found a space for it and what it replaces.

CLEANING EQUIPMENT

Ultrasound instrument-cleaning units

Ultrasound units are now considered essential for the adequate cleaning of surgical instruments.

Important factors to consider:

- Size: all that is needed is one long enough to take the longest instrument that needs sterilising.

- Turn-around: a busy skin practice will be performing biopsies, procedures and operations with a constant demand, especially, for fine forceps such as Adson's. The options are either to have sufficient forceps and such so that only one end-of-day cleaning–sterilising session is needed or to serially sterilise on-the-run.

    A cycle takes around 4 minutes. The instruments are then dried, put in an autoclave bag and sterilised. Whichever method is preferred, the ultrasonic unit should match the steriliser; it is a waste of time to have a minute ultrasound machine and a large steriliser waiting to be filled.

- Noise: ultrasound machines produce waves at 20,000 cps, ostensibly above the level of human hearing, but a high pitched whistle can be heard by some. They are, however, otherwise irritatingly noisy and this should be assessed before purchase as some seem noisier than others.

Sink

A stainless steel double-bowl sink is needed to scrub instruments in ('dirty') and for other purposes ('clean'). Good lateral stainless steel wings will provide areas for drying of instruments.

Steriliser

Autoclaves are heavy and deeper than the normal bench, necessitating a wide bench with extra support directly below the unit. They also require a water flow outlet. Instruments are hot when they come out and provision should also be made for a stacking area. Vacuum models are superior.

Distilled water maker

Autoclaves can be thirsty little devils and distilled water units can be cost effective.

GENERAL SURGERY REQUIREMENTS

Trolleys

There are two basic types of trolley: the Mayo (Figure 1.1), which is essentially a three-wheel removable tray, and the four-wheel trolley with rails and drawers (Figure 1.2). The Mayo is traditionally used for operating instruments; biopsy and even operating equipment can be stored in the drawers of four-wheel trolleys.

Tables and couches

Avoid any tables and couches with a complicated infrastructure or sharp or protruding projections (Figure 1.3).

Operating tables should be hydraulic, mobile and break to allow different postures (Figure 1.4). Many elderly patients are orthopnoeic and head/chest elevation makes the operation pleasant and possible. The shoulder can be a difficult area as it traverses three surfaces so that

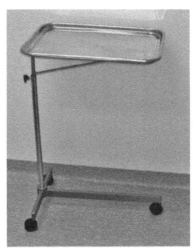

Figure 1.1 The Mayo trolley is used for operations and for minor procedures; its design allows it to slide under tables

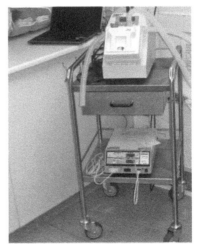

Figure 1.2 A trolley with drawer can be used for heavy equipment or to store equipment (biopsy punches etc)

the only way to gain access may be to have the patient sit up. A three-break table allows for all contingencies.

Hydraulic tables should be the type that elevates straight up; those that elongate can potentially hit other equipment and reduce available space. Castors wheels are essential and should be easily lockable and, just as importantly, easily unlockable.

Operating chairs

Operating chairs are most important for maximum comfort and ergonomics. They should be sturdy and elevate to almost standing height. Draughtsman's chairs with five legs have proven ideal.

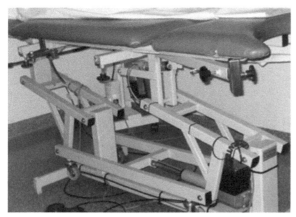

Figure 1.3 The crowded infrastructure and sharp edges of this table don't allow close contact without risking injury

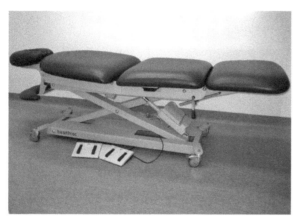

Figure 1.4 This table gets close to ideal in that it rolls easily on locking castors, breaks into three, provides for full sit-up and has minimal infrastructure

Lights

- Examination lights are best wall-mounted as floor models are intrusive and clumsy. 50-watt halogen bulbs provide very bright light, perhaps too bright. LEDs are preferable and will soon replace halogen lights.
- Dedicated OT lights are relatively expensive but an investment in the new LED range is long-term. There is very little maintenance, and they provide excellent soft, cool, shadowless light from every desired angle and can be altered by the surgeon during an operation. After using them it is hard to believe how one existed without them. The ultimate operating light has multiple sources to obviate shadows, is ceiling mounted, has an autoclavable handle that allows both positioning and focus and is fully enclosed to prevent intrusion of substances and facilitate wipe-down cleaning.

SKIN SURGERY EQUIPMENT

Hyfrecators

These are at the lower limit of 'large' equipment. If wall-mounted, they are small and not intrusive but, on a mobile stand, they occupy floor space. The latter, however, is preferable for both treatment/examination rooms and the OT as it can be easily wheeled.

Surgitron

The Surgitron uses radio-frequency wavelength to cut and coagulate and is around twice the size of a hyfrecator. It can be placed on a Mayo trolley but a fixed surface or table in the OT is probably preferable with all such procedures coming to it rather than vice versa.

Smoke exhaust units

These can usually be accommodated on a trolley along with the Surgitron or hyfrecator.

Photodynamic therapy/intense pulsed light (PDT/IPL) laser machines

All are floor units and all take up valuable space.

Automated/computerised dermatoscopes

These can be massive intrusions. Try before you buy.

OTHER EQUIPMENT

- **Refrigerators**: general practices need fridges for vaccines and such whereas skin clinics only need them for botulinum toxin if used. Unless cleared weekly they will turn into a science project scenario.
- **Waste bins**: pathology specimens, bloody gauze, used dressings and such must be placed into identified biological waste yellow bags. These can be bulldog-clipped onto the examination room trolley or opened on a dedicated frame. Operating and examination rooms necessitate wide, open bins or pedal bins. As the doctor is often staunching the blood from a biopsy or some such minor procedure (let alone a full-blown operation), the wide mouth bins one can throw into are preferable.
- **Emergency lights**: every surgeon's nightmare – a blackout! And it happens. Having a 10-million-candle power rechargeable light will get you out of trouble with an assistant focusing it on the site. New LED rechargables can work as well.
- **Alarm/help button**: when scrubbed up, a button that can be pressed with one's elbow that rings for help is needed. A battery-powered model from suppliers who service the hearing and visually impaired has been found satisfactory.

Sutures and needles

A stitch in time saves nine.

SUTURES

Good wound closure requires proper surgical technique and a thorough knowledge of the physical characteristics and properties of the suture and needle. Suture material is a foreign body and elicits a foreign body tissue reaction. Catgut, chromic, cotton, linen and silk sutures have now been supplanted, in most cases, and are not covered here.

Sutures are akin to fishing line or braided thread and what it is necessary to know about them is pretty basic albeit disguised in manufacturers' hype and blurb. Certain suture materials are better for some circumstances such as skin closure, subcuticular, tie-offs or deep sutures. Different brands have slightly different compositions so that they may impart a different 'feel' that individual clinicians may prefer, but only by trying them can any nuances be established. Fundamental practical recommendations, based on experience, are made herewith. They are not intended to be didactic but used as a start-up

---

The ideal suture

No one suture has been developed that exhibits all of these qualities:

1. Preferably monofilament
2. Synthetic
3. Strong, with a high breaking strength
4. Low tissue reaction
5. Low infection rate
6. Easy to handle, pliable
7. Secure knots
8. Predictable and reliable absorption profile (for absorbable sutures)
9. Good quality with uniform diameter evokes fewer breaks
10. Minimal tissue reaction = synthetic and monofilament (*most important* with skin)
11. Sterile
12. Ability to stretch to accommodate wound oedema and then recoil to its original length
13. Coloured sutures on hairy areas make identification and differentiation much easier
14. Absorbable sutures should hold until the wound is healed before losing their tensile strength
15. Sharper durable needles

---

help. Personal preferences will then develop by trying different ones.

The simplest generic name is used here. Some formulae may appear to be quite different but the end product for all practical purposes is the same.

Properties

- **Absorption**: defined as sutures losing the majority of their tensile strength within 60 days with progressive loss of quantity/mass. All sutures, except stainless steel, are absorbed to some degree. Some confusion may exist between loss of tensile strength and complete absorption or disappearance of the suture material from the body. Absorption is measured as the half-life of the tensile strength and not by how long some material may remain (e.g. Monoslow/PDS™ 11 is regarded as absorbable as its tensile strength has reduced by 60 days but it is not completely absorbed until 180–210 days).
- **Breaking strength**: limit of tensile strength.
- **Capillarity**: the extent fluid is transmitted along a suture. Braided sutures have higher capillary action than monofilamentous sutures, with an additional potential to harbour infection.
- **Coating**: wax was originally used to make silk sutures easier to use. Subsequently, silicon and Teflon have been used on braided sutures and, now, antibacterial and anti-tumour coatings are used. Polyglactin 910 uses triclosan, which has been shown to prevent *Staphylococcus aureus* and *S. epidermidis* infections in vitro.
- **Configuration**: monofilamentous or multifilamentous (twisted and braided). Braided sutures are easy to handle and tie, but have the potential to harbour bacteria with an increased risk of infection.
- **Drag coefficient**: friction caused by pulling sutures through tissue. The less drag, the more slippery the suture, the better.
- **Elasticity**: ability to return to its original length and configuration after stretching.
- **Knot strength/security**: the amount of force necessary to cause a knot to slip.
- **Knot breaking strain**: knotting, deformation or clamping (needle holder) weakens sutures by 10–40%.
- **Memory**: the tendency of a suture to return to its original shape after use (i.e. to its shape when it came out of the packet). A suture with a high memory is stiffer and more difficult to handle and its knots are more likely to un-tie. Nylon tends to return to the shape it had when folded into in its packet.
- **Plasticity**: ability to retain its new shape after stretching.

TABLE 1.1 USP suture classification

USP designation	Synthetic absorbable metric diameter (mm)	Non-absorbable metric diameter (mm)
11/0		0.01
10/0	0.02	0.02
9/0	0.03	0.03
8/0	0.04	0.04
7/0	0.05	0.05
6/0*	0.07*	0.07*
5/0*	0.1*	0.1*
4/0*	0.15*	0.15*
3/0*	0.2*	0.2*
2/0	0.3	0.3

*These are the sizes usually used in skin surgery.

TABLE 1.2 Modern classification of sutures

Non-absorbable	Absorbable
Monofilament	Braided
Synthetic	Natural

- **Pliability**: ease of handling – allows adjustment of knot tension.
- **Rating/size**: the US Pharmacopeia (USP) classification (see Table 1.1) provides the standard. Modern sutures range from 5 (heavy braided suture for orthopaedics) to 11/0 (fine monofilament suture for ophthalmics). For skin, 3/0 to 6/0 sutures suffice for most, if not all, operations. The actual diameter for a given USP size can differ depending on the material (wire, catgut etc).
- Suggested suture gauges for skin surgery:
  - 6/0 → face
  - 5/0 → rest of head and neck
  - 4/0 → trunk and upper limb
  - 3/0 → lower limb and back

  These, of course, are modified as the width of the wound and circumstances dictate.
- **Tensile strength**: the amount of weight required to break a suture divided by its cross-sectional area. This provides practical information as to wound support. Loss of tensile strength is not the same as, nor should it be confused with, complete absorption of the suture.
- **Tensile strength rating**: steel > polyester > nylon (monofilament) > nylon (braided) > polypropylene > silk.
- **Tissue reactivity**: the inflammatory response generated by suture material in the wound. This peaks within 2 to 7 days.
  - Non-absorbable sutures cause less reaction as they are coated in a fibrous sheath, then removed.
  - All absorbable sutures induce an immune reaction that causes their dissolution. Synthetic

sutures are dissolved by hydrolysis whereas natural sutures induce a faster, more intense proteolytic degradation and reaction.
  - Tissue reaction is minimised in sutures that are: synthetic, monofilament, non-absorbable, small diameter.
  - Most tissue reactivity: catgut > polyglactin > polyglycolic acid > poliglecaprone.
- **Tissue tear**: fat tears most easily at a force of 0.2 kg; then, in order, peritoneum, muscle (1.27 kg), skin (1.82 kg) then fascia (strongest, 3.77 kg).

Classification of sutures

The USP classification system was established in 1937. The three classes of sutures in this system were originally: 1) collagen, 2) synthetic absorbable, 3) non-absorbable. This has been updated (Table 1.2).

Non-absorbable sutures

1 **Nylon/polyamide** ('Nylon', Dafilon®, Nylene™, Ethilon™, Dermalon™): nylon was introduced to surgery in the 1940s and is the most used suture in skin surgery. It is inexpensive and has high tensile strength, minimal tissue reactivity and excellent elastic properties. Its major drawbacks are its high memory and that a greater number of throws (three or four) are required to secure the knot. Brands pre-soaked in alcohol are available with increased pliability and decreased memory but are more expensive (Surgilon™, Nurolon™). Various colours are available for hairy areas. Two nylons are used: Nylon 6 and 6.6. Nylon 6 dyes better and is more elastic. Some manufacturers use both. Nylon hydrolyses at a slow rate. Rabbit studies have shown that buried nylon retains 89% of its tensile strength at 1 year and 72% by 2 years, when degradation apparently stabilises, and retains approximately two-thirds of its original strength after 11 years. Thus, nylon could be classified as a very slowly absorbable suture. Its stability is due to gradual encapsulation by fibrous connective tissue.

2 **Polypropylene** (Prolene™, Surgilene, Surgipro™, Premilene™): polypropylene was touted to replace nylon as it is the smoothest suture surface ever, more pliable for handling and knotting than nylon with better control of stretching (extending to 30%). It is a flexible monofilament that is extremely inert with tensile strength as long as 2 years. It is especially

useful for subcuticular closures as its smooth surface, slippery lack of friction and low adherence (it does not stick to tissues) mean it can be sutured and then withdrawn easily from wounds, even after several weeks. This characteristic compromises knot security and extra throws are required. It stretches to accommodate wound oedema but remains deformed and loose when wound oedema recedes. A disadvantage is that it costs more. Surgipro II is claimed to have increased resistance to fraying with less drag, making it ideal for continuous suture closure.

Polyvinylidene fluoride (Radene™) was developed for procedures where increased contrast is required. It is a yellow suture thread that maintains all of the characteristics of the Vilene suture material.

3 **Polyester** (Ethibond™, Ethiflex®, Mersilene™, Dacron): braided polyester sutures were designed to provide the same high tensile strength and low tissue reactivity as monofilament sutures but with the added advantage of better handling and increased knot security. Mersilene and Dacron are uncoated, braided polyesters with high coefficients of friction that cause considerable tissue drag. Ethibond and TiCron™ are coated with silicon or polybutylate to minimise this problem. The relatively higher cost of these materials and the fact that the coating may 'crack' and the dislodged silicon may cause tissue reaction after the knots are tied prevent them from being frequently used, especially in skin surgery.

4 **Polybutester** (Dyloc™, Novafil™): polybutester is one of the more recent developments. Its most significant and unique property is its elasticity (sutures have the ability to elongate 50% of their length at loads of only 25% of their knot-break levels whereas nylon elongates only 25%). It is also claimed to be stronger, less stiff and induces less tissue drag than either nylon or polypropylene. This controlled elasticity at low loads has the clinical advantage of stretching with wound oedema yet restoring tension when oedema subsides, ensuring margin apposition. This property decreases the potential for suture cut-through and suture marks. It is more expensive than nylon costing approximately the same as polypropylene.

Despite its touted benefits, practice is needed to use it and some surgeons don't like it. Care must be taken not to stretch it while suturing to prevent recoil and puckering.

5 **Hexofluoropropylene-VDF** (Pronova™): Pronova is a new polymer monofilament with a very low coefficient of friction with few reports for skin use.

Refer to Table 1.3 for a summary of non-absorbable skin sutures.

Absorbable sutures

The development of synthetic substitutes for collagen sutures began in the 1960s resulting in the development of the polyglycolic acid sutures. Whereas catgut is absorbed by proteolytic degradation, synthetics are absorbed by hydrolysis, which reduces the inflammatory response. A little realised sequela of this is that, if absorbable sutures spit or surface, they are then not hydrolysed and therefore are not absorbed and must be removed. Braided sutures have a capillary action and are more likely to harbour infection than smooth monofilament. Since October 2007, plain and chromic catgut are no longer recognised by the regulatory bodies in Australia and Europe and synthetic alternatives are recommended. It should be noted that loss of even all tensile strength does not mean complete absorption or disappearance of the material from the body. 50% less tensile strength is usually taken as still providing wound support.

1 **Catgut**: plain and chromic are not used anymore because the newer synthetics have less tissue reaction, are more predictable and offer individual advantages. But they serve as a reference standard.

Braided sutures

2 **Polyglycolide or polyglycolic acid** (PGA; Dexon™, Safil®, PolySyn™, AssuCryl®): polyglycolic acid was the first synthetic absorbable suture (1954) and is the simplest, tough fibre-forming polyester. It is braided because as a monofilament it is stiff and difficult to work with but braided it is easier to handle. It provides excellent tensile and knot strength as well as delayed absorption and markedly diminished tissue reactivity compared with catgut. Absorption is about 40% after 7 days and its breaking strength is reduced to about 30% at 30 days. It is completely dissolved by 90–120 days.

3 **Polyglactic acid/polyglactin 910** (Vicryl™): polyglactic acid is a braided suture with a coating that gives it excellent handling and smooth tying properties with minimal, although occasionally some, tissue reaction. It retains 55–75% strength at 2 weeks and 20–50% at 3 weeks. Absorption is complete around 3 months. Vicryl Rapide is more rapidly hydrolysed to 50% strength in 5 days so it is used where short-term support only is wanted, such as the face, or in general soft tissue deep suture tissue approximation to close dead space and reduce wound tension or to tie off bleeders. Spitting can be a problem when superficial.

⚠	WARNING	⚠

When used in skin surgery, the dyed form can sometimes be seen beneath the skin surface.

Buried Vicryl or Dexon™ sutures may occasionally be extruded or 'spit' through the suture line.

TABLE 1.3 Characteristics of commonest non-absorbable skin sutures

Material	Brand name (manufacturer)	Uses	Memory	Handling	Knots	Strength	Drag	Reac-tivity	Colour(s)
Nylon (Monofilament)	Nylon (Assut) Nylon (Look) Dafilon (Braun) Nylene (Dynek) Ethilon (J&J) Dermalon (Syneture)	Most used suture for skin Skin closure Buried dermal support	High	Poor	Poor	High	Low	Low	Black, blue, clear
Polypropylene	(Assut) (Look) Premilene® (Braun) Prolene (J&J) Surgipro (Syneture)	Skin closure Subcuticular: slippery – aids removal Long dermal support Does not degrade Retains strength for 2 years Stronger than nylon – strongest	High	Poor	Poor	Moderate	Lowest	Low	Blue
Polyvinylidene fluoride	Vilene, Radene (Dynek)	Same as polypropylene							Blue, yellow
Polybutester	Dyloc (Dynek) Novafil (Syneture)	Closure; sub-cuticular but not if wound tension Unique elasticity	Low	Good	Fair–good	High	Very low	Low	Blue, clear
Hexofluoro-propylene-VDF	Pronova	Not many reports for skin		Good			Low	Low	

4 **Lactomer** (Polysorb™): lactomer is a braided coated copolymer with reported higher initial strength greater than Vicryl and superior knot and handling characteristics but with faster loss of strength: 80% strength at 14 days, 30% at 21 days. Polysorb reportedly has less suture spitting than Vicryl.

Monofilaments

5 **Polydioxanone** (PDS; PDS II, MonoPlus®, AssuCryl Monoslow): polydioxanone is a polyester with prolonged tensile strength that retains 70% of its original strength at 2 weeks, 50% at 4 weeks and 25–40% at 6 weeks. Thus, it is a useful suture in situations where extended wound tensile support is needed and complete absorption does not occur until 180–210 days. It is used for deep sutures on the back where it may reduce wound spread and for cartilage repair. Tissue reactions are minimal. As a monofilament it is stiffer than the braided synthetics and more difficult to handle. It is expensive costing about 14% more than Vicryl or Dexon.

6 **Polyglyconate/polytrimethylene carbonate** (Maxon™): polytrimethylene carbonate is a monofilament that was designed to combine the excellent tensile strength retention properties of PDS with improved handling characteristics and secure knots. Like PDS, Maxon provides wound support over an extended period of time but especially in the first 3 weeks, with an average strength retention of 80% at 14 days, 60% at 28 days and 30% at 40 days. Complete absorption occurs between 180 and 210 days, with minimal tissue reaction or inflammatory response. Moreover, Maxon is much more supple and easier to handle than PDS, with less drag and 60% less rigidity with good knot security. It is, however, absorbed more quickly (beginning at 60 days) than PDS II (90 days). Compared with braided sutures Maxon has a smoother knot and an excellent first-throw holding capacity, thus simplifying tissue approximation. Maxon costs slightly more than Dexon or Vicryl with superior strength and handling qualities.

7 **Poliglecaprone 25** (Monocryl™, Monosyn®): poliglecaprone 25 has the best knot strength of all absorbable sutures as it is softer with superior handling with tying, pliability, lowest stiffness and less tissue reaction. It has higher initial strength but this diminishes more quickly than Maxon or PDS II, reducing to 50–60% at 7 days, lost at 21 days with complete absorption by 3 months. Monosyn, a claimed equivalent made from glyconate, claims 50% strength at 14 days and complete absorption at 60–90 (Monosyn) compared to 90–120 days (Monocryl). Recommended for deep subcutaneous dead space closure, subcuticular suture, soft tissue approximations and ligations. Available in clear and violet.

8 **Glycomer 631** (Biosyn™): glycomer is a new monofilament not yet much used. It is similar to Monocryl but with strength retained longer during the critical healing period (75% at 2 weeks and 50% at 3 weeks) and is completely absorbed at 90–110 days. It has even less drag than Monocryl but with less secure knots.

9 **Polyglytone 621** (Caprosyn™): Caprosyn is a new monofilament that is rapidly absorbed with 50% strength at 5 days and 20–30% at 10 days (i.e. effective wound support for 10 days), lost by 21 days and completely absorbed by 56 days. Less tissue drag, minimised trauma and improved cosmesis are claimed with ease of handling and knot tying. Only available in 4/0 and 5/0.

Refer to Table 1.4 for a summary of characteristics of absorbable skin sutures.

Strength

At baseline polypropylene sutures were found to be significantly stronger than nylon ($p = 0.02$ and 0.01). Poliglecaprone was the strongest absorbable suture ($p \leq 0.001$, versus polyglactine and polydioxanone). The weakest absorbable suture at baseline has been found to be polydioxanone.

Choice of suture

The choice of suture is mostly subjective and perceived as operator 'nuances'.

Mitigating factors
- Availability
- Familiarity
- Surgeon happiness/satisfaction
- Nuances
- Tissue (skin and subcutaneous)
- Patient factors (available to return for removal of sutures [ROS], size of excision, potential for infection)
- Colour (blue for hairy areas)
- Length (75 cm for the same cost as 45 cm can halve the cost)
- Cost

Physical and biological suture characteristics
Claimed advantages for one newer material over another are difficult to assess without a lot of use and not all are suitable for skin. A fundamental knowledge of suture properties as well as recommendations based on experience should make the choice more rational. There are, arguably, better products for certain sites and situations and it is worthwhile for the practitioner to at least read or know what products are available so as to try those

TABLE 1.4 Characteristics of most used absorbable skin sutures

Material	Brand names		Manufacturer	Uses	Handling	Knots	Start strength	Late strength	Drag	Tissue reaction	Complete absorption	Colour(s)
	Monofilament	Braided										
Polyglycolic acid		Safil Dexon Polysyn AssuCryl	Braun Syneture Look Assut Ethicon	Tie off bleeders Buried sutures	Fair–good	Fair–good	Medium	35% @ 3 weeks	High	Low–moderate	90–120 days	Beige, violet, green
Polyglactin		Vicryl	Ethicon	Buried sutures	Good	Fair	High	50% @ 3 weeks	Med	Low–moderate	60–90 days	Clear, violet
Polydioxanone	PDS II Monoplus Monoslow		Ethicon Braun Assut	Extended dermal support	Poor	Poor	Medium–weakest	50% @ 4 weeks	Low	Low	90–210 days	Clear, violet
Polyglyconate/ trimethylene	Maxon		Syneture	Same as PDS but easier to handle and higher initial strength	Good	Good	V high	60% @ 4 weeks	Low	Low	60–180 days	Clear, green
Poliglecaprone	Monosyn Monocryl		Braun Ethicon	High elasticity Sub-cuticular Soft tissue approximation Minimal reaction/scar	Excellent (pliable)	Good	Highest	30% @ 2 weeks	Low	Low	91–120 days	
Lactomer			Syneture		Good	Good	High	30% @ 3 weeks			56–70 days	
Glycomer	Biosyn		Syneture					55% @ 5 days	Low		21 days	
Polyglytone	Caprosyn		Syneture	Synthetic fast absorbing								

that may suit. For example, some doctors are using monofilament poliglecaprone sutures for both subcuticular and surface skin closure. As poliglecaprone is totally absorbed, the sub-cuticular suture need not be removed and there is also greater flexibility for removal of the surface skin sutures. Fast absorbing sutures are ideal for the mucosa, which heals rapidly (usually 4 days). No claim is inferred as to the superiority or otherwise of one brand over another but, usually, the greater the cost the better the quality control and the better the product.

Absorbable sutures for skin closure

Non-absorbable, usually nylon, sutures are often preferred for skin closure because it has been thought that absorbable sutures are more inflammatory and that a braided configuration favours infection, and thus these may lead to greater likelihood of dehiscence or an inferior cosmetic outcome. This is not so and some absorbable sutures are excellent for skin closure and save the expense of opening another packet of sutures. A meta-analysis of randomised controlled trials found that there was no statistically significant difference between absorbable and non-absorbable sutures in short- or long-term cosmetic score, scar hypertrophy, infection rate, wound dehiscence or wound redness and swelling [1]. At 9- to 12-month follow-up, two blinded doctors could detect no clinically important differences in cosmetic outcome of facial skin cancers repaired by rotation and advancement flaps using buried sutures of 4/0 Monocryl, then closing half of the wound using 5/0 Prolene and the other half with 5/0 Vicryl Rapide [2]. In addition, 5/0 poliglecaprone-25 and 6/0 polypropylene were used on the face with no discernible difference [3]. The author has used polydioxanone for deep sutures on the back and limbs to then also close with no discernible difference to nylon closures. This technique obviates the need to open a new pack of sutures. 6/0 non-absorbable sutures are commonly chosen to close the superficial layer of primary closures on the face to obtain an aesthetically pleasing result. A study confirmed that using a slightly thicker 5/0 absorbable suture is a cosmetically equivalent alternative to using the traditional 6/0 non-absorbable polypropylene suture (Premilene, Prolene) to approximate the epidermis. In this study, no statistically significant differences were found in cosmetic outcomes of the 5/0 poliglecaprone-25 and 6/0 polypropylene sides of the closure. The majority of suture lines showed no difference at the 1-week and 4-month evaluations with most differences disappearing by 4 months. There were no wound complications such as infection, haematoma or dehiscence seen in the patients. In a study from the plastic surgery literature, wound complications were related to

patient characteristics (age and sex) and wound properties (location and length) rather than to suture materials or surgical techniques [4]. The deep layer closures were usually with 5/0 poliglecaprone-25 (Monocryl, Monosyn, AssuCryl Rapid).

> **NOTE**
> Sutures are absorbed by hydrolysis and exposed sutures won't degrade and should be removed.

Cost-saving measures

Being able to use a single suture type for the whole closure is cost-effective. As there is often ample 5/0 poliglecaprone-25 remaining after dermal closure, using the remaining suture material is a cost-effective alternative that does not sacrifice an excellent cosmetic result. In a previous cost analysis, using a single suture package for the deep and superficial layers saved approximately 50% of the suture cost [5]. For example, if the cost of a 6/0 polypropylene suture is $6, and the practice performs 1200 repairs, the supply savings would be $7,200 [3].

45-cm sutures are seldom long enough, frequently necessitating two packets to be opened. Assut do not charge any more for their 75-cm sutures, which also have the added benefit of being blue.

Biopsy sutures

Short biopsy sutures are available but the cost of the extra nylon is negligible so that normal sutures are often cheaper.

Thread length

Thread lengths are usually 45 cm for smaller needles to 75 cm for 3/0, but Assut make 6/0 and 5/0 in 75-cm lengths for no extra cost.

Winding in long sutures

A 75-cm thread is unwieldy, especially as nylon likes to return to its shape in the package. The surgeon cannot have it flap about to inadvertently brush against an unsterile surface. The simplest technique, when the first few sutures are inserted and drawn through leaving just enough free end to grasp and tie, is to loosely wind this excess needle end around the hand holding the needle holder until enough is wound in to give control to grasp the free end to tie. This is wound around the hand only, not the needle-holder. Practice soon ensures it is not wound too tight or too loose and can be just spooled off the hand to insert the next suture.

Recommended basic sutures for skin surgery

NON-ABSORBABLE

Everywhere:	Nylon 3/0 to 6/0	(Nylon, Nylene, Dafilon, Dermalon, Ethilon)
Face:	Polypropylene	(Prolene, Surgilene, Surgipro, Premilene)
	Polybutester	(Novafil, Dyloc)
Subcuticular:	Polypropylene	
	Polybutester	
Mucosa:	Polyester	

WARNING: grasping monofilament with instruments reduces strength by 40% and leads to breakages.

ABSORBABLE

Poliglecaprone 25	(Monocryl, Monosyn, AssuCryl Rapid)
Polydioxanone	(PDS II, Monoplus, AssuCryl Monoslow)
Polyglyconate/polytrimethylene carbonate	(Maxon)

ESSENTIALLY

Nylon gives a very good result, even on the face, but polypropylene offers an alternative.

Polybutester can offer advantages where swelling and oedema are likely.

Polypropylene is to be preferred for subcuticular sutures to be removed.

Absorbable deep suture thread can be used to close skin to save opening a new separate pack. Poliglecaprone can be used but it too should be removed. If, however, it breaks under the skin it will eventually be absorbed as it is absorbed by hydrolysis.

Exposed 'absorbable' sutures are not absorbed/degraded – they are only 'absorbed' by hydrolysis. When exposed to the air, they have to be removed.

Deep sutures are usually only needed on the back to minimise scar spread but should be used anywhere there is a wide deficit where skin sutures only would result in too much wound edge tension. The only trial to demonstrate reduced scar spread was done on polydioxanone but polymethylene may promise the same.

Ensure any braided sutures are deep as, if superficial, they tend to spit.

Braided sutures should be used to tie off bleeders as they provide better knot security.

SUITABLE FOR SKIN SURGERY
All are synthetic monofilaments:

1	Nylon	(Ethilon, Dafilon, Dermalon, Nylene, Monosof™)
2	Polypropylene	(Prolene, Surgilene, Surgipro, Vilene)
3	Polybutester	(Novafil, Dyloc)
4	Poliglecaprone	(Monocryl, Monosyn)
5	Polytrimethylene carbonate	(Maxon)
6	Polydioxanone	(PDS II, Monoplus, AssuCryl Monoslow, Monodek®)

CLAIMED EQUIVALENT SUTURE CHARACTERISTICS
Monocryl, Monosyn
Prolene, Vilene, Radene
PDS II, Monoplus, MonoSlow

TYING BLEEDERS
Braided threads are preferred as the knots are less likely to slip.

1	Lactomer	Polysorb
2	Polyglactic acid	Vicryl
3	Polyglycolic acid	Safil, Dexon

Recommended basic sutures for skin surgery continued

BAD CHOICES
1   Silk on the face (but silk now not used)
2   Polyglactic (Vicryl) subcuticular – prone to spitting
3   Dyed Vicryl on the skin – the purple stains
4   High tissue reaction material to keloid-prone patient

NEEDLES

Needle design, composition and production have progressed significantly since the 1960s with improved stainless steel amalgams creating a tougher and hence sharper needle. Cheaper needles bend more easily.

Most often the needle is made by one company and the thread by another.

Sharpness

Most manufacturers provide three needle grades of sharpness with an identifying prefix letter to code and differentiate them. Some of the highest quality needles are still hand sharpened or honed (even the 6/0), but with improving technology this will soon be a thing of the past.

Metal quality

Surgical needles are made from stainless steel alloys with a minimum of 12% chromium providing a protective coating of chromium oxide. Adding nickel and titanium produces greater resistance to bending and breaking.

Needle measurements

- Chord length: the linear distance from the point of the curved needle to the swage (bite width).
- Needle length: the distance measured along the needle from the point to the swage (the measurement supplied on suture packages).
- Radius: the distance from the body of the needle to the centre of the circle along which the needle curves (bite depth).
- Diameter: the gauge or thickness of the needle wire is considered the diameter.
- Curved body types:
  - The *⅜ semicircle* is the optimal needle path for skin surgery.
  - The *half-inch circle* was designed for confined spaces and more manipulation with increased wrist movement.

Needle design

Point

The point is not just the end tip but extends from the tip to the maximum cross-section of the body or it is the honed and bevelled, usually triangular, end. Needles can have the traditional round profile but triangular profiles are now more common, with one edge of the triangle sharpened to cut and the other two edges not sharpened and the side opposite the sharpened edge forming a flat base.

Reverse cutting needles

In effect, all needles for skin work are now 'reverse cutting' which is considered 'standard' for skin surgery (Figure 1.5). Using the triangular cross-section, the sharp cutting edge is at the back, away from the wound, and the flat base of the triangle faces the wound. The sharp cutting edge cuts through the skin and tissues at the back, furthest away from the wound. If the surgeon's palm faces the wound, a reverse cutting needle has its sharp cutting edge at the dorsum of the hand. The advantages are obvious in that the wound edges being pulled together have not been cut by a thin sharp edge, which would be more likely to initiate a tear.

Cutting needles

The cutting sharp edge of the needle triangle faces the wound (see Figure 1.5). This type is now mostly or only used for tough tissues.

Taper needles

Taper needles are essentially pointed cones with no cutting edge(s). They are used for fragile skin, especially in the elderly or those with friable skin such as patients on steroids.

Body of the needle

This part of the needle incorporates most of the curved needle length and is where the needle-holder should grab.

Swage

The thread inserts or swages to the needle either by cutting a channel or boring a hole in the needle shank or neck and then crimping them together:

- Drill swage: material is removed from the needle end (sometimes with a laser) and the needle is crimped over the suture. The diameter of the drill swage is less than the diameter of the needle body.

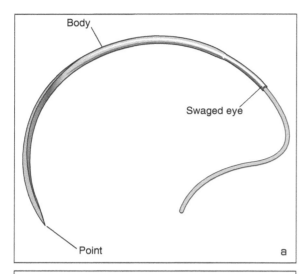

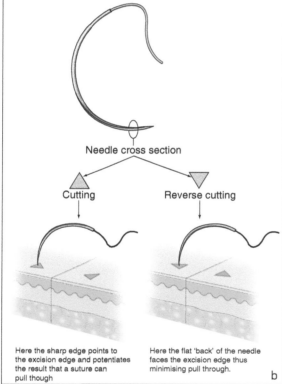

Here the sharp edge points to the excision edge and potentiates the result that a suture can pull though

Here the flat 'back' of the needle faces the excision edge thus minimising pull through.

b

Figure 1.5 Needle designs

a ⅜ Reverse cutting needles are usual for skin; blue thread helps locate sutures in hairy areas. **b** Comparison of needle shapes and cutting and reverse cutting needle designs.

- Channel swage: the needle is created with a channel, into which the suture is introduced, and the channel is crimped over the suture to secure it in place. The diameter of the channel swage is greater than the diameter of the needle body.

TABLE 1.5 USP needle pull specifications

USP suture size	Average minimum (kgf)	Individual minimum (kgf)
6/0	0.170	0.080
5/0	0.230	0.110
4/0	0.450	0.230
3/0	0.680	0.340
2/0	1.100	0.450

The highest quality needles are drill swaged, where a hole is bored in the needle to fit the diameter of the thread. The diameter of the body of the needle is then greater than this crimped shank. As wound healing is enhanced by minimising the suture hole, this design is preferred. When the needle has a channel that is crimped over the thread, the diameter of the shank is greater than the needle body, thus making a larger hole than is necessary or that the surgeon may suspect.

USP needle pull specifications

Needles may be permanently swaged to the suture or may be designed to come off the suture with a sharp straight tug (see Table 1.5). Most needles used for skin can be pulled off this way. This is recommended so that just the needle can be placed in the sharps bin without a suture thread hanging out.

Needle coating

Silicone coatings permit easier tissue passage and reduce the force needed to make initial tissue penetration and the friction as the needle passes through the tissue.

> **NOTE**
> A nickel-titanium, drill swaged, sharpest point needle represents the highest quality.

Suggested needle sizes

Various manufacturers have different identifying codes for sizes, but the most practical is the size in mm printed on the packet, and most manufacturers also provide an exact profile of the needle on the packet. The length is that along the circumference (i.e. the actual length if the needle were straightened out).

The size of the job obviously determines what needle to select:

- scalp: 19–24 mm
- face: 11–13 mm
- neck: 11–13 mm
- thorax: 18 mm
- back: 24 mm
- limbs: 18 mm.

Suggested needle circumference/circle

Needles are described as part of a circle. The standard default size for skin is a ⅜ needle (i.e. 3/8ths of a circle). For small, usually facial, flaps a half circle can be more manoeuvrable. The ⅜ needle allows for less pronation–supination but, for confined spaces, the half circle prescribes a tighter course.

Summary

A suture and needle may thus be fully described as: 6/0 nylon 45 cm, ⅜ reverse-cutting.

Surgical instruments

It has an exquisite balance, light and manoeuvrable, made of the finest materials including 'High Intensity Titanium Alloy', designed with your performance in mind to ensure the best results.

Standard advertising jargon for a golf club or a tennis racquet.

INSTRUMENT SET

The standard instrument set (Figure 1.6) consists of:
1 scalpel handle
2 forceps, fine-toothed Adson
3 needle holder
4 scissors, small/iris.

But you may also include or have on standby:
5 artery clamps
6 forceps, non-toothed Adson
7 skin hooks
8 dressing scissors (Figure 1.7).

Personal preferences will dictate types and brands but buying the best is a good investment. For the face and other fine work the instruments in Figure 1.6 are recommended.

SCALPEL HANDLES AND BLADES

Every doctor is familiar with the standard flat scalpel handle but for skin the operator would be wise to invest in the hexagonal handle as this allows it to be rotated, or twirled, between finger and thumb, ensuring better control and cosmetic result, especially on the face (Figure 1.8). The hexagonal handle is to be preferred to the round as the round can roll when the instruments are emptied onto the tray.

The small curved-end size 15 blade is used almost exclusively for skin surgery. Size 11 is pointed and good for 'stabbing', as for haematoma or abscess (Figure 1.9). It is also good for removal of sutures, cutting off difficult biopsy specimens, such as on the nose or ear, and for shave excisions. Size 23 blade may be used for very thick skin. Blades are loaded onto the scalpel handle by

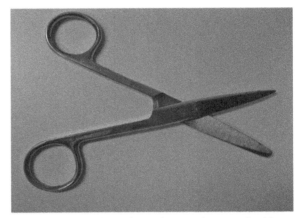

Figure 1.7 Dressing scissors have a sharp and a blunt blade – the blunt blade is placed on the skin to prevent penetration

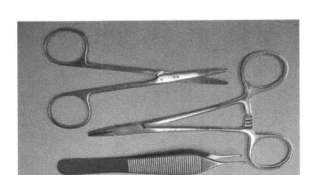

Figure 1.6 Standard skin excision operating set

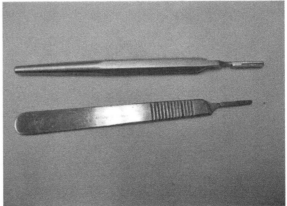

Figure 1.8 Scalpel handles

15

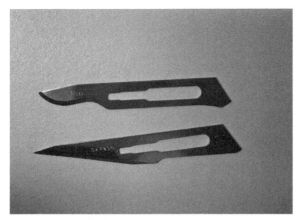

Figure 1.9 Scalpel blades

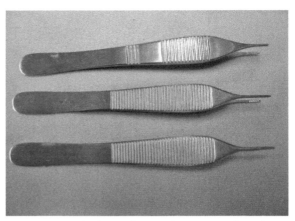

Figure 1.11 The lower forceps have more sloped shoulders and a longer tip, allowing for better vision and finer work

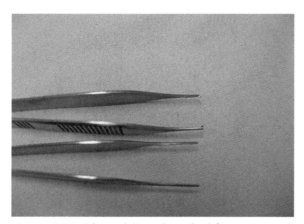

Figure 1.10 Adson plain and toothed forceps – 'one' tooth is best for fine work

grasping the blade at its neck, from behind (blunt side) with the needle holder and using the needle holder to slot it on the handle. If there is difficulty loading the blade onto the handle, it means it is not in the handle groove. Loading the blade using a loupe or magnification facilitates locating the groove.

FORCEPS
Excisions can require both plain and toothed forceps, but toothed are essential (see Figures 1.10 and 1.11).

Toothed forceps
Toothed forceps grab the skin securely but, in doing so, penetrate and leave a mark. Use mostly on skin that is being excised ('skin to go') and minimise use on skin remaining ('skin to stay'). They do not hold the thread well.

Plain forceps
Plain forceps contact larger areas of tissue and hold the thread when needed. They are not good holding skin to go but they don't penetrate and are less damaging to the skin although increased use and pressure nullify this.

Bipolar forceps
Bipolar forceps are used to provide electrical haemostasis/ cautery and are not used for grasping tissue. The electrical current passes only between the two tips and not, as with monopolar, through the body. This ensures more discrete haemostatic cautery with better blood supply to the wound and especially the tips of flaps, thus helping prevent tip necrosis. The tips are placed either side of the bleeding point but are not closed so the spark can jump across. The autoclavable leads fit into most standard hyfrecators.

NEEDLE HOLDERS
Buy the best instruments, but especially needle holders, you can afford. Get the 'feel' you are happy with. The prices increase with better materials. A fine neck just before where the arms pivot yields a more sensitive feel (Figure 1.12). Tungsten tips (Figure 1.13) are preferable and are usually denoted by gold ends (finger holes). All-tungsten needle holders are also made. For fine and facial work even models with the same specification differ from manufacturer to manufacturer.

The needle holder jaws are meant to hold the needle securely, which smooth jaws don't (Figure 1.14). Grooved or toothed jaws are a minimum requirement.

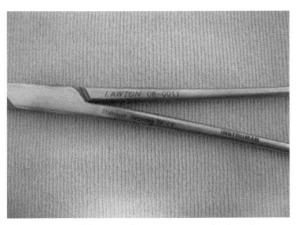

Figure 1.12 Thin arms impart greater feel and sensitivity

Needle holder selection

The jaws of the needle holder must be appropriate or matched to the needle size. The needle needs to be held securely without twisting, rocking or turning (Figure 1.15). It is also important to ensure that the needle holder does not deform a small needle because it is too large.

The needle-holder handle must be appropriate for the depth needed for placement of the suture. The difference between the lengths of the handle and the jaw creates a mechanical advantage for exerting force through the needle point. Some needle holders incorporate scissors (Figure 1.16).

For facial work using small needles (11 to 13 mm) and 5/0 to 6/0 sutures, a 13-cm needle holder is appropriate. A larger 24-mm needle and 3/0 sutures require a larger needle holder. Larger needle holders should never be used on smaller needles as their jaws will flatten, distort and deform the smaller diameter needle, and a

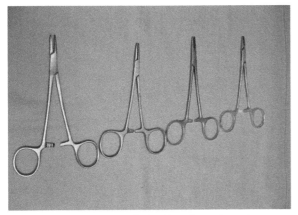

Figure 1.13 Mayo needle holders in various sizes – gold identifies tungsten tips

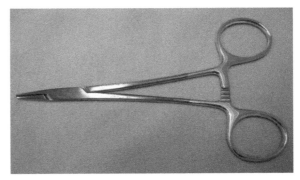

Figure 1.15 Mayo needle holders are most used as they are simple, effective and secure

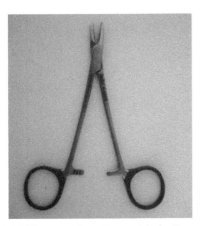

Figure 1.14 Tungsten inserts provide better grip with ceramic inserts claiming to provide many of the same benefits but at a cheaper cost

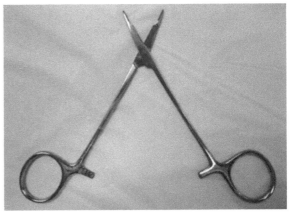

Figure 1.16 Olsen Hagar (and Gilles) have scissors proximal to their tips making solo surgery simpler – once the operator gets used to them (by not inadvertently cutting the thread), they may be preferred

bent needle takes a relatively traumatic path through soft tissue and may cause increased soft tissue injury. Smaller needle holders should never be used with larger needles as this splays their jaws, and they then will not grasp fine sutures such as 6/0.

The jaws of the needle holder contact a curved needle at one point on the outer curvature and two points along the inner curvature.

It has been shown that the sharp edges of smooth needle holder jaws can cut the smooth surface of monofilament sutures, weakening their strength [6].

SCISSORS

Scissors are mostly used for cutting sutures during operations. Some surgeons use them for dissecting, undermining or snipping off biopsy specimens. There are, of course, dressing and even specific suture removal scissors but the latter, while invariably excellent, may occasionally be found to be too coarse for removal of fine 6/0 facial sutures, when an 11 blade or even a 23G needle prove their worth. The problem is that, by repeatedly cutting nylon (especially 3/0), scissors blunt quickly and sharpening services may not be handy.

Scissors may be divided into those with pointed, sharp ends or blunt, rounded ends and are either curved or straight. A curve provides better visibility of the exact area being cut.

The usual scissors for skin surgery are 6-inch curved iris scissors, but the same size Metzenbaum have rounded ends making undermining and dissection safer (Figures 1.17 and 1.18).

The sharp-blunt scissors as seen in Figure 1.7 are used with the round/blunt end down on the skin/tissues as a safety guard against stabbing or cutting inadvertently, as is the knob on suture scissors (Figure 1.20).

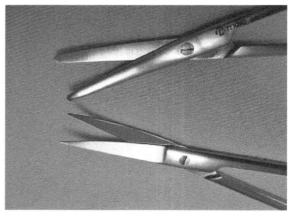

Figure 1.18 Round end Metzenbaum scissors (top); sharp point iris scissors (bottom)

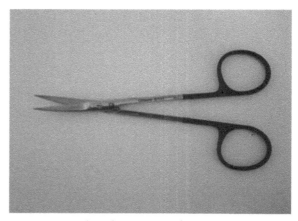

Figure 1.19 Ultra-sharp scissors (identified by black handles) are a revelation – recommended!

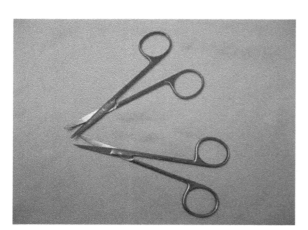

Figure 1.17 Curved round-end Metzenbaum scissors (top); sharp iris scissors (bottom)

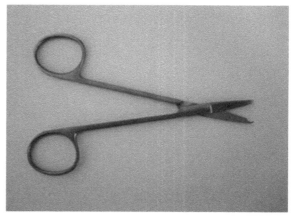

Figure 1.20 Suture removal scissors work – recommended!

Even for tight, fine sutures the hooked end slips under and makes ROS easier.

SKIN HOOKS AND CURVED ARTERY FORCEPS

Skin hooks were eschewed by some as causing damage but they are useful, especially for retracting a flap to find the bleeder underneath (the 'artery of Sod'); see Figure 1.21.

Other stand-by equipment includes:

- Artery clamps – small curved mosquito clamps (Figure 1.22). Seldom needed but must be on stand-by. They can also be used to secure the end of a subcuticular suture to stop it accidentally pulling through.
- Dressing scissors if dressings/gauze is to be cut (ears/nose).

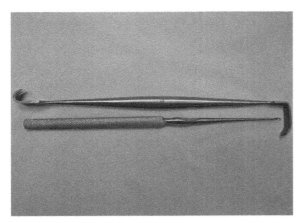

Figure 1.21 A cat's paw retractor, here shown with a skin hook, is also useful to have handy

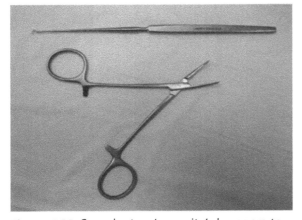

Figure 1.22 Curved artery 'mosquito' clamps are to be preferred to straight as they provide a better view of what has to be clamped

BUYING INSTRUMENTS

Nothing can beat handling the actual instruments to be purchased. Unfortunately, most instrument suppliers are now located in one city and ordering by catalogue has most often to be resorted to. It then comes down to finding a good brand and a reliable supplier. German instruments, with good reason, have earned the overall best reputation. The other irrefutable advice is to 'buy the best'. A good source of instrument information is *Health Devices*, published monthly by the ECRI Institute, a non-profit independent organisation that applies scientific, objective, evidence-based research to evaluate medical procedures, devices, drugs and processes.

INSTRUMENT CARE

Instruments can corrode and become deformed if not looked after. They represent both a considerable investment and a great deal of bother to obtain. If instruments are to be maintained correctly and sterility/hygiene ensured, it is essential the staff member responsible understands the importance of caring for and maintaining these delicate and expensive instruments. This is an educational process. The advantage of a small clinic and having one's own staff is that doctors can have close and personal control over their instruments. However, once an instrument develops problems it should be replaced. Forceps can end up in the sharps bin so a weekly stocktake reinforces greater diligence.

Stainless steel

Most surgical instruments and equipment are made from stainless steel. However, there is actually no such thing as stainless steel. Rather, it is 'corrosion resistant' steel and can rust if scratched, cracked or abused by chemicals or electrolysis. There are two basic grades of stainless steel: 1) one with higher nickel and lower carbon content, which resists corrosion but is too soft to grind an edge and is used for bowls and dishes, and 2) that which is used in instruments that is tougher but corrodes more. Surface chromium oxidation provides a protective 'passive oxide layer' preventing rusting unless broken. This layer increases with time so older instruments are more protected. Scratching, abrasives and using different metals in the ultrasound bath or chemicals at the wrong pH break this protective coat.

- Tarnishing/rust: the key is to preserve the chromium oxide passive protective layer by using the correct cleaning solutions, demineralised/distilled water, meticulous cleaning and drying and avoiding scratching, abrasives, bleaches or any non-recommended 'cleaners'.
- Pitting: always use demineralised/distilled water on instruments. Never use tap water.

Instrument maintenance

- Needle holders: the cause of most damage to needle holders is the use of small needle holders on large needles and then closing them too tightly. The result is that the jaws now don't close completely. This becomes most obvious when fine sutures such as 6/0 slip through jaws that don't grab the thread securely. Looking at the jaws with a binocular loupe will show if they are bent or deformed. It is recommended with all needle holders that the first 'click' be used.
- Forceps: the most common problem with forceps is that one of the teeth is bent, causing the forceps to stick.
- Scissors: scissors should only be used to cut tissue or fine sutures. Cutting anything else, especially dressings, is the most common problem and cause of blunting. The days of having them sharpened seem over. Replacing them at the first sign of bluntness will save inevitable later frustrations.
- Needles and sutures: occasionally needles will pull out of their swage. Make a note of the box and batch number and, if it happens again, report it. Similarly, sutures may break. This is most usually due to the suture having been grabbed inadvertently by the needle holder, which reduces its tensile strength alarmingly (by up to 40%). Check your technique.

REFERENCES

[1] Al-Abdullah T, Plint AC, Fergusson D. Absorbable versus nonabsorbable sutures in the management of traumatic lacerations and surgical wounds: a meta-analysis. Pediatr Emerg Care 2007;23:339–44.

[2] Parell GJ, Becker GD. Comparison of absorbable with nonabsorbable sutures in closure of facial skin wounds. Arch Facial Plast Surg 2003;5:488–90.

[3] Rosenzweig LB, Abdelmalek M, Ho J, et al. Equal cosmetic outcomes with 5-0 poliglecaprone-25 versus 6-0 polypropylene for superficial closures. Derm Surg 2010;36(7):1126–9.

[4] Gabrielli F, Potenza C, Puddu P, et al. Suture materials and other factors associated with tissue reactivity, infection, and wound dehiscence among plastic surgery outpatients. Plast Reconstr Surg 2001;107:38–45.

[5] Fosko SW, Heap D. Surgical pearl: an economical means of skin closure with absorbable suture. J Am Acad Dermatol 1998;39:248–50.

[6] Abidin MR, Towler MA, Thacker JG, et al. New atraumatic rounded-edge surgical needle holder jaws. Am J Surg 1989;157:241–2.

Essential anatomy for skin surgery

The deplorable method of instruction which is used today demands that one person – generally a surgeon or barber – should carry out the dissection of the human body, while the lecturer reads a description of the different parts of the body derived from books. ... Those who are actually performing the dissection are so ignorant that they are in fact not in a position to demonstrate to the students the parts they are preparing, or to explain them, as the professor never touches the body ...

Andreas Vesalius (1515–64), De Humani
Corporis Fabrica

The essential anatomy is that of the head and neck. The facial nerve is the main motor nerve and the facial artery is the main blood supply. There are three danger zones where either the facial nerve or the facial artery crosses bone, becomes superficial and is vulnerable to injury. Cutting one of these results in paralysis or dangerous bleeding. Knowing the anatomy of the danger zones and the layers in which these vital structures run is mandatory. The peroneal nerve where it runs across the head of the fibula is also superficial.

Hydrodissection – using local anaesthetic to blow the lesion up and away from any underlying neurovascular bundles – is strongly recommended (see Chapter 3, 'Local anaesthesia'). The trigeminal nerve is the main sensory nerve that can be blocked to provide total anaesthesia to the face.

Incisions on the limbs are best done vertically as blood vessels run lengthways and hence there is less chance of cutting across them.

Undermining (see Chapter 5, 'Basic rules') in the superficial fat is the 'Golden Rule'.

FACIAL TISSUE LAYERS

The cheek is comprised of the epidermis, dermis and subcutaneous tissue that overlie the fibrous superficial muscular aponeurotic system (SMAS; see Figure 2.1).

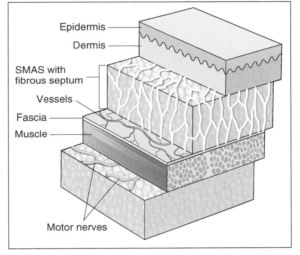

Figure 2.1 Facial tissue layers
Adapted from Larrabee WF, Makielski KH, Hendersen JL. *Surgical anatomy of the face,* 2nd edn. Philadelphia: Lippincott, Williams & Wilkins, 2003.

The SMAS is the superficial fascia of the face and neck. More accurately, it is a fibromuscular layer and is a continuous, superficial net-like fascial layer that extends throughout the cervical facial region. Superiorly, it is continuous with the posterior portion of the frontalis muscle. Inferiorly, it becomes part of the platysma; laterally, it invests the parotid fascia over the parotid gland. It sends fibrous septae extensions into the dermis and to all the facial muscles and thus transmits the contractions of the facial muscles to the overlying skin.

In general, the nerves and vessels on the face run in or below the SMAS. However, the temporal branches of the (motor) facial nerve over the zygomatic arch and the mandibular branch of the (motor) facial nerve immediately anterior to the masseter muscle on the mandible are superficial to the SMAS and are thus highly vulnerable.

THE FOUR DANGER ZONES

It is essential to know the anatomy of the four danger areas (see Figure 2.2 and the box below):

1 Zygomatic arch – temporal
   A Temporal branch of the facial nerve crosses the arch
   B Superficial temporal artery lies above the fascia in this area

2 Facial artery
   A Mandible in front of the masseter muscle insertion where the facial artery crosses

3 Inner canthus

4 Erb's point

All of these must be approached with care to remain as superficial as possible just below the dermis in the superficial fat layer.

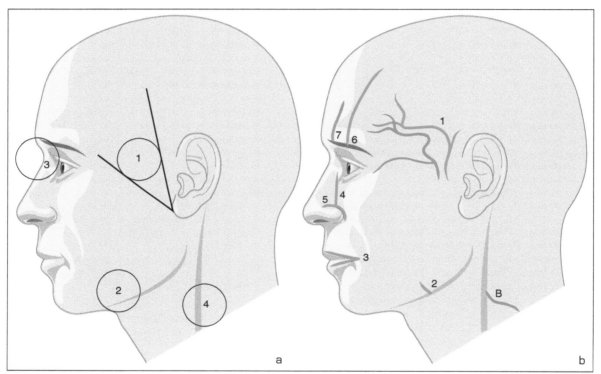

Figure 2.2 The four danger zones

a 1 The temporal zone: may be identified by drawing a *lower line* from the ear lobule to the lateral eyebrow and an *upper line* to 4 cm (+) above the lateral eyebrow. Then a 3-cm (+) circle or rectangle centred over the zygomatic arch between these lines is the danger zone.
  2 The facial artery zone: is located directly in front of the masseter muscle and may be palpated as it superficially traverses the mandible.
  3 The inner canthus zone: the lacrimal (tear) duct runs relatively superficially here. Careful dissection in the fat layer usually avoids it.
  4 Erb's point: the sensory nerves are superficial and the motor accessory nerve is deeper.
b 1 Superficial temporal artery (red), nerve (green)
  2 Facial artery
  3 Lingual artery
  4 External nasal artery
  5 Ala artery
  6 Supraorbital artery
  7 Supratrochlear artery
  B Accessory nerve (green)

Temporal danger zone

Draw a line from the ear lobe to the lateral eyebrow and upper forehead crease (Figure 2.2). Here, both the superficial temporal artery and the motor temporal branch(es) of the facial nerve cross over the zygomatic arch, lie in the superficial fat (not deeper as elsewhere) and are highly vulnerable.

Facial artery/mandibular danger zone

Immediately in front of the insertion of the masseter on the mandible (get the patient to clench teeth), the facial artery winds from under the jaw to cross the over the mandible, lying superficially on bone, and is vulnerable.

Inner canthus danger zone

The tear duct lies relatively superficial in the inner canthus.

Erb's point danger zone

The motor accessory nerve lies deeper to the sensory nerves of the cervical plexus at Erb's point on the posterior order of the sternomastoid muscle and, although not as vulnerable, Erb's point must be identified and care taken when excising in this area. **Erb's point** is located by drawing a line from the mastoid process to the angle of the jaw, then taking a vertical line from the midpoint to the posterior border of the sternomastoid muscle.

Motor nerves are most important as severing them leads to muscle paralysis whereas sensory nerves can partially recover. The recommended procedure is to be aware of and palpate the arteries, if possible, and draw their course preoperatively, as well as having tie-off sutures at the ready. Then keep to the superficial fat and proceed with care and delicacy.

Essential anatomy, danger zones and structures

NERVES

Motor (paralysis)
1 Temporal branch facial nerve (CN VII)[a]
2 Accessory nerve (CN XI)[b]

Sensory (anaesthetic block)
3 Trigeminal nerve (CN V)

ARTERIES
1 Superficial temporal artery (of the facial artery)[a]
2 Facial artery winding over mandible in front of masseter muscle[c]

Lesser arteries
3 Labial arteries
4 Angular artery
5 Lateral nasal
6 Supraorbital
7 Supratrochlear

STRUCTURES
Inner canthus (lacrimal duct)[d]

In practical surgery, if dissection is done superficially, these are the only elements to worry about. The areas of maximum concern are where they cross bone on the zygomatic arch or mandible.

The lateral nasal artery runs in the ala groove and must be planned for (tie-off sutures) in addition to the arteries on the forehead.

[a]Temporal danger zone
[b]Erb's point danger zone
[c]Mandibular danger zone
[d]Inner canthus danger zone

TABLE 2.1 Characteristics of the facial nerves

Nerve or vessel	Danger zone	Innervation	Injury
Facial – main trunk (VII)	Exits at stylomastoid foramen into parotid	Muscles of facial expression	Protected by SMAS
Temporal branch (VII)	Area between lines from the ear lobe to lateral eyebrow and hair line	Frontalis and corrugators	Ipsilateral frontalis paresis, ptosis
Zygomatic branch (VII)	Anterior to parotid	Orbicularis oris, procerus, lip elevators nasalis (OPEN*)	Can't close lids tight, ?ectropion, can't show upper teeth
Buccal branch (VII)	Same as above	Orbicularis oris, buccinator	Food trapping between gums and teeth
Marginal mandibular branch (VII)	Anterior to masseter insertion	Depressor anguli oris, depressor labii inferioris, mentalis, risorius	Can't show lower teeth
Erb's point		Great auricular nerve Lesser occipital, transverse cervical, spinal accessory	
Great auricular nerve	Erb's point:** A vertical line dropped from the midpoint of a line from the angle of the jaw to the mastoid process to the posterior border of the sternomastoid	Sensory Numbness inferior 2/3 ear, lateral neck, angle jaw	Numbness of these areas
Spinal accessory (XI)	Erb's point Covered only by skin and superficial fascia not platysma	Trapezius	Dropped shoulder, scapula winging, inability to shrug, impeded arm abduction, chronic pain (shoulder)
Peroneal nerve	Superficial inferio-lateral to knee where it lies on the head of the fibula	Peroneus longus, peroneus brevis, and the short head of the biceps femoris muscles	Foot drop Sensory loss dorsum foot

*OPEN: **o**rbicularis oris, **p**rocerus, **e**levators alaqui, **n**asalis
**Erb's point alternative: A line drawn from the top of the thyroid cartilage to the posterior of the sternomastoid.

NERVES – MOTOR

The motor supply of the face is essentially via the **facial nerve** (CN VII). Knowing its course and where it is likely to be vulnerable are mandatory (see Table 2.1). The facial nerve supplies the muscles of facial expressions.

Facial nerve (CN VII)

Zygomatic arch where the temporal branch of the facial nerve crosses

The temporal branch of the facial nerve exits the parotid gland usually as a single ramus and runs within the SMAS over the zygomatic arch into the temple region. The frontal branch of the temporal nerve usually has four (three to five) rami that cross the zygomatic arch [1] within the superficial layer of the temporal fascia where they are very superficial and vulnerable. It enters the undersurface of the frontalis muscle where it is then not vulnerable and lies superficial to the deep temporalis fascia. Endoscopic studies have revealed the relationship of the temporal fascial layers to the facial nerve – the frontal branch lies in the deep layer of the fatty tissue interposed between the suprazygomatic extension of the SMAS and the superficial leaflet of the temporal aponeurosis [2].

NOTE

If fat is seen on the floor of the excision, the nerve should not have been cut. Excise and dissect in the superficial fat layer.

Cutting this nerve results in ipsilateral frontalis paresis and the inability to wrinkle the forehead, raise the eyebrow or open the eye completely. To avoid injury to the frontal branch during elevation of facial flaps, the surgeon should elevate either in a (superficial) subcutaneous plane, the superficial fat layer or, only if very experienced, deep to the SMAS.

 CAUTION

Clearly, get informed consent in that permanent nerve damage can occur in this area.

Surface markings may be made to delineate the danger zone where undermining must be done with great circumspection (see Figure 2.2). The superficial temporal artery is even more superficial than the temporal nerve. The surgeon may be well advised to ink these lines before operating.

 WARNING

A glistening white membrane firmly bound down (not movable to the finger tip) means the fascia over the temporalis muscle has been reached and the nerve is likely to have been cut.

The level of the depth of the hair follicles may help when dissecting in the temporal area as the superficial temporal fascia lies immediately deep to the hair follicles and is part of, and continuous in all directions with, other structures belonging to that layer, including the galea above and the SMAS layer of the face below.

Mandibular branch
The mandibular division lies along the body of the mandible (80%) or within 1–2 cm below (20%). This is a critical landmark to observe. The marginal branch lies deep to the platysma throughout much of its course. *It becomes more superficial approximately 2 cm lateral to the corner of the mouth.* Injury results in paralysis of the muscles that depress the corner of the mouth. As the facial nerve runs in the SMAS, excising above the SMAS in the fatty subcutaneous tissue layer is the safest approach. If a cancer invades the fascia/SMAS, referral to an appropriate specialist may be indicated.

 NOTE

The facial nerve (CN VII) also supplies the anterior two-thirds of the tongue, the external auditory meatus, soft palate and pharynx, which are not encountered in cutaneous surgery.

Accessory nerve (CN XI)
The **accessory nerve** supplies the trapezius muscle and damage results in a dropped shoulder. It emerges from the posterior border of the sternomastoid at Erb's point. Although it is deeper than the sensory cervical plexus nerves and not usually affected by local anaesthetic/nerve blocks, it is relatively superficial and care must be exercised.

Damage to this nerve typically results in **foot drop**, where dorsiflexion of the foot is compromised and the foot drags (the toe points) during walking, and in sensory loss to the dorsal surface of the foot and portions of the anterior, lower-lateral leg.

NERVES – SENSORY
Sensory nerves travel as part of the neurovascular bundle and are more superficial than motor nerves. Being superficial perineural invasion is possible with skin cancers and the nerves are readily subject to damage. The resulting sensory dysfunction is not debilitating because of collateral sprouting of nearby sensory nerves and recovery should occur. Knowledge of sensory nerve anatomy is useful for nerve blocks (see Chapter 3, 'Local anaesthesia').

Trigeminal nerve (CN V)
The sensory innervation of the face, excluding the ramus, is essentially via the trigeminal (CN V) nerve and its three branches [ophthalmic or supraorbital (V1), maxillary or infraorbital (V2), mandibular (V3)]. They all emerge in a vertical line drawn as running through the pupil (looking straight ahead). Learning how to 'block and tackle' the face makes life more pleasant for both the patient and the surgeon. The anatomy for these nerve blocks is detailed in Chapter 3, 'Local anaesthesia'. There is no area of the head and neck that cannot be (nerve) blocked. The **trigeminal nerve** supplies the muscles of mastication.

Cervical plexus
Sensation to the posterior scalp, neck and ramus is supplied by the cervical plexus, which has three sensory branches. They emerge from behind the sternomastoid muscle and curl around its posterior border at Erb's point where they can be blocked (see Chapter 3, 'Local anaesthesia') but are also superficial and vulnerable. When operating in the posterior triangle, Erb's point must be identified and marked (if necessary). Nerve blocks can anaesthetise large areas including the ear.

NERVE DAMAGE – ALTERED SENSATION
Small superficial sensory nerves are frequently cut in skin surgery resulting in altered sensation to numbness distal

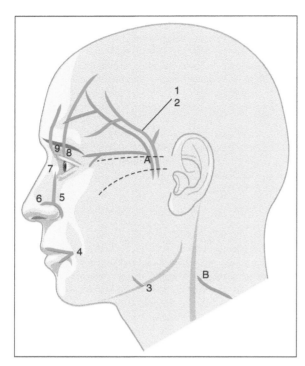

Figure 2.3 Facial and superficial temporal arteries

1   Superficial temporal artery (red)
2   Superficial temporal nerve (green)
3   Facial artery
4   Lingual artery at corner of mouth
5   Nasal artery
6   Ala artery
7   External nasal artery
8   Supraorbital artery
9   Supratrochlear artery
B   Accessory nerve (green)

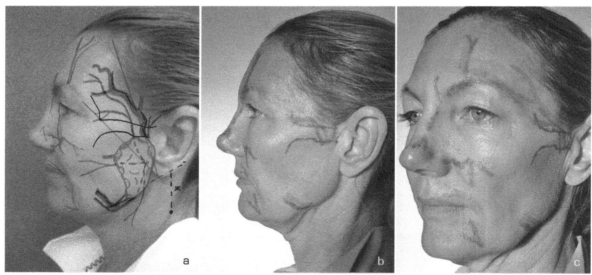

Figure 2.4 Overview of the nerves and blood vessels of the head and neck

Red = arteries; blue = veins; green = motor nerves; brown = sensory nerves; purple = danger zone; solid black = zygomatic arch; dotted black = Erb's point.

Essential components: 1) the zygomatic arch, 2) anterior to the masseter muscle and 3) the three sensory nerves in the mid-pupillary line. The anatomy of the superior labial and nasal arteries, the supra- and infratrochlear and external nasal nerves should also be known as well as the lacrimal apparatus.

1   The facial nerve runs very superficially over the zygomatic arch.
2   The superficial temporal artery has a main branch that runs forward across the temple.
3   The facial artery and nerve curve over the mandible immediately anterior to the masseter muscle. Hydrodissection should be done and great care taken in these areas.
4   Nerve blocks are done at supraorbital, maxillary and mandibular foramens, which are all in a straight mid-pupillary line, but also the supratrochlear and external nasal branches.

to the incision, but recovery almost always occurs from collateral reinnervation. Reassure the patient it will take 6 months to a year. The commonest sites are the forehead (by placing the incision horizontal in a corrugator furrow) or on the dorsum of the hand.

ARTERIES

The vessels and motor nerves that pose most risk for facial skin surgery travel together. The blood supply to the face is via the external carotid artery's facial and superficial temporal branches, both of which wind over bone (mandible and zygoma) to become superficial and vulnerable (Figure 2.3).

Superficial temporal artery

The superficial temporal artery is the terminal branch of the external carotid and emerges between the condyle of the mandible and the external auditory meatus from deep in the parotid gland. As it nears the zygomatic arch it lies just deep to the dermis within the substance of the temporoparietal fascia or SMAS, which also contains the facial nerve, but the artery is even more superficial. It can usually be palpated as it emerges from the parotid, on the zygomatic arch and seen on the temples of older people. It lies in the fat and great care must be taken excising temporal lesions and undermining. It divides into anterior and posterior branches. Palpating it out, drawing it and then hydrodissection (see Chapter 3, 'Local anaesthesia') are recommended.

Facial artery

The facial artery winds over the inferior border of the mandible directly in front of the masseter muscle and it too can be palpated. It frequently has a bony groove or notch and is prone to damage in this exposed site.

WARNING

Facial veins lack valves and allow bi-directional flow.

The facial vein communicates with the cavernous sinus via the ophthalmic vein and pterygoid plexus (upper lip and paranasal drainage).

Thus, glabella and paranasal wound infections have the potential to spread to the cavernous sinus with serious consequences. Treat vigorously.

INNER CANTHUS

The caruncle of the eye has superior and inferior lacrimal ducts that connect to the tear duct at the inner canthus.

Again, dissecting in the superficial fat layer avoids damage to these structures.

NOTE

This area heals well by secondary intention.

REFERENCES

[1] Bernstein L, Nelson RH. Surgical anatomy of the extraparotid distribution of the facial nerve. Arch Otolaryngol 1984;110:177–83.

[2] Campiglio GL, Candiani P. Anatomical study on the temporal fascial layers and their relationships with the facial nerve. Aesthetic Plast Surg 1997;21(2):69–74.

Local anaesthesia

3

Gentility is the best anaesthetic.

Probably a traditional medical observation but taught to me by my father, G S Hayes

For this relief much thanks.

W Shakespeare, Hamlet, *Act I, Scene 1, 1601*

There was a faith healer of Deal,
Who said, 'Although pain isn't real,
If I sit on a pin
And it punctures my skin,
I dislike what I fancy I feel'.

Anonymous

Local anaesthesia encompasses infiltrative and topical anaesthesia, nerve blocks, field blocks and hydrodissection.

Procaine, an ester of para-aminobenzoic acid (PABA), was developed in 1906 and became the standard local anaesthetic but was associated with allergenic side effects. Lignocaine introduced a new family of local anaesthetics in 1948–49, the amides, which had far fewer side effects, and is still the most used local anaesthetic though others have been developed. Lignocaine needs preservatives, which acidify the solution and make it sting; sodium bicarbonate reduces this sting. Adrenaline can be added to promote a bloodless field and longer action; however, it is the cause of most adverse reactions and interactions. Nevertheless, local anaesthesia is safer than general anaesthesia.

The advent of more extensive facial procedures and laser facial surgery has further increased the demand and the need for local anaesthesia. Eight fail-safe nerve-blocks can provide profound full facial anaesthesia, and practically every skin cancer operation can be done under 'local'.

CLASSIFICATION

There are now two major groups of anaesthetics: amides and esters (Table 3.1).

TABLE 3.1 Classification of local anaesthetics

Group	Generic name	Trade name
Amides	Lignocaine (lidocaine) Bupivacaine Prilocaine	Xylocaine® Marcain™ Citanest®
Esters	Benzocaine Amethocaine (tetracaine)	Hurricaine® Minims Amethocaine

Lignocaine is far and away the most used. The only contraindication to lignocaine is if the patient has an allergy to it. Then, prilocaine (Citanest) or bupivacaine (Marcain) is usually used even though they too are amides. The esters have a higher allergenic potential than the amides.

Most have similar times of onset (lignocaine being the quickest) and varying durations. The esters have a shorter duration as they are rapidly hydrolysed. The duration of all local anaesthetics is effectively doubled or more by combining with adrenaline (epinephrine). Bupivacaine is stronger but with a longer time to onset and longer duration. Vascular areas such as the nose and scalp lead to increased absorption and decreased duration whereas poorly vascularised areas such as fat are affected for much longer. The usual advice to patients as to how long their anaesthetic or pain-free time will be is that lignocaine with adrenaline will last about 4 hours.

Lignocaine is almost entirely metabolised in the liver and its metabolites excreted by the kidneys. A history of hepatic or renal disease should be obtained.

Others are used as topicals (e.g. benzocaine), and a mixture of lignocaine and prilocaine constitutes EMLA® topical anaesthetic cream. Some cosmetic surgeons have their other favourites; some have compounding chemists make up their own formula but they are all much the same.

MODE OF EFFECT

Nerve electrical impulse is caused by membrane depolarisation of the sodium–potassium ionic gradient when the critical action potential threshold is reached. Local anaesthetics are lipophilic and diffuse through the highly lipophilic nerve membrane and block the influx of sodium ions into the cells so the threshold of the action potential is not reached, there is no impulse and conduction does not occur.

Nerve fibres are classified by diameter:

1 type A = largest (motor and pressure)
2 type B = myelinated and mid-size
3 type C = unmyelinated and smallest (pain and temperature).

Local anaesthetics block the smaller type C pain and temperature sensory fibres but the patient will still discern touch and pressure from the larger fibres. Motor fibres can also be temporarily paralysed.

LIGNOCAINE (XYLOCAINE)

Available in concentrations of 0.5%, 1% and 2% with or without adrenaline ('plain'), where 1% = 10 mg/mL = 50-mg/5-mL ampoule.

In Australia, following the transmission of HIV to other patients by a surgeon using a multi-dose vial, only 5-mL ampoules are now usually supplied. 20-mL 'theatre packs' are, however, still available. 2.2 mL 'Lignospan' dental vials are also available.

Dose

Maximum doses:

- Plain = 4 mg/kg (200–300 mg). (The product information recommends a maximum dose of 200 mg plain lignocaine.)
- With adrenaline = 7 mg/kg (~500 mg)

1% lignocaine with 1:200,000 adrenaline produces optimal vasoconstriction and duration of anaesthesia. 1% lignocaine with 1:100,000 adrenaline is what is invariably supplied (Figure 3.1).

2% lignocaine (plain) is only of use for nerve blocks where it provides a greater concentration around the target nerve.

1:80,000 adrenaline is what dental vials contain but this offers no advances or advantages as far as anaesthesia or vasoconstriction. Sealed Lignospan 2-mL dental vials are, however, much more economical than 5-mL Xylocaine ampoules for small biopsy injections, usually using insulin syringes. The rubber plunger may resist the insulin syringe withdrawal, which can easily be solved by pushing it down with a swab stick.

Interactions

There is no reported drug interaction that totally precludes using lignocaine for local anaesthesia.

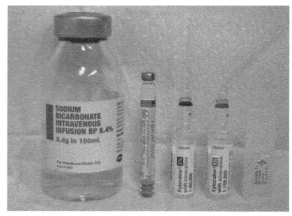

Figure 3.1 Local anaesthetics
Sodium bicarbonate 8.4%; Lignospan dental vial, 2.2-mL (lignocaine + adrenaline); Xylocaine 2% (green and yellow band) with 1:80,000 adrenaline; Xylocaine 1% (red and yellow band, now red and white) with 1:100,000 adrenaline (which does the job just as well); and plain Xylocaine, which used to be recommended for terminal tissues but is now used on ears, noses and fingers

Toxicity

Allergic reactions are idiosyncratic, not dose dependent, and extremely rare.

Know the safe dose and don't exceed:

- The usual 5-mL ampoule contains 50 mg of 1% lignocaine. Plain lignocaine should not exceed a dose of 300 mg or 6 ampoules. (The product information recommends a maximum dose of 200 mg plain lignocaine.)
- As the maximum dose with adrenaline is 7 mg/kg, the standard 75-kg man could have 525 mg or 10.5 × 5-mL ampoules.
- Keep a count of the ampoules used and stay below 10 for men and 7 for women.

The 75-kg standard man in these days of obesity is somewhat antediluvian, and elsewhere a maximum dose of 100 mL of 1:100,000 or 20 × 5-mL ampoules is recommended but reduced to a fifth (20 mL) for those with heart problems due to the effect of adrenaline. Use less for those with hepatic damage, heart failure or on interacting drugs. Refer to Table 3.2.

Toxic dosage is usually the result of inadvertent intravenous injection.

At-risk patients

- Children
- Elderly
- Heart failure
- Renal failure
- Chronic hepatic disease
- Drug interactions (see Table 3.3)

Pregnancy

Lignocaine is not contraindicated and adrenaline can be used in mid to late pregnancy. Obviously, non-urgent cases should wait till after the first trimester. Lignocaine is excreted in the breast milk but in such small concentrations the mother can continue to feed.

Heart effects

Lignocaine became the drug of choice for preventing ventricular arrhythmias (and used to treat President Eisenhower after his heart attack) and is still supplied in emergency injection packs of 100 mg in 5 mL.

Technique

After drawing up the bicarb and lignocaine, the most used needle is a 30-mm 25G, which is then bent at ~30° to facilitate easier subcutaneous injecting (Figure 3.2). Bend the needle with the covering keeper.

Snapping open an ampoule can be quite terrifying to those who haven't done it. If the surgeon is scrubbed up and has to ask an ingénue to do so, clear advice must be issued viz: *'Hold the ampoule with the non-dominant*

hand by its main bulb with the blue spot (Figure 3.3) *on the ampoule neck to your chest, then snap it away from your body with your dominant thumb and index finger'* (Figure 3.4). Sounds pedantic? Just wait until you have to do it.

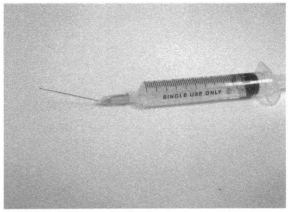

Figure 3.2 Lignocaine syringe with bent needle

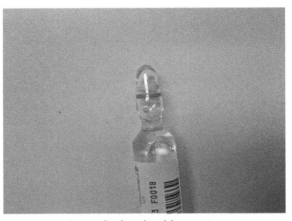

Figure 3.3 Ampoule showing blue spot

TABLE 3.2 Symptoms and signs of lignocaine toxicity

Low blood levels (1–5 microg/mL)	Moderate levels (5–8 microg/mL)	High levels (8–12 microg/mL)
Increased anxiety Talkativeness Tinnitus Paraesthesia lips and tongue Nausea and vomiting Metallic taste Diplopia	Nystagmus Twitching Tremor	Focal seizures Generalised convulsions Respiratory arrest

TABLE 3.3 Drugs that interact with local amide anaesthetics

Antibiotics	Antiarrhythmics	Antidepressants	Antiepileptics	Antifungals
Erythromycin* Tetracycline	Amiodarone	Citalopram Fluoxetine Paroxetine Sertraline	Carbamazepine Valproic acid	Fluconazole Itraconazole Ketoconazole* Metronidazole
Anti-TB	**Anti-ulcer**	**Benzodiazepams**	**Beta/Ca channel blockers**	**Immunosuppressives**
Isoniazid	Cimetidine	Midazolam Triazolam	All beta-blockers esp. propranolol Diltiazem* Nifedipine Verapamil	Cyclosporin* Dexamethasone Methylprednisolone

*Those most commonly implicated as causing problems are ketoconazole, erythromycin, cyclosporin and diltiazem.

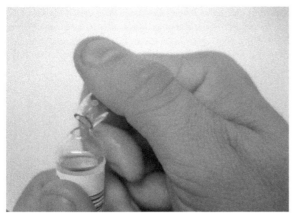

Figure 3.4 Remember: 'blue spot to the body, snap away'

BUPIVACAINE (MARCAIN)

Bupivacaine is classed as a membrane stabilising agent of the amide type. It is some four times more potent than lignocaine and with a much longer duration of anaesthetic action of 4–8 hours. Its main disadvantage is its slow onset of action, which may be as long as 30 minutes. This can be overcome by mixing it with equal amounts of lignocaine. Adrenaline extends its duration. It is available in 0.25% and 0.5% with or without adrenaline.

PRILOCAINE (CITANEST) 0.5%

Developed in 1960 it had approximately the same properties as lignocaine but with less toxicity. In high doses, however, especially in very small children, it can cause methaemoglobinaemia.

Its main use is for patients who are unable to tolerate lignocaine.

INTERACTIONS

The amide anaesthetics are metabolised in the liver. Any liver disease or drugs interfering with cytochrome P-450 3A4 (CYP450) can cause clinical problems. Interactions and problems with lignocaine are very rare. It is, however, circumspect to keep the major drug groups in mind, especially for operations where larger doses may be needed, and to observe for the first signs of toxicity. Concurrent use of the drugs listed in Table 3.3 may inhibit the enzyme and toxic levels may result.

Metabolism of the ester anaesthetics is reduced in patients with pseudocholinesterase activity.

> **NOTE**
> People can faint lying down (i.e. a vaso-vagal episode).

LOCAL COMPLICATIONS

Poor injecting technique is the main cause of problems. Most of these can be avoided by keeping in mind the following;

- Hitting a vessel will result in bruising or a haematoma. These are invariably minor and immediate pressure over the area solves or reduces the problem. If resistance is felt, draw back. Do not proceed if blood drawn back. Withdraw and start again or slide to side (and draw back).
- Ecchymoses are common with anticoagulants and steroids.
- Tissue irritation is mostly due to the acidity of the anaesthetic. This can be neutralised with sodium bicarbonate 8.4%.
- Adrenaline focuses and contains the anaesthetic better, as well as prolonging its action.
- Blanching from the adrenaline usually defines the anaesthetised area but not always! If a blanched area is not anaesthetised, wait longer and massage the area to better disperse the anaesthetic.
- On acral areas shallow injections may balloon the site as the local disperses through epidermal channels.
- There is little or no evidence that an alcohol swab is necessary to sterilise the site but it has become a ritual few can discard.
- Infections should be almost unknown from anaesthetic injections but, obviously, neighbouring sores and infections increase the risks and demand optimum sterile technique.
- Don't let the patient rub the injected site.
- Blocks carry the extra risk of nerve and tendon laceration – see the section on 'Blocks' below.

PAINLESS INJECTIONS

Injection phobia (belonephobia) affects 3.5% of the population in the USA [1]. This can make them avoid donating blood, dental treatment and, sadly, even excision of a malignant skin lesion. Real needle phobias probably won't attend but there is a descending hierarchy from those who suffer genuine vaso-vagal responses to those who seem to feel they must complain.

Accordingly, there are a number of ways of minimising any pain for mutual benefit:

1 Know the anatomy and levels. There are two levels to infiltrate with different results:
   A dermal – painful and distorting, fast-acting
   B subcutaneous – less painful, diffuse swelling, level of choice, slower onset.
2 Have the injection prepared and hide the syringe.
3 Keep a diversionary banter going/ask questions.

4 Use a 30G or smallest possible needle.

5 Warming reduces pain, even when the anaesthetic is buffered.

6 Sodium bicarbonate neutralises the anaesthetic pH and reduces pain.

7 Hyaluronidase expedites the spread of anaesthetic.

8 Skittish or phobic patients may need ice, EMLA or even diazepam.

9 Warn the patient you are about to inject.

10 Reassure them you will be 'gentle as possible'.

11 Instruct the patient to look away [2].

12 Ensure anaesthetic is at room temperature.

13 Gentility and calm reassurance.

14 Place the needle with slight pressure, preferably in a pore, but don't insert.

15 Inject slowly – rapid infiltration hurts.

16 Advance injection through previously anaesthetised areas.

17 Massage the area.

18 For really nervous patients, an ice block before and after may help.

Redheads

The difference in local anaesthetic requirements between people with red hair and a control group of people with black or brown hair showed that subcutaneous lignocaine (lidocaine) was significantly less efficacious in the red-haired cohort, who were also more sensitive to the perception of pain from cold and heat than the control group [3].

SEDATION

Some apprehensive patients may benefit from a preoperative anxiolytic:

- relaxes
- amnesia effect
- reduces vaso-vagal episodes
- minimises toxic reaction(s)
- preoperative.

For nervous patients 10 mg oral diazepam is usually effective but make sure it is a 'good' 2 hours prior.

IV diazepam is even more effective, with the added benefit of usually providing amnesia for the operation.

HINTS AND TIPS

Biopsies

For biopsies where only a minute dose is needed, 2-mL dental ampoules are more economical.

Use needle-on insulin syringes. 0.3-mL are usually adequate for at least five punch biopsies.

Buy bicarb (sodium bicarbonate 8.4%) in the smallest or most economical size and watch expiry date.

Draw bicarb up first with virgin syringe.

Don't inject air into bicarb vial.

Ratio of bicarb to lignocaine = 1:10 (with or without adrenaline).

Operations

1% lignocaine with 1:200,000 adrenaline produces optimal vasoconstriction and duration of anaesthesia.

Use anaesthetic to pump up lesions away from underlying neurovascular bundles.

Bend long needles to suit. Use longest to minimise injections.

Use the finest needle possible (30G).

Warn, place, don't rush but be quick, don't push or force.

If multiple injections needed ensure the subsequent ones are done through anaesthetised areas.

Blanching from adrenaline usually, but not always, defines anaesthetised area.

Wait and massage.

Adrenaline takes 15 minutes to effect optimum vasoconstriction. If you want a bloodless field – wait!

Stay below 10 × 5 mL, 1:200,000 ampoules or 20 mL with patients with heart problems, then monitor.

Don't use more than 4 × 5 mL ampoules (20 mL in toto) in other patients at risk.

Don't use adrenaline in patients on propranolol (Inderal®/Deralin) without extreme caution.

Finally:

Gentility is the best anaesthetic

and

Give it your best shot!

ADDITIVES

Adrenaline (epinephrine)

Most local anaesthetics are vasodilators and increase bleeding, thus the addition of adrenaline with its vasoconstrictive effect is of great benefit as it provides a less bloody field for longer.

Lignocaine works almost immediately as anyone who does biopsies will testify. Adrenaline, however, takes some 15 minutes to maximise its vasoconstrictive effect, so the informed advice is to inject the patient as soon as possible and then go and have a cup of tea or do the other preparation. Most bleeding problems are from the surgeon cutting too soon before the adrenaline has had time to act.

1:200,000 (5 microg/mL) adrenaline produces optimal vasoconstriction [4] and is available in theatre packs of 20-mL vials.

1:100,000 is supplied in 5-mL ampoules.

1:80,000 does not enhance vasoconstriction nor increase duration, but 2.2-mL dental ampoules are ideal for biopsies.

The adrenaline vasoconstrictive–necrosis myth

Lignocaine with adrenaline can be used on the ears, nose, digits and penis. Care should be taken with patients with peripheral vascular disease and diabetes. It is medical folk lore that adrenaline is so vasoconstrictive as to cause necrosis when used with lignocaine for the fingers, ears, nose or penis. Many practitioners still believe this and this myth is being perpetuated throughout medical training institutions and even in current major textbooks. However, many studies support the safe use of lignocaine and adrenaline for infiltrative and block anaesthesia as one recent review article, appropriately titled 'Mythbusters', stated: 'The oft-repeated dogma that epinephrine (adrenaline) should never be used in digital blockade is based on very scant, old and misleading evidence. Moreover its safe and effective use is supported by nearly a quarter of a million documented cases with no ischemic or gangrenous outcome. However, despite the drive towards increased use of evidence-based medicine, this may be a challenging practice to change. The reason that this myth is so engrained is not entirely clear in the face of the evidence' [5].

The author has used lignocaine with adrenaline on noses, ears and flaps for decades without any necrosis.

Risks of vasoconstriction

Impaired peripheral circulation and diabetics pose risks.

Systemic risks

Systemic effects can occur after only 2 mL of lignocaine 1:100,000 and care must be taken with patients at risk:

- Angina
- Arrhythmias
- Severe hypertension
- Patients on non-selective beta-blockers
- Severe peripheral vascular disease
- Myocardial infarct within 6 months
- Coronary bypass surgery within 3 months
- Hyperthyroidism
- Phaeochromocytoma
- Psychiatric instability (acute psychosis)
- Pregnant

Symptoms and signs

Transient tachycardia, palpitations, angina, tremor, nervousness and hypertension.

Maximum dose

The maximum recommended dose is 4 mg/kg (although the product information recommends a maximum of 3 mg/kg of plain lignocaine) plain or 7 mg/kg with adrenaline.

For patients at risk, especially those with angina or arrhythmias, the maximum dose should be reduced and not exceed 20 mL of 1% plain or 40 mL of a 1:200,000 solution.

Interactions

- Beta-blockers, especially propranolol
- Tricyclics
- Phenothiazines
- Butyrophenones (e.g. haloperidol)

Non-selective beta-blockers, especially propranolol, cause vasoconstriction by blocking the beta-2 receptors but non-selectives also block the beta-1 receptors, thus decreasing the heart rate. Adrenaline stimulates alpha-receptors causing vasoconstriction and increased vascular resistance. With propranolol the effect of adrenaline on alpha-receptors is not balanced and only alpha stimulation results with consequent severe hypertension and bradycardia with myocardial infarcts and cerebrovascular events being recorded. The smallest dose reported to cause such interaction was 8 mL of 1:200,000 adrenaline. Other non-selective beta-blockers include alprenolol and sotalol but no adverse interactions with these have thus far been reported.

> **To achieve a 'bloodless' field**
>
> Inject lignocaine with adrenaline ASAP.
> Wait at least 15 minutes for the adrenaline to act.
> Go and have a cup of tea: don't cut too soon.

Sodium bicarbonate

Adrenaline mixed with lignocaine is preserved with sodium metabisulfite or bisulfite (and parabens may also be used) making it acidic and hence painful. These are the cause of most allergic reactions. The acid can be neutralised with sodium bicarbonate 8.4%, significantly reducing acidic pain and stinging. The patient, however, won't thank you unless he has experienced the alternative. Also, don't believe doctors who say, 'It doesn't make a difference' – they should try both themselves.

Hyaluronidase

Hyaluronidase helps diffuse and spread local anaesthetic by hydrolysing the hyaluronic acid in connective tissue.

It is most useful in nerve blocks around the eyes where site distortion needs to be minimised.

The resultant increased absorption and consequent increased blood levels have the potential for increased toxic reactions. As a foreign protein it can cause allergic reactions, especially in patients allergic to bee stings. Its preservative, thiomersal, is also an allergen. Intradermal test pricks should be done. If urticarial wheals occur it is contraindicated.

The usual dilution is 150 units hyaluronidase to 30 mL lignocaine.

HEAD/NECK NERVE BLOCKS

Total head and neck anaesthesia is possible via nerve blocks. Sensory nerves, however, are often multi-branched and so a single ramus seldom presents and multiple local injections may also be needed.

Regional nerve blocks produce anaesthesia in the distribution of that nerve. Distribution and areas supplied vary slightly and any anaesthesia must be tested at the limits of known distribution.

Unless otherwise stated all following descriptions of distribution and supply are ipsilateral.

With nerve blocks large areas can be anaesthetised with small volumes of anaesthetic. Blocks are useful when distortion needs to be minimised and/or where a large area, as supplied by the nerve, can be anaesthetised with just the one injection.

Lignocaine 2% plain is preferred here as its greater concentration promotes diffusion into the nerve.

Essential anatomy for anaesthesia

The trigeminal nerve (CN V) has three main branches that convey sensation from the face (Figure 3.5):

1 V1 = ophthalmic
2 V2 = maxillary
3 V3 = mandibular.

The three essential foramina are:

1 supraorbital
2 maxillary (infraorbital)
3 mental.

These are in a straight mid-pupillary line (Figure 3.6). The supraorbital and maxillary notches can usually be palpated. Here can also be seen where the nasal bones end and where the external nasal nerve exits.

Total facial anaesthesia

Total facial anaesthesia is possible via these eight blocks (refer to Figures 3.6 and 3.7):

1 supraorbital – supratrochlear
2 external/dorsal nasal

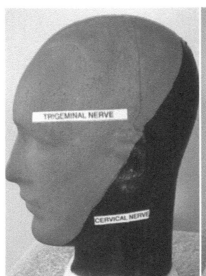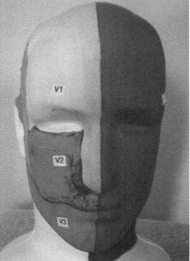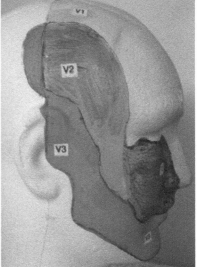

Figure 3.5 Main branches of the trigeminal nerve (V1, V2, V3)

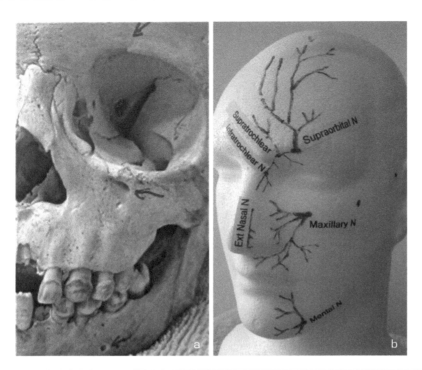

Figure 3.6 Three essential foramina (**a**) and the nerves that pass through them (**b**)

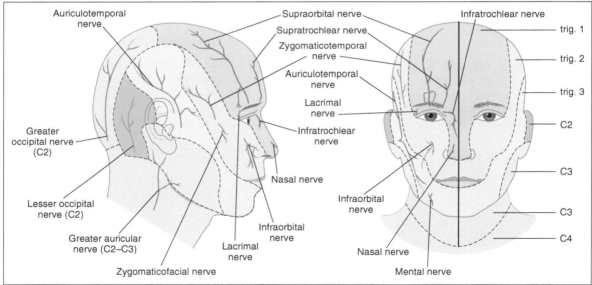

Figure 3.7 Branches of the ophthalmic, maxillary and mandibular nerves
Adapted from Fewkes JL, Pollack SV, Cheney ML (eds). *Illustrated atlas of cutaneous surgery.* Philadelphia: JB Lippingcott, 1992.

3 infraorbital

4 mental

5 zygomaticotemporal

6 zygomaticofacial

7 V3 block (mandibular)

8 great auricular.

Technique
The correct technique involves the following:

- Use 2% plain lignocaine and, usually, a longer needle (30 mm and 30G).
- Infiltrate around the nerve and not into it.
- Do not enter the foramina as this risks nerve laceration and entrapment oedema.

- Bevel at 90°.
- Always aspirate (especially with mental blocks – high vessel hit rate with dentists).
- Withdraw if any shooting pain (nerve hit).
- Check for any nerve damage before injecting and at review.

  2–3 mL of anaesthesia is the usual dose.

All except the infraorbital and mental blocks are through the skin surface. The infraorbital block can also be done this way too. The mental block is done inside the mouth via the mucosal surface.

There are no guaranteed distinct areas of distribution. They are variable and not dependable such that either a local touch-up or another adjoining block is needed.

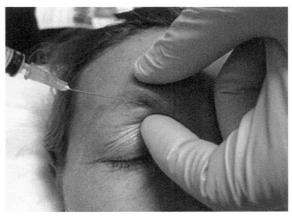

Figure 3.8 Blocking the supraorbital and supratrochlear nerves

HINTS AND TIPS

Studies suggest that the medial iris, as opposed to the mid-pupillary line, serves as a reliable topographical landmark for the course of the supraorbital nerve at the supraorbital rim [6]. (To the author this would seem to assume the iris is in its contracted state.)

Supraorbital and supratrochlear nerve blocks

The supraorbital nerves (Figure 3.7) supply the forehead and frontal scalp and emerge in the mid-pupillary line from the supraorbital rim via the supraorbital foramina, usually easily felt as a notch. Usually 1–2 mL of 2% lignocaine is used.

Techniques

- Technique 1: get the patient to look straight ahead. Feel along the superior orbit to the supraorbital notch. Inject lateral to this sliding inframedially along the curve of the supraorbital rim to its medial corner, about 1 cm from the supraorbital notch medially towards the glabella as this will also get the supratrochlear nerve at the supratrochlear notch, which is also palpable, should anaesthesia in this region also be desired.
- Technique 2: approach from behind the patient and grasp their eyebrow between the non-injecting index finger under the supraorbital rim and the thumb above it and stretch the eyebrow laterally. The needle enters lateral to the mid third of the eyebrow and is aimed at the supraorbital notch (see Figure 3.8). It is then slid under the corrugator muscle depositing 1–1.5 mL at the supraorbital notch and 0.7–1 mL at the supratrochlear notch.
- Technique 3: in some patients the lateral branch of the supraorbital nerve exits through their own foramen above the rim and 1 mL of lignocaine is then needed as a separate injection 1 cm above the rim.

Excess anaesthetic may result in swelling of the upper eye. The vein runs next to the nerve so always aspirate. Hitting a cutaneous vessel can result in severe bruising and swelling of the upper eyelid. Reassure the patient this will resolve in 10 days. Bruising/ecchymosis may result and the patient should be forewarned.

Supratrochlear and infratrochlear nerve block

The supratrochlear nerve supplies the midline of the forehead whereas the infratrochlear (see Figure 3.7) can supply the glabella to the tip of the nose. The three nerves, supraorbital, supratrochlear and infratrochlear, can all be anaesthetised with one injection starting at the supraorbital notch then sliding a long needle medially. Often, the supraorbital notch can be palpated; otherwise, locate it at the mid-pupillary line with the patient looking straight ahead. The fingertip rests on the medial orbital bone.

Bruising may result – warn the patient.

Dorsal/external nasal branch block

Painful nasal tip injections can be avoided with this block.

The dorsal/external nasal branch of the ethmoid nerve supplies the nasal dorsum, tip and columella (Figure 3.9). It emerges at the junction between the nasal bone and cartilage and is easily felt by wiggling the cartilage.

Blockade anaesthetises the cartilaginous dorsum and tip and should be done to avoid the more painful local infiltration of the tip.

Technique

- Palpate where the nasal bone finishes and cartilage begins. Insert the needle to run inferolaterally some 6–10 mm off the midline.
- Inject 1 mL lignocaine (bilaterally if necessary – withdraw and do the other side) 1 cm (6–10 mm) lateral to the midline (Figure 3.10).

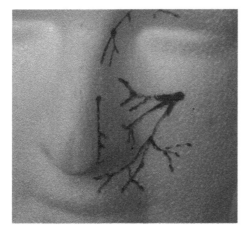

Figure 3.9 Dorsal/external nasal branch

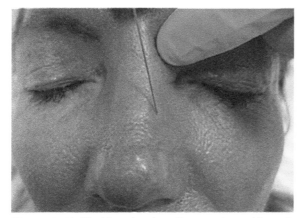

Figure 3.10 Blocking the dorsal/external nasal branch

Note: the external nasal nerve does not innervate the whole alar. A maxillary (infraorbital) block is also needed.

Maxillary branch of the trigeminal nerve (the infraorbital nerve) blocks

The infraorbital nerve (see Figure 3.7), or the maxillary nerve (V2), is the largest branch of the trigeminal nerve (CN V). It emerges at the mid-pupillary line from the infraorbital foramen and supplies the lower eyelid, medial cheek, side of the nose, alar (to a variable degree) and the upper lip. The infraorbital foramen is usually palpable about 1 cm below the orbital rim in the mid-pupillary line.

Technique
Locate the infraorbital foramina 1 cm below the infraorbital rim in mid-pupillary line (see Figure 3.6).

Four approaches are possible; each has its advocates. Three are through the skin (trans/percutaneous) using slightly different approaches (medial nasolabial, perpendicular and lateral) and one is inside the mouth (intraoral).

There may be some alarm issued at entering the foramen, which points downwards and medially. Approaching laterally and perpendicularly minimises this. However, very skilled practitioners do inject the foramen with a '100% success rate using this approach'. They imply that entering the foramen is preferable and that all other approaches prevent this [7].

1 Medial nasolabial approach (provides a direct face-on approach to the foramen):

A Inject medial to the nasolabial groove lateral to the alar in the triangle so defined by the nasolabial fold and the alar base (Figure 3.11).

B Place the non-injecting index finger on the infraorbital rim; ask the patient to look straight ahead and advance the needle towards the foramen some 4–7 mm below the rim. Often the needle tip goes straight into the foramen but, otherwise, the foramen can always be found.

C Inject in the centre of the triangle directing the needle superolaterally (Figure 3.12).

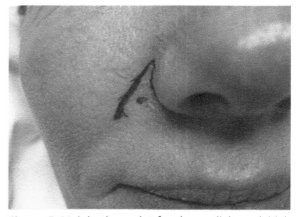

Figure 3.11 Injection point for the medial nasolabial approach

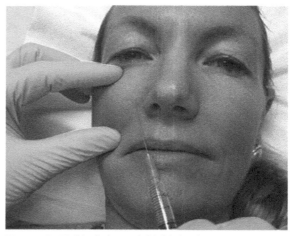

Figure 3.12 Medial nasolabial injection

2 Perpendicular approach (arguably the simplest and most practical approach):

  A Place the non-injecting index finger next to the patient's alar, then place the middle finger one finger's breadth away and stretch the skin between.

  B Inject slowly down to the bone (Figure 3.13). Resistance will be progressively felt. This is a minor variation to approach 1.

3 Lateral approach:

  A Get the patient to look straight ahead.

  B Feel the infraorbital foramen 1 cm below the orbital rim. Approach laterally (bevel); do not push straight in as this 'improves' the chance of entering the foramen (Figure 3.14).

  C Withdraw a tad if and when periosteum is hit, aspirate, deposit 1–2 mL lignocaine.

4 Intraoral approach:

  A This is easier if the patient is lying down or the surgeon's line of vision is lower so (s)he can look up to see the buccal sulcus. Get the patient to look straight ahead.

  B Place the middle finger of the non-injecting hand on the infraorbital foramen. Lift the upper lip up and out with the thumb (of the same hand) inside the cheek supported by the index finger on the outside cheek, which rests on the infraorbital foramen.

  C Advance the needle to the buccal sulcus where the mucosa is reflected to the cheek at the mid-pupillary line and at the apex of the canine fossa (Figure 3.15).

  D Advance through the mucosa to the periosteum, withdraw a tad, aspirate, slowly deposit 1–2 mL 2% lignocaine.

Dose
1.5–3 mL lignocaine.

Complications
- Puncture of area vessels can cause a black eye/bruising for 2–10 days.
- Entering the foramen can cause significant pain.

Blocking the mental nerve
The mental nerve is a terminal branch of the mandibular nerve (V3). Age and mandibular atrophy can make the foramen closer to the upper mandible margin.

Technique
The mental foramen is usually slightly medial to the mid-pupillary line, some 2.5 cm from the midline. The nerve supplies ipsilateral chin and lower lip. The percutaneous route can be used but is unreliable as the mental nerve exits as two to three fascicles, and locating it intraorally by traction on the lower lip is usual and easier. The nerve itself is only covered by mucosa when it exits and can often be palpated.

  Get the patient to look straight ahead. By pulling the lower lip with the thumb of one hand lateral to the lower canine tooth, then squeezing the lip and sliding the thumb outwards to evert the lip, the nerve is visible

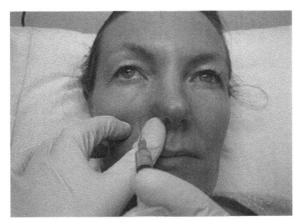

Figure 3.13 Perpendicular approach

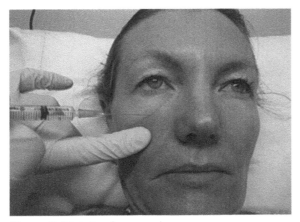

Figure 3.14 Lateral approach

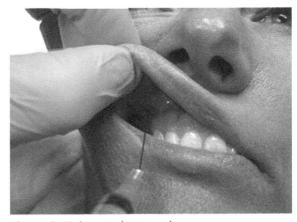

Figure 3.15 Intraoral approach

some 85% of the time as a white band just under the mucosa as it transits to the cheek; for the other 15%, the nerve is still in the same area but is just not visible (Figure 3.16).

- Foramen block: locate the second lower bicuspid or between the first and second premolars, place the tip of the needle in the buccal sulcus and inject 1–2 mL of lignocaine. Aspiration should be performed as a vessel hit-rate of some 10% has been recorded in dental practice with consequent systemic adrenaline side effects. This anaesthetises the lower lip to the labio-mental fold but usually not the chin pad or laterally.
- Mental plus or premandibular block: to block the whole chin an end branch of the mental nerve and the terminal branches of the mylo-hyoid need to be blocked. Do the mental block as above, then move behind the patient and aim the needle more anteriorly and fan out towards the lip just below the skin. Use a long needle (25G × 38 mm).

Zygomaticotemporal nerve block

The zygomaticotemporal nerve (see Figure 3.7) is one of two terminal branches of the zygomatic nerve and provides sensation to a fan-shaped area from the orbit up to the scalp and along the zygomatic ridge. It passes from the orbit through a foramen on the posterior orbital rim to enter the temporal fossa where it can be anaesthetised.

Technique
1 Palpate the zygomaticofrontal suture and insert a long (38 mm) needle along the posterior wall to 1 cm below the external canthus (Figure 3.17).
2 Inject 1–2 mL lignocaine when withdrawing.

Zygomaticofacial nerve block

The zygomaticofacial nerve is the other terminal branch of the zygomatic nerve and emerges through a foramen at the anterior of the zygoma just posterior to the orbital rim (Figure 3.7), where it is prone to being cut when flaps are elevated here. However, it is also thus available to be anaesthetised, covering an area of an inverted isosceles triangle with a base of some 3 cm along the superior border of the zygoma and its apex at the angle of the ramus.

Technique
This is always done following the zygomaticotemporal block by injecting just lateral to the junction of the lateral and inferior orbital rim into a 1.5-cm area (Figure 3.18). Hyaluronidase ensures efficacy.

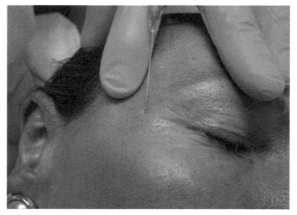

Figure 3.17 Blocking the zygomaticotemporal nerve

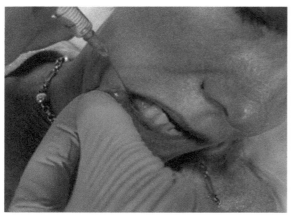

Figure 3.16 Blocking the mental nerve
The needle here is bevel up and pushing at least 1 cm anteriorly out towards the bottom lip and down to the inferior mandible border. Aspirate.

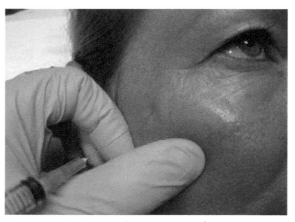

Figure 3.18 Blocking the zygomaticofacial nerve

Auriculotemporal nerve (mandibular nerve V3) block

The auriculotemporal nerve emerges from behind the temporomandibular joint (Figure 3.7) but is best blocked 1 cm above this where it crosses the zygomatic arch and runs with the superficial temporal artery. Aspirating is mandatory. Anaesthesia can be effected to the anterior auricle, lateral temple and temporal scalp.

Technique
1 Have the patient open their jaw. Palpate the temporomandibular joint; feel the zygomatic arch. The nerve runs superficial here across the arch with the superficial temporal artery.
2 Bevel the needle obliquely, aspirate, deposit 2–3 mL above the periosteum.

Greater auricular and transverse cervical nerve (Erb's point) block

These nerves emerge near the midpoint of the sternomastoid posterior border at Erb's point (see Chapter 2, 'Essential anatomy for skin surgery'). The great auricular emerges 1 cm above and the lesser occipital 1 cm below Erb's point, but 2 mL of 2% lignocaine will usually anaesthetise both.

The great auricular nerve (Figure 3.7) rounds the posterior border of the sternomastoid and passes almost vertically on the surface of the muscle then traverses towards the ramus to supply the lower third of the ear, the lower posterior auricular skin, the angle of the jaw and the submandibular area. It is approximately 6.5 cm below the external auditory meatus.

Technique
1 Define the sternomastoid by getting the patient to push against a hand and draw its edges. Mark a point midway between these two lines.
2 Measure 6.5 cm down from the lower edge of the external auditory meatus. Inject into a 2-cm area on the muscle fascia.

The transverse cervical nerve emerges 1 cm below the great auricular and passes anteriorly to supply the inferior middle border of the mandible and the anterior neck.

> **WARNING**
>
> The accessory nerve (CN XI) also exits at Erb's point but deeper to the sensory auricular and occipital nerves. Nevertheless, it is a motor nerve that supplies the trapezius and cutting it results in a dropped shoulder. Always be aware and careful in the posterior triangle.

WRIST BLOCKS

Wrist blocks are particularly useful for palmar operations; the dorsum is usually best done with local infiltration. The ulnar, median and radial nerves all contribute innervation to the hand (Figure 3.19).

Median nerve block

The median nerve supplies most of the palm from the distal thumb to half the ring finger. It lies between the tendons of palmaris longus and flexor carpi radialis

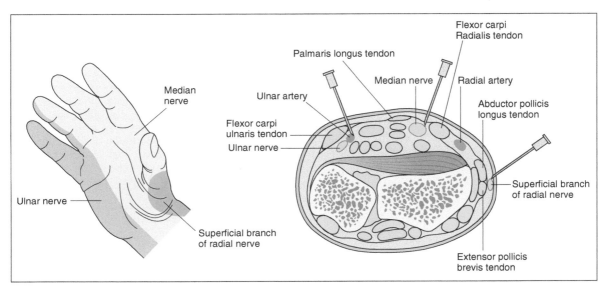

Figure 3.19 Palmar innervation and wrist nerve block
Adapted from Robinson JK, Hanke WC, Sengelmann R et al (eds). *Surgery of the skin*. Philadelphia: Mosby, 2005;50 (Fig 3.8).

(Figure 3.20). Making a claw mostly demonstrates and locates palmaris longus.

Technique
Inject 3–5 mL 2% lignocaine immediately lateral (thumb/radial) to this tendon at the proximal wrist crease and through the flexor retinaculum.

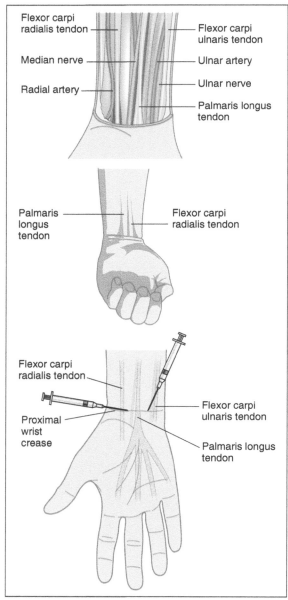

Figure 3.20 Landmarks for the median and ulnar nerves
Adapted from Robinson JK, Hanke WC, Sengelmann R et al (eds). *Surgery of the skin*. Philadelphia: Mosby, 2005; Fig 3.9.

Ulnar nerve block
The ulnar nerve runs under or slightly lateral (central) to the flexor carpi ulnaris tendon, which is best located by asking the patient to make a fist (Figure 3.20).

Technique
Inject 3–5 mL lignocaine at the proximal wrist crease (ulnar styloid process) just on the lateral/radial/central side of flexor carpi ulnaris tendon. Be sure to aspirate as the ulnar artery is juxtapositioned laterally.

Radial nerve block
The *superficial branch* of the radial nerve supplies the palmar surface of the thumb usually proximal from the metacarpophalangeal joint.

Technique
With the patient's palm up, inject slightly above half-way up the lateral side of the wrist but angled down (dorsal) at 30–45°. The nerve is superficial and 3 mL 2% lignocaine should be enough. Its location, however, is variable.

DIGITAL BLOCKS
Four digital nerves that run both dorsal and ventral on both sides of the fingers can be blocked to give total digital anaesthesia. For a bloodless field, a tourniquet is easily fashioned from a spare rubber glove but ensure it is fully removed.

Tourniquet for the finger
1 Anaesthetise the finger, then put on a glove leaving the end longer (Figure 3.21a).
2 Cut the tip off (Figure 3.21b, c).
3 Roll it down to the web (Figure 3.21d).

Tourniquet dangers

Tourniquets are used in hand and foot surgery because of the need for a bloodless field. Once the tourniquet has been removed, check for adequate perfusion of finger or toe. Ensure patients know to look for later signs of tissue ischaemia (skin discolouration or a pulseless, painful, paralysed, paraesthetic and cold digit) [8].

Technique
1 Use 2% plain lignocaine so as to minimise volume and maximise concentration gradient. Large volumes may strangulate and compromise the circulation. Be careful in those with small vessel disease such as diabetics, those with peripheral vascular disease and smokers.

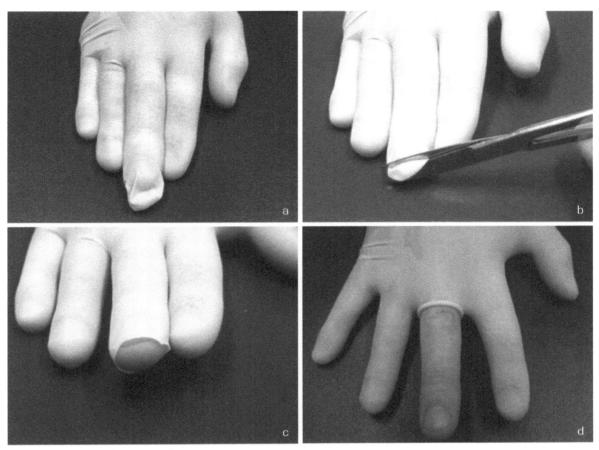

Figure 3.21 Preparing a tourniquet

2 Lay the hand palm down, which helps secure the site and the dorsum is less painful than the palmar approach (Figure 3.22).

3 Inject 1 mL near the web space sloping it at some 30–40°, withdraw and push slowly to the palm, depositing another 1 mL around the inferior border of the flexor tendons.

4 Repeat on the other side.

ANKLE BLOCKS

Peroneal block
Refer to Figures 3.23 and 3.24.

FIELD BLOCKS
Field blocks are essentially anaesthetising an enclosed square or triangle by advancing a needle subcutaneously along each edge. This technique accounts for an area that is being supplied from various nerves and cannot be anaesthetised by just one infiltration or nerve block.

Technique
1 Use a long needle that hopefully will reach right along one side. Inject at the proximal area that should account for most sensory innervation.

2 Withdraw and, using the same hole, advance along the adjacent side at either right angles for a square area or some 30–60° for a triangle. Inject slowly and only move on when the area distal to the needle is anaesthetised. Only inject into anaesthetised areas and minimise injections.

3 Move to the next anaesthetised corner and proceed until the three or four sides have been completed, thus enclosing an anaesthetised field.

SCALP BLOCKS
A deeper injection is needed to infiltrate the cutaneous, subcutaneous and aponeurosis (galea) layers.

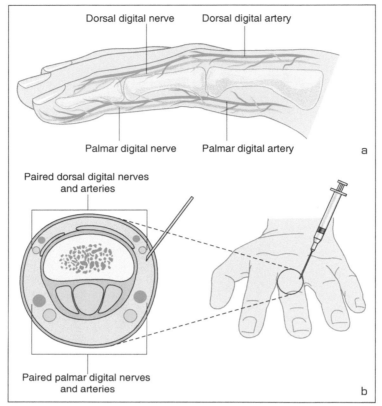

Figure 3.22 Digital innervation and nerve block

a Dorsal and palmar digital arteries and nerves run together. **b** Dorsal approach in administering digital nerve block allows anaesthesia of dorsal and palmar bundle with one puncture.
Adapted from Robinson JK, Hanke WC, Sengelmann R et al (eds). *Surgery of the skin*. Philadelphia: Mosby, 2005; Fig 3.7.

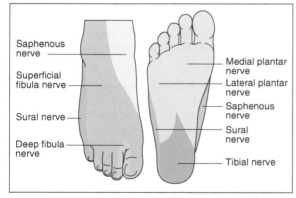

Figure 3.23 Sensory innervation of the foot

Adapted from Robinson JK, Hanke WC, Sengelmann R et al (eds). *Surgery of the skin*. Philadelphia: Mosby, 2005; Fig 3.10.

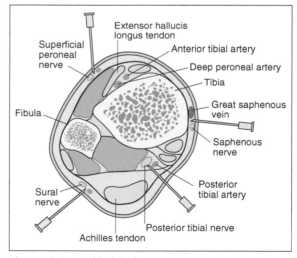

Figure 3.24 Ankle block

Transverse section of the right leg above malleoli to show location of the sensory nerves – the sural, superficial fibular, posterior tibial and saphenous nerves.
Adapted from Robinson JK, Hanke WC, Sengelmann R et al (eds). *Surgery of the skin*. Philadelphia: Mosby, 2005; Fig 3.11.

TOPICAL BLOCKS

Topical anaesthetics diffuse through the superficial layers of the skin to the nerve ends in the dermis. Anaesthesia is achieved to an average depth of 2.9 mm [9]. The anaesthetic effect is inversely related to the stratum corneum thickness and, hence, less effective in such areas as the palms and soles.

The best known and most used topical anaesthetics are EMLA – a combination of lignocaine 2.5% and prilocaine 2.5% as a cream – and amethocaine (tetracaine), most usually used as eye drops. Many different compounded formulas are available (e.g. benzocaine, lignocaine, amethocaine (tetracaine) or BLT) but have been implicated in four deaths after being applied to a large surface area [10]. LMX4 is a cream that contains lignocaine in a liposomal delivery system that facilitates penetration of the anaesthetic into the skin while protecting the drug from being rapidly metabolised and does not need an occlusive dressing.

There is an increasing demand for cosmetic procedures with no or little post-procedural recovery time. This has led to increasing use and development of topical anaesthetics. Two topical local anaesthetics, a gel containing 4% amethocaine (tetracaine) and a patch containing 7% lignocaine and 7% amethocaine (tetracaine), appear to work equally well [11]. A lignocaine/prilocaine cream has been shown to significantly decrease the pain induced by injection and infiltration, particularly on sensitive areas of the face, lower limbs and genitals, but is not effective on thick skin such as the soles [1].

Precautions

Dangers, risks and side effects increase when anaesthetic is applied to a large surface area, for longer than the manufacturer's recommendation and under occlusion. On mucous membrane absorption and anaesthesia is rapid; on the skin, however, an occlusive polythene cover is needed. A wad of EMLA is needed but only a smear of amethocaine (tetracaine). EMLA needs some 2 hours to be effective; amethocaine (tetracaine) needs 1 hour. If left on longer, amethocaine (tetracaine) can cause an allergic reaction. Neither provides complete anaesthesia but can dull the needle prick, especially on mucosal surfaces.

Indications

- Needles
- Injectable fillers
- Laser and IPL procedures
- Radiofrequency (RF)
- RF tissue tightening [12]
- Chemical peels [13]

Topical anaesthesia is *not recommended* for PDT as the high acidity of topicals can inactivate the photosensitisers.

Preparation

Ensure the area is thoroughly cleansed. Benzoyl peroxide decreases the effect of topical anaesthetics [14].

Topical anaesthesia technique

1. Pre-application: wash the area with 'no soap wash' and water.
2. Apply the anaesthetic cream to a uniform 1–2-mm thickness with a tongue depressor.
3. Leave on for 30–60 minutes. Quicker onset is achieved by occlusion with plastic wrap and/or by massaging into the skin with a gloved finger.
4. Immediately preceding the procedure remove the cream with a water-dampened gauze, then dry.

ANALGESIA

For most skin excisions patients report remarkably little pain, not even necessitating paracetamol. Paracetamol is the drug of choice and effective in most. Thereafter, the usual range of analgesics can be used by adding codeine, but it is extremely rare and concerning if stronger analgesics such as pethidine and morphine are requested.

HYDRODISSECTION

Local anaesthetic is very useful to pump up a pathological lesion to be excised up and away from deeper vital structures or, on the ear, to assess if the cancer has invaded the cartilage. If the cancer raises easily off the cartilage it usually has not invaded, and so the cartilage need not be excised. Hydrodissection is most useful in the four danger zones but aberrant vessels and nerves make it a useful standard/default technique to use anywhere.

The area between lines from the ear lobe to the eyebrow, from the tragus to the hair line, is highly dangerous with the facial nerve very superficial over the zygomatic arch and, as in Figure 3.25a, a main branch of the superficial temporal artery. The pumped-in anaesthetic raises a mound of tissue elevating the cancer away from the underlying dangerous structures (Figure 3.25b). Despite this seemingly large amount it was only a 5-mL syringe – well within the safe toxic levels for lignocaine and adrenaline – as well as providing excellent anaesthesia. Although the patient was warned that he might develop a black eye this did not occur. On the helix (Figure 3.26), if pumping up under the lesion easily raises it, this suggests that the cancer has not invaded and is not bound to the cartilage. This then allows for a simple ellipse rather than a wedge resection or flap.

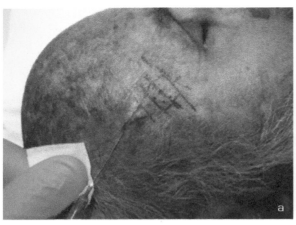
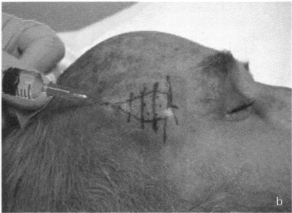

Figure 3.25 Hydrodissection

a Injecting just into the subcutis elevates the cancer up and away from deeper dangerous vessels and nerves, here a main branch of the superficial temporal artery. **b** This is more than adequately pumped up with only 5 mL or less of local anaesthetic.

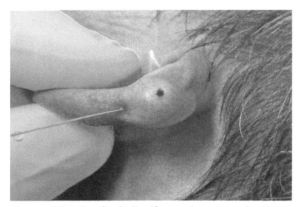

Figure 3.26 On the helix, if pumping up under the lesion easily raises it, this suggests that the cancer has not invaded and is not bound to the cartilage

REFERENCES

[1] Shaikh FM, Naqvi SA, Grace PA. The influence of a eutectic mixture of lidocaine and prilocaine on minor surgical procedures: a randomized controlled double-blind trial. Dermatol Surg 2009;35:948–51.

[2] Höfle M, Hauck M, Engel AK, et al. Viewing a needle pricking a hand that you perceive as yours enhances unpleasantness of pain. Pain 2012;153(5):1074–81.

[3] Liem EB, Joiner TV, Tsueda K, et al. Increased sensitivity to thermal pain and reduced subcutaneous lidocaine efficacy in redheads. Anesthesiology 2005;102:509–14.

[4] Cassidy JP, Phero JC, Grau WH. Epinephrine: systemic effects and varying concentrations in local anesthesia. Anesth Prog 1986;33(6):289–97.

[5] Gratenstein K, McCally C. The use of epinephrine-containing local anesthetics for digital blockade. The American Society of Regional Anesthesia and Pain Medicine ASRA NEWS May 2011:10–12.

[6] Cuzalina AL, Holmes JD. A simple and reliable landmark for identification of the supraorbital nerve in surgery of the forehead: an in vivo anatomical study. J Oral Maxillofac Surg 2005;63(1):25–7.

[7] Zide BM, Swift R. How to block and tackle the face. Plast Reconstr Surg 1998;101:840–51.

[8] Lamont T, Watts F, Stanley J, et al. Reducing risks of tourniquets left on after finger and toe surgery: summary of a safety report from the National Patient Safety Agency. BMJ 2010;340:c1981.

[9] Wahlgren CF, Quiding H. Depth of cutaneous analgesia after application of a eutectic mixture of the local anesthetics lidocaine and prilocaine (EMLA cream). J Am Acad Dermatol 2000;42:584–8.

[10] Kapes B. Media microscope analyzes misuse of topicals. Dermatol Times 2005;26:22.

[11] Ravishankar N, Elliot SC, Beardow Z, et al. A comparison of Rapydan® patch and Ametop® gel for venous cannulation. Anaesthesia 2012; 67(4):367–70.

[12] Alster TS, Tanzi E. Improvement of neck and cheek laxity with a nonablative radiofrequency device: a lifting experience. Dermatol Surg 2004;30:503–7.

[13] Koppel RA, Coleman KM, Coleman WP. The efficacy of EMLA versus Ela-max for pain relief in medium-depth chemical peeling: a clinical and histopathologic evaluation. Dermatol Surg 2000;26:61–4.

[14] Burkhart CG, Burkhart CN. Decreased efficacy of topical anesthetic creams in presence of benzoyl peroxide. Dermatol Surg 2005;31:1479–80.

Haemostasis

4

If you prick us, do we not bleed?

W Shakespeare, The Merchant of Venice,
Act III, Scene 1

Yet who would have thought the old man to have had so much blood in him?

W Shakespeare, Macbeth, *Act V, Scene 1, 43*

Don't panic! Don't PANIC! **DON'T PANIC!**

Corporal Jones, Dad's Army

If bleeding occurs it does so two-thirds of the time in simple ellipses and one-third in flaps. Never stop aspirin or warfarin or anticoagulants, especially within 3 months of a thrombotic episode. Thrombosis–embolus risk increases after 67 years of age.

Haemostasis usually follows a logical sequence

1 Anatomy
   a Be aware of and avoid significant vessels, especially: subdermal plexus, facial artery at mandible crossing, superficial temporal artery, ears, nose, lips (labial artery).
   b Monitor for secondary bleeding and consider hydrostatic pressure.
2 Patience – inject the anaesthetic with adrenaline, wait, then go for a cup of tea, and then wait some more. Adrenaline takes 15 minutes to start to reach optimum vasoconstrictive effect.
3 Pressure – pressure, pressure, then more pressure. Most bleeding stops with pressure, especially on areas such as the nose. To control bleeding constant pressure is needed for 10 minutes.
4 Topical styptics – these are only effective in superficial lesions where a light fulguration arguably gives a better result. Most often quoted are: Monsel's solution (20% ferric sulfate), which can pigment the lesion; aluminium chloride hexahydrate (not meant to be as effective as Monsel's but available as a roll-on deodorant that doesn't stain); silver nitrate sticks (not very effective).
5 Surgical technique – see 'Surgical techniques to minimise bleeding' below.
6 Electrosurgery/cautery – see 'Electro-haemostasis' below.
7 Haemostatic dressings – these are needed for the open excision site for slow Mohs, when the excised lesion is sent to the pathologist to analyse and the site is then closed or extended depending on the results.
8 Tying off – see 'Tying off – suture ligation' below.

SURGICAL TECHNIQUES TO MINIMISE BLEEDING

1 Preparation: ensure adequate lighting to obviate shadows and see under flaps/undermining. Always prepare for the unexpected/worst. Have extra gauze swabs, skin hooks/retractors, small artery forceps, tie-off absorbable sutures, bipolar electrocautery on standby.
2 Position, position and position: above all, position the patient so that the surgeon has optimum access, vision and comfort. Awkward positioning can lead to long-term musculoskeletal damage to the surgeon but, above all, it makes technique difficult and can result in an inferior job or worse, such as a bleeder being missed.
3 Do the simplest operation.
4 Vertical incisions are less likely to cut across vessels.
5 Know the patient's bleeding profile. Even if they are not on any medications or supplements they may still be 'little Aussie bleeders'. A previous diagnostic biopsy may alert.
6 Ensure normotensive BP – high BP exacerbates bleeding.
7 Minimise undermining.
8 Minimise dead space. Use deep sutures where needed.
9 Open wounds/healing by secondary intention: Consider purse-string closures, such as absorbable 5/0 Monocryl®, continuously around the wound edges to minimise postoperative haemorrhage. A purse-string closure does not require undermining and serves to tamponade peripheral wound bleeding. The centre of the wound remains open and acts as a drain.
10 Fenestrated full thickness skin grafts with a tie-over bolster provide wound tamponade and a collagen substrate for haemostasis.

Postoperative

1 Gelfoam® or Kaltostat® to the wound and securing a pressure dressing also helps.
2 Pressure bandages – wherever possible – foreheads, forearms but especially lower legs. Cushions to press into back wounds.
3 Rest, elevate (legs on heels, nothing under calves). No lifting, stretching, stooping or bending for 3 days. Then slowly mobilise but avoid over-activity for 1 week.
4 Be aware of possible rebound when vasoconstriction of adrenaline wears off.
5 It used to be said that postoperative bleeding occurred at 6 and 48 hours. Urge extra rest then.
6 Drains: often forgotten but of use, especially with coagulopathies, where bleeding continues as a slow ooze. A Penrose drain into the wound and withdraw after 48 hours.
7 Analgesics but not NSAIDs.
8 Issue written instructions and insist they read them.
9 Leave dressings on (see the 'Dressings' section in Chapter 12, 'Postoperative care').

ELECTRO-HAEMOSTASIS

Monoterminal ('monopolar')

A hyfrecator (Figure 4.1) provides low-powered, high-frequency AC. It does not need a grounding pad and is intended for use in conscious patients in an office setting. The current passes through the patient's body, which you will feel if you touch the patient. If held above the field, its use is called fulguration and, if applied to the surface, it is cauterisation or desiccation and provides quick and convenient haemostasis for superficial vessels usually <1–2 mm diameter. This is not coagulation per se, which is only provided by biterminal electrodes, but rather a heat-induced desiccation/destruction/thrombosis. If used for coagulation, don't be afraid to turn it up to even Hi-30. The cause of most inadequate haemostasis is using power that is too low.

Biterminal ('bipolar')

Biterminal electrosurgery is coagulation and uses a lower current. The current passes from one electrode to the other and not through the patient's body and, as such, is safer with the least tissue destruction and three times less tissue necrosis than a monopolar electrode (Figure 4.2). It is safe with pacemakers and defibrillators.

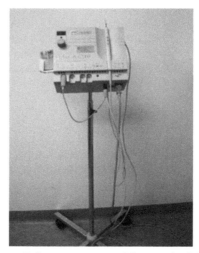

Figure 4.1 Hyfrecator on a mobile stand minimises hassles with multiple room usage

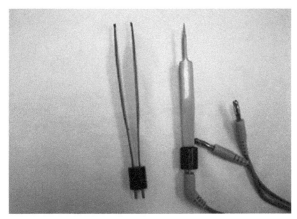

Figure 4.2 Bipolar forceps blunt and sharp with autoclavable lead

With both mono- and biterminal use, direct and collateral tissue damage with charring occurs. Accurate application is essential but *do not close the tips of the forceps – a gap must be left for the spark to jump.*

> ### HINTS AND TIPS
>
> Place bipolar forceps either side of the bleeding point, not on it.

Identification and location of bleeding points

Arteriolar bleeding from under flaps can be profuse and difficult to locate. Here, a skin hook is strongly recommended with the assistant retracting the flap allowing the sub-flap surface to be fully exposed, dried and the bleeding spot identified. Give yourself the best chance and optimise the view of the site.

Ensure the area is dry as fluid/blood disperses the current, increases charring and prevents pinpointing the target.

Technique: roll, don't dab; visualise, then cauterise

1 Cotton buds or dental rolls are used to press the bleeding point. A cotton bud allows better accuracy and vision. Gauze swabs may be used initially to dab the area but, when a pinpoint or bleeding spot reveals itself, press the cotton bud on it.
2 Roll the tip either away from or towards the surgeon, whichever gives the best vision, while maintaining pressure and with the coagulation tips poised to zap the first sign of bleeding.

If a mosquito clamp has been used it usually grasps a swathe of perivascular other tissue. Using forceps or two forceps it may be possible to isolate the vessel and just coagulate it rather than blitz, blast and damage excessive tissue.

Nose tips

- Bleeding with excisions of the tip of the nose is best controlled by thumb and index pressure on either side intermittently released to reveal the bleeding points.
- Chalazion clamps and scissor finger holes can be used as 'field blocks' to stem bleeding from all around.

Lips

A sufficiently large chalazion clamp can clamp both the vermillion actual lip and the supra- or infralabial skin.

TYING OFF – SUTURE LIGATION

Vessels >2 mm should always be ligated. The usual technique is to use braided absorbable sutures. The braiding gives greater knot security (see Chapter 1, 'Equipment, sutures and design').

There are two basic suture ligation techniques: the stick tie and the figure-of-eight/crisscross stitch.

The stick tie

This is used when the open bleeding/squirting end of the vessel can be seen and grasped.

1 Use a fine curved mosquito haemostat forceps to grasp the vessel (Figure 4.3).
2 Insert the needle across and behind the grasping/securing forceps. Ensure there is no traction and minimal movement on this forceps as you do not want it to slip off the vessel, which will then retract and be lost (i.e. hold the mosquito still and work around it).
3 Either tie off in front of the clamp or make another pass into the tissue in front (closest to the surgeon) and tie off.
4 Remove haemostat.
5 Check for bleeding, cut on knot.

Figure-of-eight

This is used when the vessel end cannot be seen to grasp.

1 Nevertheless, clamp the bleeding site, again with a fine curved mosquito clamp, until the bleeding reduces significantly or stops. Avoid taking too big a grasp of tissue.
2 Mentally mark four points to form a small square or rectangle around the central vessel/clamp. Then suture diagonally, across the base, back on the other diagonal, such that the clamp/vessel is now between these two diagonals (Figure 4.4), and tie off.

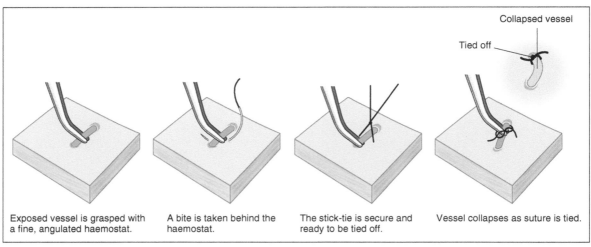

Figure 4.3 The stitch tie
Adapted from Salasche S, Orengo IF, Siegle RJ. Dermatologic surgery tips and techniques. Philadelphia: Mosby Elsevier, 2007; Figs 7.1–7.4.

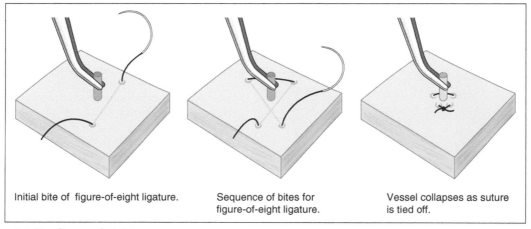

Figure 4.4 The figure-of-eight
Adapted from Salasche S, Orengo IF, Siegle RJ. Dermatologic surgery tips and techniques. Philadelphia: Mosby Elsevier, 2007; Figs 7.5–7.8.

The mattress and square or U suture

The mattress suture is useful as an epidermal suture for nonspecific oozing along the wound edge (Figure 4.5). The square or U suture is used for the same purpose but can be placed deep with an absorbable suture (Figure 4.6).

Running lock stitch

The running lock stitch also provides good haemostasis (Figure 4.7). The deeper the stitch, the greater the

haemostasis. An assistant to hold the tension while the next needle entry is made is very helpful.

Technique

Both ends of the vessel should have a simple loop suture tied around them. Sutures should be tied 'on the knot' to minimise any foreign material.

When the vessels cannot be found, a bigger bite must be taken to embrace the vessel(s) by suturing a wider grab. Then, by drawing them in, this wider area is compressed along with the vessels therein (as with a

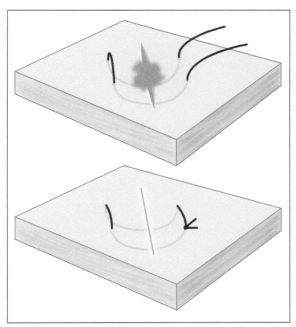

Figure 4.5 Horizontal mattress suture
Adapted from Robinson JK, Hanke WC, Sengelmann R et al (eds). Surgery of the skin. Philadelphia: Mosby, 2005; Fig 17.6.

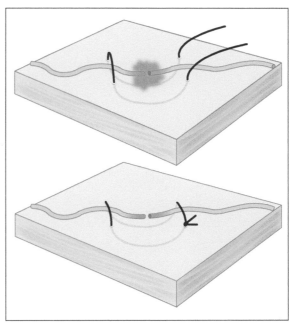

Figure 4.6 Square or U suture
Adapted from Robinson JK, Hanke WC, Sengelmann R et al (eds). Surgery of the skin. Philadelphia: Mosby, 2005; Fig 17.9.

figure-of-eight or square stitch). For bigger more copious bleeding, a double imbricating suture can be very effective (Figure 4.8).

Causes of excessive bleeding
1 Anticoagulants
2 Other medications, supplements and herbs
3 Missed bleeding vessel not tied off/ cauterised
4 Vessel that had gone into spasm or was constricted by adrenaline and then relaxes and dilates
5 Medical conditions a Coagulation defects/bleeding dyscrasias/ platelet defects b Hypertension

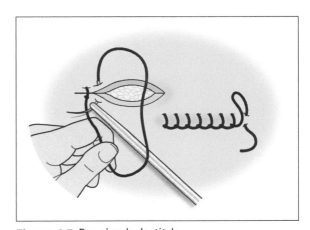

Figure 4.7 Running lock stitch
Adapted from Salasche S, Orengo IF, Siegle RJ. Dermatologic surgery tips and techniques. Philadelphia: Mosby Elsevier, 2007; Fig 11.2.

ANTICOAGULATION THERAPY

Maintain anticoagulants

Do not cease prescribed anticoagulants.

For skin surgery, general surgery practice guidelines in managing blood thinning medicines prior to and during cutaneous procedures have usually been implemented and patients advised thus. However, based on this previous medical advice, some patients may stop anticoagulation medicines without consulting a doctor.

Patients on long-term anticoagulation should maintain this protection and the practitioner should check that they have not stopped it. Thromboembolic events have been reported in cutaneous procedure patients whose anticoagulants were stopped in order to limit ostensible perioperative bleeding [1–3].

TABLE 4.1 Generic and trade names of anticoagulants

Aspirin	Aspirin + dipyridamole	Dipyridamole	Clopidogrel	Warfarin	Heparins	Antithrombotics
Astrix™ Cardiprin Cartia®	Asasantin®	Persantin®	Iscover® Plavix®	Coumadin® Marevan®	Clexane, Fragmin, Heparin sodium and Orgaran	Eliquis, Pradaxa and Xarelto

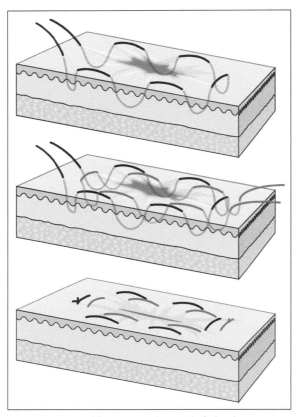

Figure 4.8 Double purse-string or imbrication suture
Adapted from Robinson JK, Hanke WC, Sengelmann R et al (eds). Surgery of the skin. Philadelphia: Mosby, 2005; Fig 17.7.

Although one study showed that cutaneous surgeons are unable to accurately predict blood thinner status of the patient based on intraoperative oozing [4], this has not been the experience of the author, and the risk of encountering copious bleeding can make a simple operation more than difficult.

If there are any bleeding problems, refer the patient to a hospital where resuscitation facilities are in place.

Four independent risks for postoperative bleeding are:

1 older than 67 years
2 ears
3 grafts
4 warfarin.

Relative risks compared to warfarin monotherapy [5]:

- aspirin, 0.96
- clopidogrel, 1.45
- clopidogrel + aspirin, 1.91
- warfarin + aspirin, 1.75
- warfarin + clopidogrel, 3.57
- warfarin + clopidogrel + aspirin, 4.03.

Clopidogrel is associated with significantly increased risk for severe postoperative wound complications whereas the risk for severe complications after skin surgery does not increase in patients on aspirin or warfarin [6].

Warfarin (Coumadin)

Warfarin, which inhibits vitamin K dependent coagulation factors, is the most widely used oral anticoagulant and has been available for more than 65 years [7]. Obtaining an INR of 3 immediately preoperatively is recommended. Warfarin users exposed to any of the six antibiotic drug classes in the previous 60 days were twice as likely to experience a bleeding event that required hospital admission as those who were not exposed. The adjusted ORs for bleeding were 4.57 for azole antifungals; 2.70 for cotrimoxazole; 2.45 for cephalosporins; 1.92 for penicillins; 1.86 for macrolides; and 1.69 for quinolones [8].

Aspirin

Primary prevention
Numerous studies have concluded that evidence of net benefit is insufficient to recommend routine aspirin for primary cardiovascular prevention in any patient subgroup. The new USPSTF guidelines implicitly embrace this view; they recommend that middle-aged and older men (age range 45–79) and women (age range 55–79) take aspirin only if an individualised quantitative risk assessment shows that risk for adverse cardiovascular events exceeds risk for serious bleeding. This recommendation requires calculations for each patient, but it might be the best approach to a question that remains very close to clinical equipoise.

Secondary prevention
For patients with cardiovascular risks or disease aspirin should not be stopped [9].

A PubMed and Medline literature search strongly supports continued perioperative use of aspirin in patients taking it for secondary prevention of coronary artery disease, cerebrovascular disease and peripheral vascular disease. Stopping aspirin can cause a platelet rebound phenomenon and prothrombotic state leading to major adverse cardiac events. However, nearly all of the available data are observational and retrospective [10]. There is a need for prospective randomised trials to evaluate the optimal management strategy of perioperative aspirin therapy.

Clopidogrel (Plavix/Clovix)

Clopidogrel is a platelet aggregation inhibitor.

One study concluded that, as the risk for severe wound complications increases with the size of the surgical defect, a prudent approach might be to continue clopidogrel in small surgical cases and to consider holding it, after consultation with the patient's cardiologist or internist, for 5 to 7 days before surgery for large tumours. If clopidogrel is stopped, other anticoagulants should be continued or substituted in the perioperative period [6].

New anticoagulants

The main advantages are rapid onset, more predictable pharmacokinetics and potentially lower interactions with other drugs, food and lifestyle with less routine monitoring required.

The main disadvantage is that there are no antidotes.

Dabigatran (Pradaxa)

This newer thrombin inhibitor has a half-life of 14–17 hours in healthy volunteers but persists for 168 hours (7 days) according to the product monograph. The recommended discontinuation times before surgery are 24 hours for a standard risk of bleeding (skin surgery) to 2–4 days for a high risk of bleeding (invasive surgery) with a renal function creatinine clearance CrCl >80 mL/min, but other factors such as age, comorbid conditions and concomitant use of antiplatelet agent therapy modify the risk of bleeding [11].

Apixaban (Eliquis) and Rivaroxaban (Xarelto)

Apixaban and rivaroxaban are direct inhibitors of Factor Xa. Rivaroxaban has a half-life of 4–9 hours and was approved in November 2011 by the FDA for prevention of stroke in patients with nonvalvular atrial fibrillation.

Discontinuation

No prescribed anticoagulant should be discontinued. The only exception may be those patients who are on aspirin for some vague reason, usually 'to protect their hearts', but who have no cardiovascular risks.

The times to achieve normal coagulation after discontinuation are:

- Warfarin = 4–5 days (reduction of INR to <3 recommended for skin surgery) [12]

- Aspirin = 5 days [13]
- Clopidogrel = 5–7 days (manufacturer's recommendation)
- Dabigatran = 24 hours (manufacturer's recommendation)

Note: antibiotics in the preceding 60 days prolong the effect of warfarin [8].

HINTS AND TIPS

Despite the numerous reassurances that aspirin does not affect cutaneous surgery, it is my practical experience that it does, especially on noses, causing blood to 'sheet' from innumerable un-cauterisable points. Similar bleeding is found with fish oil, which many patients self-medicate.

MEDICATIONS, ALTERNATIVE MEDICATIONS, SUPPLEMENTS AND FOODS

Prescribed drugs, herbs and supplements can cause both bleeding and coagulation problems.

Medications

- Anticoagulants
- NSAIDs
- SSRIs appear to raise bleeding risk in patients with coronary disease who are taking antiplatelet drugs [14].

Foods, herbs and supplements

The increased awareness and availability of herbs and supplements can cause increased bleeding. In the author's experience fish oil has proven the most common and problematical. Others include:

- Alcohol
- Angelica
- Anise
- Capsicum
- Celery
- Cloves
- Fish oil
- Fenugreek
- Garlic
- Ginger
- Ginkgo
- Ginseng
- Onion
- Turmeric
- Vitamin E

POSTOPERATIVE

It used to be said that postoperative bleeding occurs mostly at 6 or 48 hours. What this probably means is that the vasoconstrictive effect of adrenaline has worn off and rebound bleeding is noticed at 6 hours or that bleeding hasn't stopped and it's 48 hours before the patient complains. In any event, the risk of postoperative bleeding is greatest during the first 48 hours. Rest, elevation, pressure and cold packs are important in this period. Patients should be advised to lie down, elevate the site and apply direct pressure constantly for a minimum of 15 minutes if they suspect bleeding.

Rest

All activity should be reduced and patients need specific instructions to do so. Common sense must prevail as to avoiding stretching the wound but specific instructions as to 'elbows in' and 'avoid stretching to put on shoes' help alert patients with back excisions.

Any activity that stretches the wound is to be avoided. No bending and lift only light objects. No twisting both limbs and body.

Avoid activity that increases heart rate, hence BP.

Elevation

Avoid bending over after facial surgery. A figure of eight bandage for lower arm lesions to keep hand to shoulder is helpful for those patients on anticoagulants.

After all leg operations patients should put their feet up above their nipple line. Rest on heels. Do not compress calf muscles (DVT).

Pressure dressings

Conforming bandages are a great help especially around the forehead, arms and legs.

Surgifix®/tube for scalp, fingers and lower legs is excellent.

Backs may present a problem but advising the patient to watch TV with a cushion pressing over the wound is advice seemingly followed.

Hydrostatic pressure

From the heart to the ankle is a long drop with a large pressure gradient, especially in the elderly with incompetent venous valves or those on anticoagulants. Even when the wound looks super-dry, ensure a pressure dressing before the patient stands up.

Secondary bleeding

This is most likely oozing that builds up to where the patient notices it. As documented in Chapter 12, 'Postoperative care', wounds heal best under waterproof occlusion and many patients and their relatives get most alarmed at even a mildly blood-stained dressing. There is no need to remove this unless there is pain, inflammation and fluctuance. An opaque cover over the intact original dressing is the best treatment.

Alcohol

Alcohol is a vasodilator and 2 days abstinence is good advice.

Trauma

Situations such as sport, where the wound may be subjected to trauma, should be avoided.

Patients who turn and twist in their sleep may need tape-strips as extra insurance and protection.

HAEMATOMAS

Continued bleeding and haematomas are rare in dermatological surgery but are always a potential risk in those patients on anticoagulants. Periorbital haematomas are an emergency as are those in the neck if they compress the trachea.

Haematoma stages

1 **Accumulation:** the wound becomes swollen and is warm and fluctuant. Removal of suture(s) may be all that is necessary to allow release of the accumulated blood with the wound or part thereof left open. If ongoing bleeding is suspected the whole wound should be opened and explored, the bleeding site(s) found and haemostasis established. Then irrigate with normal saline and observe until haemostasis guaranteed. The wound can now be resutured or left open. There is no hard and fast rule but infection would mandate leaving it open and antibiotic cover to heal by secondary intention.
2 **Clots:** form quite quickly with the site becoming more spongy than fluctuant. The skin may now have a purple hue. A small clot may be left to resorb but evacuation by squeezing is usually preferable.
3 **Organisation:** clots organise into adhesive, harder, rubber-like structures and the wound feels firm. These adhesive clots are now difficult to evacuate by squeezing or even exploration and instrument-aided removal. It is better not to do anything but wait for clot lysis.
4 **Lysis:** between 7 and 10 days the wound again feels fluctuant. This is because fibrinolysis is liquifying the clot(s) to be resorbed. Aspiration with an 18G needle is possible rather than opening the wound. Resorption can take many months.

REFERENCES

[1] Schanbacher CF, Bennett RG. Postoperative stroke after stopping warfarin for cutaneous surgery. Dermatol Surg 2000;26(8):785–9.
[2] Alam M, Goldberg LH. Serious adverse vascular events associated with perioperative interruption of antiplatelet and anticoagulant therapy. Dermatol Surg 2002;28(11): 992–8.
[3] Kovich O, Otley CC. Thrombotic complications related to discontinuation of warfarin and aspirin therapy

perioperatively for cutaneous operation. J Am Acad Dermatol 2003;48(2):233–7.

[4] West SW, Otley CC, Nguyen TH, et al. Cutaneous surgeons cannot predict blood-thinner status by intraoperative visual inspection. Plast Reconstr Surg 2002;110(1):98–103.

[5] Hansen ML, Sørensen R, Clausen MT, et al. Risk of bleeding with single, dual, or triple therapy with warfarin, aspirin, and clopidogrel in patients with atrial fibrillation. Arch Intern Med 2010;170(16): 1433–41.

[6] Tey HL, Tan AS, Chan YC. Meta-analysis of randomized, controlled trials comparing griseofulvin and terbinafine in the treatment of tinea capitis. J Am Acad Dermatol 2011;64(4):663–70.

[7] Schulman S. Is the warfarin saga over? J R Coll Physicians Edinb 2012;42:51–5.

[8] Baillargeon J, Holmes HM, Lin YL, et al. Concurrent use of warfarin and antibiotics and the risk of bleeding in older adults. Am J Med 2012; 125:183–9.

[9] Biondi-Zoccai G, Landoni G. Discontinuation of aspirin for secondary prevention. BMJ 2011;343:d3942.

[10] Gerstein NS, Schulman PM, Gerstein WH, et al. Should more patients continue aspirin therapy perioperatively?: clinical impact of aspirin withdrawal syndrome. Ann Surg 2012;255(5):811–19.

[11] van Ryn J, Stangier J, Haertter S, et al. Dabigatran etexilate – a novel, reversible, oral direct thrombin inhibitor: interpretation of coagulation assays and reversal of anticoagulant activity. Thromb Haemost 2010;103:1116–27.

[12] Kearon C, Hirsh J. Management of anticoagulation before and after elective surgery. N Eng J Med 1997;336:1506–11.

[13] Cahill RA, McGreal GT, Crowe BH, et al. Duration of increased bleeding tendency after cessation of aspirin therapy. J Am Coll Surg 2005;200(4):564–73.

[14] Labos C, Dasgupta K, Nedjar H, et al. Risk of bleeding associated with combined use of selective serotonin reuptake inhibitors and antiplatelet therapy following acute myocardial infarction. CMAJ 2011;183:1835–43.

The basics 5

A man's hands and a woman's face are their fortune.

The Author

The fundamental principles of wound closure have changed little over 4000 years. However, unlike most other operations where wound edges approximate to be easily sutured together, the excision of skin cancers results in large defects that have to, somehow, be closed. Because of this wide distance between wound edges, it is often impossible to pull one edge to the other. This has led to the evolution of flap surgery, which has progressed exponentially in recent times. The simple ellipse or side-to-side, however, remains the basic excision technique that can be used in most instances and heals better.

Overview of skin surgery

Always remember the first operation is the best chance to effect a cure and never compromise correct margins.

The surgeon aims to:

1 completely excise the lesion (with histological confirmation – Mohs pathology for all melanoma and cancers of the face)

2 preserve function

3 maximise and optimise wound edge apposition

4 restore appearance (cosmesis – desirable cosmetic result)

5 minimise operative risk (infection, DVT, hypertrophic scars and other complications).

Any deficit imposes varying problems determined by size and site:

1 Is there enough skin elsewhere to close the hole?
  a By undermining and ellipse
  b By moving skin from elsewhere (flaps)

2 Can the closure remain vital?
  a No tension
  b Adequate blood supply

Practical difficulties arise on the face, hand, lower leg and foot from cosmesis, lack of skin or poor circulation.

The essential feature of skin cancer surgery is to ensure a cure by excising the lesion with adequate, evidenced recommended margins. These margins may often result in quite large defects. Nevertheless, the surgeon must not take closer margins to optimise cosmesis in preference to adequate margins. The latter may impose greater technical difficulties with a larger hole or one that is much harder to close. However, an ugly scar is better than a patient dying from metastases or later having a far more disfiguring operation due to a recurrence because the original margins were too close.

Terminology

Traditionally, the simplest excision was called a **simple fusiform ellipse** or a **side-to-side**. However, a **rhomboid** or **diamond** shape is the best technique in that it is more tissue sparing, technically easier and precise. Although this text may use 'ellipse' or 'side-by-side', as they are the entrenched terms, the rhomboid/diamond shape should be performed. Note that the term rhomboid also refers to a well-documented flap and so, to avoid any confusion, this text will use and recommend the diamond shape (i.e. simple ellipse or side by side = diamond).

Dog-ears seem to have different meanings to different surgeons. They are often used to describe the raised triangles made from excess tissue lumped up at the end(s) of a lesion excision because the incision was too short with too wide a terminal angle, and the term will be used in this text in this sense. This is also called a 'cone'.

MARGINS
Above all, skin cancer surgery demands that correct margins be obtained so as to maximise cure rates and survival. Excising a lesion is effectively blind. All that can be done, as best as possible, including dermoscopy, is to identify the visual edges and then take the recommended margins to ensure excised clearance of a lesion and do follow-up pathology. The following sections list recommended margins.

Excisional biopsy
Suspicious pigmented naevus = 2 mm.

Dysplastic naevus/atypical mole
- Mild = no need to excise
- Moderate = 2 mm
- Severe = 5 mm

Note: A recent editorial in *Dermatology Practical and Conceptual* [1] points out that the word 'dysplasia' has never been lucidly defined in pathology and that there is no step between naevus and melanoma, which has erroneously led to the over-treatment (excision) of what are normal melanocytic naevi ('the so-called dysplastic nevus is not dysplastic at all'). They propose that the term 'dysplastic naevus' be lapsed and replaced by 'melanocytic naevus'. To the author this would seem a problem for the dermopathologist. For the clinician, if such naevi are still reported as 'moderate' or 'severe' dysplastic naevi, there is the medico-legal obligation that these need treatment, either by sequential dermoscopic digital imaging (SDDI) or by excision as above.

Melanoma
The AJCC/UICC TNM (2009) [2] system has been recommended for melanoma staging. After initial excision biopsy, the recommended excision margins, measured clinically from the edge of the melanoma, are listed in Table 5.1.

TABLE 5.1 Excision margins for melanoma

Melanoma	Margin lateral	Margin deep
Non-invasive (above the basement membrane): melanoma-in-situ (MIS), lentigo maligna (LM) or superficial spreading melanoma (SSM), <1 mm, Clark Level 1, <1 cm diameter		
pTis, in situ	5 mm (9 mm)*	5 mm (9 mm/deep fascia)*
Invasive (through the basement membrane): superficial spreading, nodular melanoma		
pT1, <1.0 mm	10 mm/1 cm	Deep fascia
pT2, 1.0–2.0 mm	1–2 cm	Deep fascia
pT3, 2.0–4.0 mm	1–2 cm	Deep fascia
pT4, >4.0 mm	2 cm	Deep fascia

*A recent study found 9-mm margins give the best results (Kunishige et al. 2012 [34]).
Adapted from the Union for International Cancer Control, TNM Classification of malignant tumours, 7th edn. 2009. Online. Available: TNM_Classification_of_Malignant_Tumours_Website_15May2011(1).pdf.

TABLE 5.2 Recurrence rates: the significance of a close margin varies depending on the subtype of BCC

BCC type	<0.38 mm	0.38–0.75 mm	>0.75 mm
Solid	40%	10%	4%
Multifocal Sclerosing Infiltrative (micronodular)	80%	45%	20%

Adapted from Dixon AY et al, J Cutan Pathol 1993;20:137–42.

Basal cell carcinoma (BCC)

Lateral margins
- Superficial, nodular (solid) = 4 mm
- Micronodular, morphoeic/infiltrative = 5–6 mm
- Recurrent or difficult clinical margin = Mohs on face; at least 6-mm elsewhere

Deep margins
It is unusual for small primary BCC to penetrate into the fat. Thus, if excision is carried into fat, the depth of excision is usually adequate [3].

Squamous cell carcinoma (SCC)
- Well differentiated, <10 mm = 4 mm
- Undifferentiated
  - <10 mm = 4 mm
  - >10 mm = 6–10 mm
- Dangerous
  - Histology: poorly differentiated, perineural or lymphovascular invasion, acantholytic features, spindle cell
  - Site: ear, lip, previously damaged skin (burns, radiation), arising in Bowen's disease
  - Size: >2 cm diameter
  - Invasion: >4 mm depth (but only 8% of dermatopathologists measured tumour thickness)
  - Fast growth
  - Recurrence

Note: it is the author's recommendation that slow Mohs pathology be used for all SCC on head, neck, hands, lower leg, the undifferentiated and the dangerous. The above margins are recommended because they have been shown to provide clearance in most cases, but slow Mohs pathology will *confirm* clearance. SCCs kill and complete clearance is mandatory.

Recurrence/clearance rates
BCC and SCC clinical margin measurements:
- 2 mm = 70% clearance: 30% recurrence
- 3 mm = 85% clearance: 15% recurrence
- 4 mm = 98% clearance: 2% recurrence [4]

As well as being clinical measurements some experienced clinicians argue that, with an excellent light and a loupe, the edge of a lesion can be better identified and more carefully mapped and the 4-mm margins are not needed as 'out is out'. They argue that the Wolfe margins (above) are a 'fail safe' guide not necessary if the margin edge can be confidently seen and that a 2-mm margin will suffice. This may well be the case for a nodular BCC. The margins in the pathology report (if it measures them) will be significantly less because of shrinkage. The present best advice is that a pathological margin of more than 1 mm confers clearance whereas a margin of less than 1 mm may be cause for concern (see Table 5.2).

The usual recommendation is that a histological margin <1 mm for an SCC (not a BCC) should require re-excision. The inference is that the margins for a BCC are less, as above.

Mohs or en face pathology
Mohs surgery involves the surgeon freezing and staining the excised lesion, then examining all margins and extending the excision until clearance is obtained. The surgeon has to be trained and accredited. It also has the inherent weakness that freezing does not provide as good a specimen as paraffin.

Mohs pathology embeds the lesion in paraffin but instead of breadloafing, which may miss an involved margin, turns the lesion over to examine all of the lateral and deep margins.

Slow Mohs was introduced wherein the lesion is excised, the wound left open with haemostasis obtained, then packed and dressed. The site is then addressed and closed on obtaining the pathology report.

After witnessing this done by very competent colleagues, the author decided to close and not leave the wound open. The rationale was that most patients could not tolerate an open wound, especially on the face. But further, most excisions were in fact clear and hence the delay was unnecessary. Finally, even if the excision was not clear, the involved margin was now exquisitely identified and invariably required minimal 'trimming' and not a complete new full operation. In view of this, the author routinely requests Mohs pathology on all melanomas and all facial, hand and lower leg cancers as well as any that appear difficult and sinister.

Specimen shrinkage

Specimens sent for pathology shrink. This is not due to the formalin but the drying process. This is of medico-legal importance when claiming the size of a lesion.

- Length = 21% (20.66% ± 2.15%)
- Width = 12% (11.79% ± 2.35%)
- Area = 16%
- Range of shrinkage: 0 to 41.18% for length and −18.75% (indicating expansion) to 37.50% for width [5].

Margins and quality control

The following is documented to reinforce and encourage the need for correct margins (Table 5.3).

In previous retrospective audit studies, rates of incomplete excisions of BCCs ranged from 4% to 16.6% [6–16]. Incomplete excision has been associated with

TABLE 5.3 Victorian statistics for melanoma margins

Wide excision performance	Adequate margins = 31% Margins too narrow = 37% Margins too large = 32%
Location and margin adequacy	Face = 78% too narrow Trunk = 57% too large With no prior biopsy = 58% too narrow
In situ melanoma margins	36% <3 mm This is considered inexcusable. In situ melanoma treatment (excision) should be curative with 5-mm margins. Narrow margins can result in residual tumour, high recurrence rates, metastasis and death

Adapted from Kelly et al. 2007 [35].

Summary: correct diagnosis, excision, correct margins

- Biopsy → diagnosis
- Surgery is the gold standard – the only sure way of ensuring margin control
- Ensure correct margins – get a dermopathologist to check them
- Do slow Mohs where necessary
- Know the danger areas for metastasis (lips, nose, ears)
- Know the more dangerous lesions needing wider excision and ?Mohs
  - Lentigo maligna on faces
  - Nodular melanoma
  - BCC: multinodular, morphoeic/infiltrative; 'H' zone of face
  - SCC: high-risk SCC 'bell ringers':
    - □ Histology: poorly differentiated, perineural or lymphovascular invasion, acantholytic features
    - □ Site: ear, lip, previously damaged skin (burns, radiation), arising in Bowen's disease
    - □ Size: >2 cm diameter
    - □ Invasion: >4 mm depth
    - □ Fast growth
    - □ Recurrence
    - □ Immunosupression: renal transplants have ≈250-fold risk
- Ensure adequate margins and complete clearance – this is someone's life!

---

various recurrence rates from 26% to 67% [6, 17, 18] with an estimated median interval to recurrence of 18.5 months [6].

In one study, 179 non-melanoma skin cancers of the head and neck were excised and histopathologically confirmed in 160 patients. Histology included 125 BCCs and 54 SCCs. Excision with 5-mm margins was performed in every case, and the defects were closed mainly using local flaps. Incomplete excision was limited to 3.9% of cases, and the recurrence rate was 1.7% [19].

From the above it would seem 5-mm margins minimise the recurrence of BCC and SCC to 1.7%. 5-mm margins on the nose, however, are a daunting prospect (in all surveys the nose and ears had the greatest recurrence rates – obviously as the surgeon tried to minimise technical difficulties and maximise cosmesis). It is the author's practice to do slow Mohs on all facial and otherwise difficult cancers, which minimises the margins needed to be taken.

SHAVE AND SNIP EXCISIONS

Experience is the name that everyone gives to their mistakes.

Oscar Wilde

So the best way to be happy is to make the other person happy.

Dalai Lama

Please refer to Figures 5.1 and 5.2 for examples of this technique.

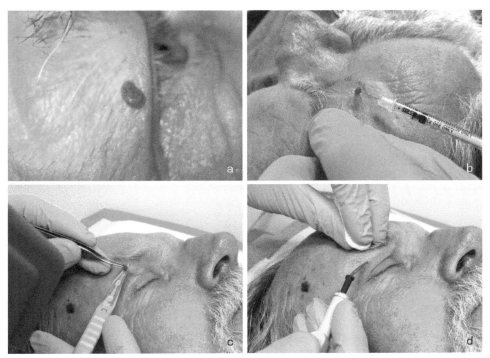

Figure 5.1 Shave excision of a lesion on the right orbit

a A presumably benign lesion R orbit. **b** The lesion is not only anaesthetised but pumped up, which helps define the base or any pedicle. **c** An 11 scalpel or a stitch cutter allows the best vision to cut just below the pigmented or naevus margins. **d** A zap of hyfrecation to cauterise.

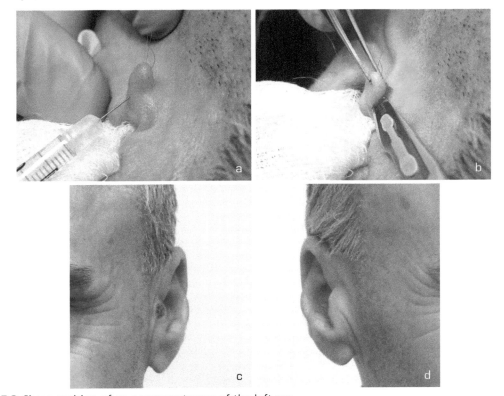

Figure 5.2 Shave excision of an accessory tragus of the left ear

a An accessory tragus local anaesthetic to the base. **b** Shaved off parallel to the skin surface. **c** Cauterised. **d** Most important – compare it to other side. Now no discernable difference – patient happy.

OPTIMISING EXCISION TECHNIQUE

The fundamentals are too often glossed over resulting in quite bizarre scars by a well-meaning operator who, with a few basic hints as follows, could have done a much better, and frequently much easier, operation.

Halsted's principles of surgery

- Handle tissue gently
- Use strict aseptic technique
- Sharp anatomical dissection
- Haemostasis
- Avoid dead space
- Avoid tension in tissue

William Stuart Halsted (1852–1922)

Incision technique

- Incisions can be made with a variety of surgical blades, most usually a number 15 (small curved) or occasionally an 11 sharp point.
- The angle of the blade relative to the skin has traditionally been recommended to always be 90° (i.e. a vertical scalpel, see Figure 5.3). However, it is the experience of the author that angling the blade out and away from the lesion, up to 45°, not only provides a wider sub-epidermal excision (and hence enhances clearance) but also provides a desirable default eversion of the wound edges (Figure 5.4).
- Incise to the same depth from start to finish. First cut one side then the other, starting at the same point. Make one incision, not multiple cuts, and avoid over-runs or cross-hatching ends.
- The floor of the excision should be the same depth and flat from edge to edge and end to end. This then results in vertical wound edges or, as proposed, edges that slope out and away. The edges should not

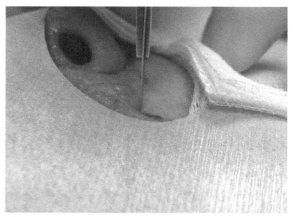

Figure 5.3 Here the scalpel blade is vertical, the usual recommended technique

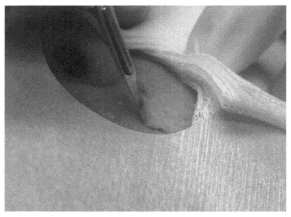

Figure 5.4 Here the blade is angled out and away, which provides a wider subepidermal margin and a natural desirable default eversion when it comes to suturing of the edges

Note: the glistening nostril is from instilled chloramphenicol as prophylaxis against surgical site infection (SSI) as the nostrils are repositories of germs.

slope in or be bevelled inwards or of uneven depth (especially rising at the ends) such that it is now easiest to suture.
- The thumb and forefinger of the other hand can steady or even slightly stretch the skin while incising. Avoid 'wedging' – making the excision shallow at the ends; this means there is more tissue at the ends and hence more compression with closure, forcing this excess up and forming a 'dog-ear'.
- If the incision is an ellipse, the narrower or more acute the ends the less chance of a puckering dog-ear. 30° ends are considered maximum (see Figure 5.5). A diamond excision not only ensures this but spares more tissue than the traditional fusiform ellipse.
- The length of these excisions should be, at minimum, three times the width but four times longer is optimum. Do not make the mistake of a too short excision and never be afraid to extend one – longer excisions are easier to close and thus heal better with less tension.
- For a scalp incision (Figure 5.6), angle the blade at 45° and parallel to the hair follicles so as to preserve them and not leave a bald scar (see Figure 5.7).

HINTS AND TIPS

Excising outwards (i.e. angling the blade slightly out and away from the vertical centre) both gives a wider clearance of the lesion and facilitates better eversion even in non-hair bearing skin.

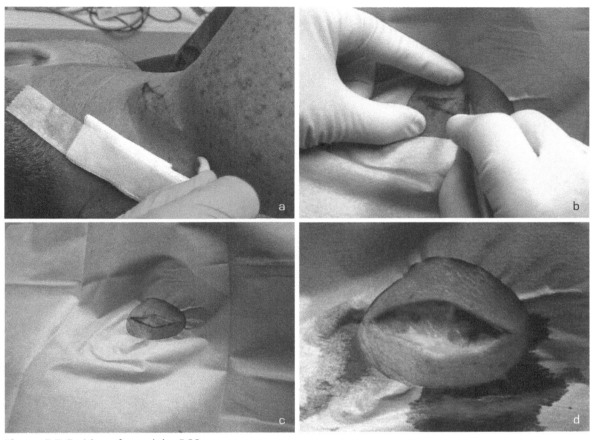

Figure 5.5 Excision of a nodular BCC

a The lesion has been marked with 4-mm rhomboid margins and prepped. **b** The skin is stretched and the incision started at the far end. The scalpel blade is angled out. **c** The completed initial margin excision. One incision either side deep to the fat layer. **d** The completed excision where the walls are vertical or preferably angled out (best seen at the superior margin as the lower one has dropped down) and the base is the same depth right to the ends to prevent dog-ears. The length of the incision is four times the maximum width – this also prevents dog-ears.

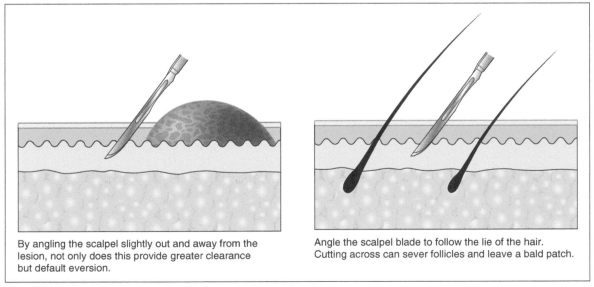

By angling the scalpel slightly out and away from the lesion, not only does this provide greater clearance but default eversion.

Angle the scalpel blade to follow the lie of the hair. Cutting across can sever follicles and leave a bald patch.

Figure 5.6 A scalp incision

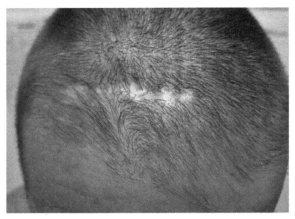

Figure 5.7 Results of a 'biopsy' (according to the patient)

It cuts across the hairs and has left an ugly scar. One wonders if a smaller hair-sparing biopsy could not have been done.

Types of excisions

Punch

- Punch excisions (Figure 5.8) are excellent and quick for small lesions if an adequate margin can be obtained. Punches up to 12 mm are available.
- Stretch the skin at 90° to the intended line of closure. Use interrupted figure-of-eight sutures.
- A punch is also the way to go for skin grafts on the finger as it is again quick and there is no need for a template for the harvest/donor site, which is usually the medial aspect of the upper arm.
- For larger circular defects wide undermining allows the circle to best relax into the relaxed skin tension line (RSTL) ellipse orientation.

Simple fusiform ellipses or diamonds and rhomboids

- The 'ellipse' should more accurately be called fusiform as the ends are never rounded but pointed (Figure 5.9) [20, 21].
- Rhomboid excision is simplest and less wasteful of tissue (Figure 5.10).

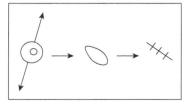

Figure 5.8 Punch excision

- It has been taught that to avoid dog-ears the distal angles of the ellipse must be <30°. This is correct but this also can mean the ratio should increase to 4:1 (i.e. the length of the incision should be four times its width). Do not hesitate to lengthen an incision to facilitate better closure with less tension and no dog-ears.
- To minimise a dog-ear deformity during closure, the angle of the apex should be less than 30°, and the lengths of each side of the incision should be made equal to each other. When such an angle cannot be made, an M-plasty can be made at the apex to minimise a dog-ear deformity.

HINTS AND TIPS

A diamond is better than an ellipse. When 'simple ellipse' is used, please read 'diamond'.

Diamond excisions need to be long and thin – when in doubt extend.

The length of the excision should be three times its width *at a minimum*. If the apex is 30°, it is better to make it 4:1. In fact, make it practice to go 4:1.

Do not hesitate to go longer to reduce the tension at the middle and to be able to do an ellipse rather than a flap as an ellipse (a straight line) heals better.

Diamond (ellipse) excisions are frequently 'overlooked' when they could be used.

Keep the scalpel blade angled out or at least vertical, especially in thick skin, right to the end.

No wedging.

Ideal for subcuticular sutures.

Better results on large lesions if deep sutures are also used.

If the centre is too wide closure can usually be obtained by moving in equally from the ends.

Pre-excision markers then help alignment.

Undermining is not always necessary but usual to minimise tension.

Preoperative planning

Preoperative planning of the actual operation (as distinct from the anaesthetic/medical risks) to achieve optimal cosmetic and functional results is essential. The goals should be to completely excise the cancer but also to re-establish functional soft tissue structural support and to give the most natural aesthetic appearance with minimal distortion after healing has occurred. Wound healing involves contraction and scarring, which can compromise function and appearance and must also be taken into consideration in planning.

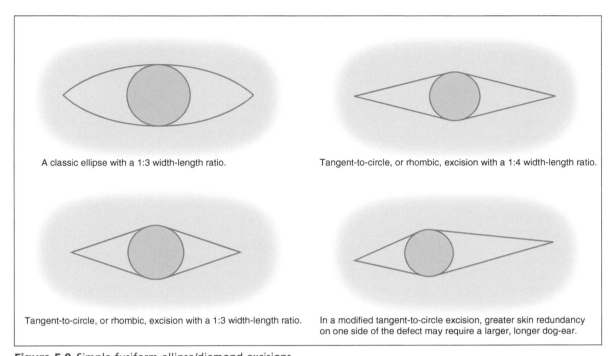

A classic ellipse with a 1:3 width-length ratio.

Tangent-to-circle, or rhombic, excision with a 1:4 width-length ratio.

Tangent-to-circle, or rhombic, excision with a 1:3 width-length ratio.

In a modified tangent-to-circle excision, greater skin redundancy on one side of the defect may require a larger, longer dog-ear.

Figure 5.9 Simple fusiform ellipse/diamond excisions

Adapted from Goldberg LH, Alam M. Elliptical excisions variations and the eccentric parallelogram. Dermatol 2004;140(2):176–80.

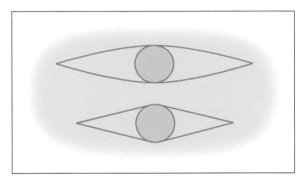

Figure 5.10 Comparison of a fusiform ellipse (top) and a rhomboid excision (bottom)

The rhomboid excision conserves more tissue (lower skin waste-to-lesion ratio) and has a smaller vertex angle (28°) compared to the fusiform ellipse (33°).

Adapted from Buchen D. *Skin flaps in facial surgery.* New York: McGraw Hill, 2007; (Fig 1.4).

It is a surgical axiom that there should be 'four possible alternative operations'. This usually includes a simple ellipse and secondary intention and, in reality, means that the surgeon should only have two others, plan A and plan B if and when flaps are needed. What was the most likely choice at the pre-op consultation may not prove to be the optimal choice when it comes to the actual operation, so preferences may be adjusted at the last minute according to the variety of skills at the operator's disposal. For the author it has been of immense help to see the patient the day before so that the lesion and the plan(s) are fresh in the operator's mind. There are then no nasty surprises as when the patient has not been seen for some time and the lesion has grown dramatically or the patient has had a pacemaker inserted in the interim, is on anticoagulants and has developed diabetes.

'When the only tool you own is a hammer, everything starts to look like a nail.' While this observation applies mostly to equipment or lack thereof, it also applies if the practitioner is limited to just the one operation. Although it is inevitable that each practitioner develops personal preferences for some flaps, there are some operations that are definitely superior in certain sites and some that are better avoided. An O-S flap across a joint, for example, has an inherent expansion 'spring' that compensates for the up to 30% scar contraction and allows free joint mobility. Some surgeons seem, if not oblivious to the cosmetic result, more interested in the excision without due thought as to the cosmesis. Excision with adequate margins to effect a cure is mandatory and the essential goal, but some flaps result in ugly scars. Hence, some surgeons avoid rhomboid flaps on the face, and it is hard to envisage a facial lesion that could not be adequately excised with a different flap, which provided a better cosmetic, less ugly scar. Learning and mastering the flaps described later will provide the practitioner with the variety to execute the best operation.

PRE-OP PREPARATIONS

Drawing in the defect
• Bright light
• Magnification
• Three-finger stretch
• Draw or dot in the tumour edge
• Measure and draw in excision margins
• Photograph if over 10 mm

Marking skin for excisions

Commercially available Sharpie pens or the equivalents almost never harbour enough bacteria to show up in a culture because their ink is alcohol-based. On the other hand, pens specifically designed for surgical use – and meant to be used only once – harboured a range of pathogens for several hours. These findings imply that surgeons could keep an alcohol-based marker with them and use it on all of their patients until the ink runs out [22].

Preoperatively marking the sitting patient helps determine the effect of gravity on the surrounding tissue around the planned incision. Furthermore, it helps give a more accurate assessment of the planned incision with respect to the relaxed skin tension lines before local anaesthetic is injected.

Hairy areas

- Shaving the site is now *not recommended* as minute abrasions/cuts promote infection. Hair trimmers (Figures 5.11 and 5.12) can be used the day of the operation, not before; otherwise, germs are more likely to accumulate and contaminate. Depilatory cream is arguably to be preferred.

- Ensure the area is wide enough.
- Tape away long hair or use clips to hold hair that may fall into or across the excision site.
- Large tubular gauze also holds the hair back (Figure 5.13).

Catchers

Gauze squares held by paper tape can be placed where wound blood will run, thus preventing staining of further skin, clothes, operation table or even the floor (Figures 5.14 and 5.15). Make sure these are far enough away so as not to intrude into the hole in the sterile drape to prevent inadvertent touching and contamination. If this is impossible, as around the eye or nose, place sterile gauze swabs over these catchers.

Drapes/undersheets

Waterproof absorbent undersheets should obviously be placed under any possible drip areas.

'Use-once' fluid impervious drapes have been developed and are recommended. They have adhesive around

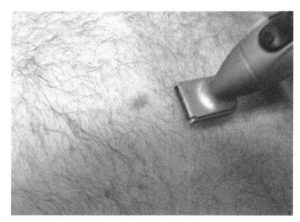

Figure 5.11 Hair trimmer

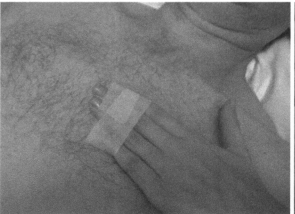
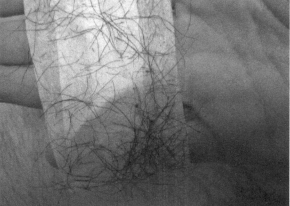

Figure 5.12 Loose trimmed hair is best picked up by dabbing the area with the sticky side of a paper tape strip

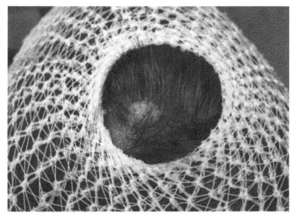

Figure 5.13 Tubular gauze holds back the hair

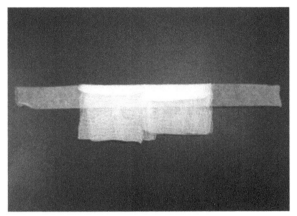

Figure 5.14 Gauze squares folded over and held by paper tape

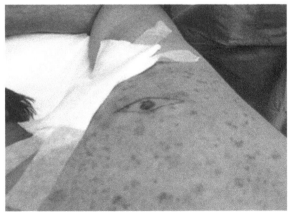

Figure 5.15 Blood follows the easiest path but the body also has creases

Note: this photo does not show how the patient's body was angled down and all blood ran towards these catchers.

the fenestration as well as at the tabbed corners. As they are impervious, blood can run down gutters and needs to be watched. The plastic drapes supplied in disposable packs are, if not useless, then an annoying compromise as they lift up when instruments are picked up. Some practitioners just sterilise a paper towel and cut a hole in it to suit the excision. The paper absorbs most excess blood. The material/cotton drapes used in hospitals are too expensive and impractical for private general practices.

 CAUTION

Cover any hairy areas, especially the eyebrows, if using an adhesive drape to avoid painful depilation.

INCISION LINES

Surface anatomy – Langer's and other lines and orientating incision lines

Skin tension lines (STLs) of the face are in effect the wrinkles. The elasticity of young skin rebounds against the contortions and contractions of the muscles of expression, but with age the elastin and collagen degrade and wrinkles form along the attachment of the SMAS to the skin and usually run across or perpendicular to the underlying muscle contractions (e.g. the frontalis muscle contracts vertically but the forehead wrinkles are horizontal).

Relaxed skin tension lines (RSTLs) are formed during relaxation and often follow a different direction than age and contracting wrinkles. Relaxed skin tension lines are created by the natural tension on the skin from underlying structures (see Figures 5.16 and 5.17). They were thought to provide a guide to the best incision lines but now some 36 differently named guidelines have developed as surgeons have searched for an ideal guide for elective incisions [23].

There are no single recommendations as to incision lines in all circumstances and sometimes even contradictory incisions, such as a vertical mid-forehead incision, work very well if not best. The medical practitioner faced with the responsibility of having to excise a lesion on a live body should get the patient to move and contort the excision area as much as possible. Often the incision is best placed in the 'action' – movement or 'favourable' lines. Active movement means getting the patient to move the area, whereas passive movement means the examiner pinches the site from various angles to find where the skin moves together most easily (i.e. where it is looser and there is laxity and 'harvest' areas make approximating the deficit edges as easy as possible). These proposed lines are therefore only a guide and the operator should study the individual, observe the RSTLs then the

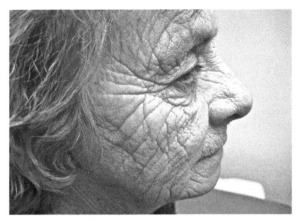

Figure 5.16 RSTLs in a patient who claimed to be a non-smoker, showing where the natural wrinkle lines are

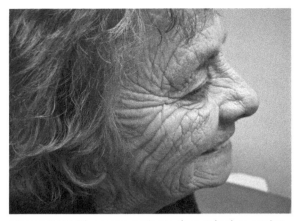

Figure 5.17 The same patient when asked to squint and grimace – these are often the best wrinkle furrows in which to place incisions – most patients have these same lines

action lines and predict any cosmetic deformation or anatomical impediment that may result, such as eyebrow elevation, ectropion or scars across joints. Obvious wrinkles should always be used for incision lines where possible and cosmetic units utilised.

HINTS AND TIPS

Pinch test

On the contralateral, non-lesional side, pinch up the amount of skin needed to excise the lesion and see which skin is the loosest and also which pulls apart most when the patient moves. This orientates the optimum incision line. Then try and hide it in a crease.

Face

Cosmetic units

The face is divided into cosmetic units that have the same skin type in terms of colour, pigmentation, texture, elasticity, thickness, pore size, sebaceous characteristics, hair and even response to blush stimuli (Figure 5.18). They are defined by anatomical areas and each can usually be subdivided into smaller units (Figures 5.19 and 5.20). Surgical results are best if confined to the same unit or incisions placed in the natural division line.

The face consists of six major aesthetic units comprised of the forehead, eye/eyebrow, nose, lips, chin and cheek. These can be subdivided into additional anatomical subunits (e.g. the nose can be divided into nasal tip, dorsum, columella, soft tissue triangles, sidewalls and nasal alar regions). Facial aesthetic units and subunits are the obvious visual anatomical boundaries. Light reflections and shadows along these facial aesthetic borders help hide scars.

Key functional and aesthetic structures are: eyelids, nasal alae, nasal tip, auricle, vermilion, commissures and philtral ridges. Correct orientation of planned incisions next to these mobile functional and aesthetic facial structures and free edges is important to avoid distortion when closing wounds. The closer an incision comes to lying within a 'favourable' line, the better the ultimate cosmetic appearance of the scar. If possible, avoid making incisions perpendicular to RSTLs because the greatest amount of lax skin lies perpendicular to RSTLs. Always consider the potential defect that will result after excision. Evaluate the planned skin incision in its relationship to the facial subunits in attempting, as much as possible, to achieve symmetry with the contralateral normal face.

The contralateral normal facial region can serve as a helpful visual template for comparison.

Avoid crossing anatomical boundaries with a flap. The obliteration of folds and creases that occur naturally will lead to an undesirable result. Try and stay within the same cosmetic unit to maximise tissue match and minimise distortion.

Experimental studies showed twice as much tension is needed to close a wound made across or perpendicular to an RSTL as compared to one made along it. There is a clear-cut inverse relationship between flap tension and blood flow in these flaps, which correlated well with the experimental flap necrosis seen [24].

Get the patient to grimace, contort, frown, squint and so on. Crows' feet, brow corrugations and other wrinkles may not be obvious at rest but demonstrate great grooves or gutters to hide an incision when the patient so contorts.

The danger of causing an ectropion or eyebrow lift must always be kept in mind and can be avoided by vertical incisions on the brow and infraorbital. The long axis of a fusiform excision should follow favourable/obvious

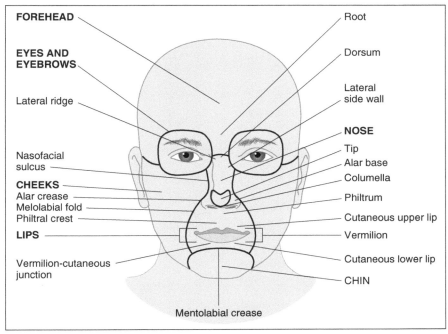

Figure 5.18 The boundaries of the five cosmetic units of the face (forehead, cheeks, eyes, nose, lips and chin)
They are defined by the contour lines of the nose, lips and chin.
Adapted from Robinson JK, Hanke WC, Sengelmann R et al (eds). Surgery of the skin. Philadelphia: Mosby, 2005; Fig 1.4.

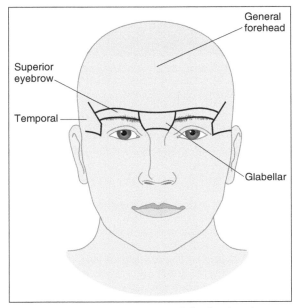

Figure 5.19 Four components of the forehead
Adapted from Robinson JK, Hanke WC, Sengelmann R et al (eds). Surgery of the skin. Philadelphia: Mosby, 2005; Fig 1.5.

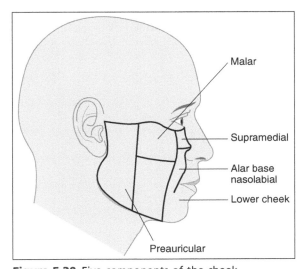

Figure 5.20 Five components of the cheek
Adapted from Robinson JK, Hanke WC, Sengelmann R et al (eds). Surgery of the skin. Philadelphia: Mosby, 2005; Fig 1.6.

RSTLs. Facial scarring can be minimised by adherence to meticulous techniques of tensionless incision closure, wound edge eversion and placement of incisions within FSTLs. Preoperatively identify and map vital structures (e.g. zygomatic arch, temple – temporal nerve and artery, marginal mandibular nerve, CN IX at Erb's point).

Free margins

Free margins are unopposed and hence wound contraction or tension can cause distortion. Free margins occur at the nostril – alar rim, helices of the ears, eyelids, columella and lips. All technique should be directed at minimising any tension or contraction.

Loose skin – harvest areas

A good reservoir on the face is the skin near the ramus and the pre-auricular area, the temple and the neck. Assess skin laxity surrounding the planned incision. Undermine lax areas that can donate to a more fixed area that maintains the original anatomical architecture, thus causing minimal distortion as with the nasolabial groove.

Although using the nasolabial fold may be obvious, Figures 5.21, 5.22 and 5.23 illustrate a case in which, by pinching up the other side, it was evident that continuing this on inferiorly would result in elevation or distortion of the lateral left lip. This exemplifies the need to use every available help/wrinkle/fold but to also be prepared to modify with the end result in mind. A resulting sneer would not have been appreciated had the lip been pulled up by strictly adhering to the obvious nasolabial groove.

Nasolabial groove

Usually, if an incision is made in the nasolabial fold it should lie (straight) in it whereas any ellipse should be incised laterally in a semicircle from it. This lateral

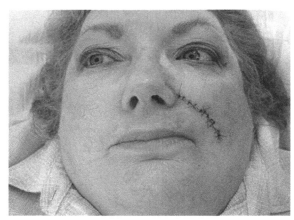

Figure 5.22 No undermining was done on the medial aspect but extensive undermining was done laterally plus a deliberate attempt to fold the cheek over to recreate the nasolabial fold

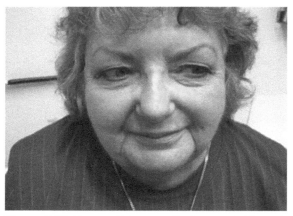

Figure 5.23 The result is cosmetically acceptable such that friends 'don't know it's been done', a very happy patient and complete clearance

semicircle edge is then extensively undermined but the medial edge in the nasolabial groove is not undermined (Figures 5.24 to 5.27).

Back

Ask the patient to raise their arms above their heads Then the actual *functional skin lines* can be seen as well as where and what skin is loose so as to provide the most skin, thus reducing tension on the excision wound as much as possible (Figures 5.28 and 5.29). As with the pinch test above, ask the patient to cross arms as this provides the greatest stretch the potential wound will have to survive.

Scar spread

The back skin is 'different' and scars tend to spread ('burst'). The best that can be done to try and prevent

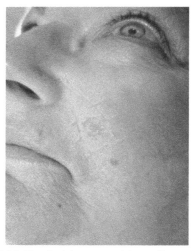

Figure 5.21 The incision veered laterally away from the nasolabial groove inferiorly

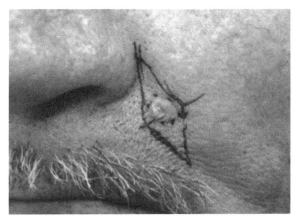

Figure 5.24 NBCC with 4-mm excision margins marked but roll of nasolabial fold distorts this until flattened out

Note: proximity of the BCC to the nasolabial fold meant the excision had to extend either side.

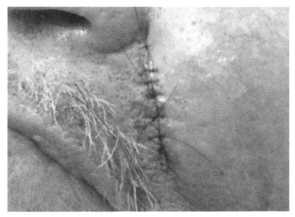

Figure 5.26 Excision sutured in a straight line re-forming the normal nasolabial groove

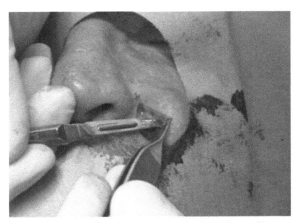

Figure 5.25 Undermining is mostly done laterally to free this side, allowing it to move over to the fixed medial side, thus re-establishing the straight nasolabial fold

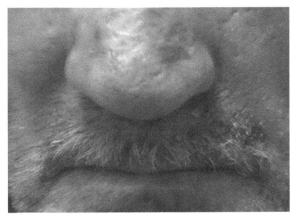

Figure 5.27 One week later at removal of sutures (ROS) – excision complete

Unlike the example in the section 'Loose skin – harvest areas', this was a smaller incision and the pinch test suggested that there would be no lip elevation if the incision stuck to the nasolabial groove. Assess all incisions individually and use suggested incision lines and maps only as guides. Think of the end result.

this scar spread is to place the incision in the most favourable 'action' lines and use deep long duration sutures with minimal tension on the skin sutures. Despite all these efforts, scars can still spontaneously spread months to even years later.

Limbs

On the limbs the cadaver or theoretical lines would suggest horizontal incisions as do some, if not most, surgical texts. However, such horizontal incisions have a greater chance of cutting across nerves and vessels. More

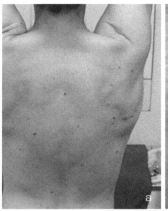 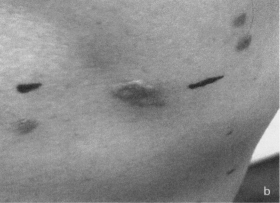

Figure 5.28 Planning an excision on the back

a Getting the patient to raise his arms demonstrates the functional skin lines where the incision is best made to reduce stretching/tension with movement. **b** Fortunately, the NBCC lined up along this axis as well.

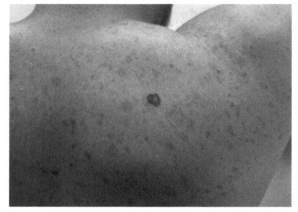

Figure 5.29 Another male back but, again, by getting the patient to stand and elevate his arms the skin and incision line can best be seen

Note that it is completely different from the example in Figure 5.28. Assess each patient individually.

than that, passive movement invariably allows more skin movement vertically than horizontally. Vertical incisions are recommended on limbs where possible.

Scars can contract by up to 30% of their length so an 'S' scar allows for it to extend more. An O-S flap over a joint with the arms of the S going down the limb also provides this. Avoid a straight incision on the dorsum of the hand if it has to cross the wrist; the resulting scar may limit future flexion.

Nerve blocks

Perform wherever possible to minimise field distortion. Refer to Chapter 3, 'Local anaesthesia'.

HINTS AND GEMS

Make yourself as comfortable as possible so you can do the best job. Avoid having to stretch, reach or bend.

The operation site should sit comfortably under your hands.

Two lights eliminate shadows. Three are even better.

Use magnification (Loupe etc).

A wall clock behind the patient will keep you in touch.

Use 'the arc' wherein you can pick up instruments and throw away swabs without twisting.

Use the simplest procedures that will get the job done.

A straight side-to-side ellipse/diamond heals better than a flap.

On the limbs, incise proximal to distal to minimise cutting across nerves and vessels.

Pinch up the skin to find where most loose skin is. Your fingerprints indicate the lateral edges of the excision.

Illustrations of skin lines are only of theoretical help. Look at your patient. Get them to grimace, squint and furrow their brow for lesions on the face and elevate their arms for lesions on the trunk. This will reveal the creases to use.

Know the face and neck danger areas.

Draw the tumour edge.

Measure appropriate margins and mark your excision. Cut outside the marks.

You need to know the defect size, not the tumour size, to plan closure.

Plan the operation based on this defect size.

Hydrodissection is a good technique, achieved by pumping up the area with local anaesthetic or 10–20 mL of normal saline so as to elevate the cancer to be excised up and away from the underlying danger, and should be routine.

Palpating and mapping of underlying arteries may also be prudent and helpful, especially the facial

artery anterior to the masseter and the superficial temporal artery.

For nerve blocks, know the distribution of the fifth cranial nerve and others and where they can be blocked. See Chapter 3, 'Local anaesthesia'.

Always have a plan B.

Remember most wounds will heal by secondary intention.

Remember there is always a colleague in a hospital who can retrieve the situation.

Use a check list.

Use good instruments. Get the best, especially needle holders, you can afford.

Know your suture materials and get used to ones to rely on. Needles have different grades of quality/sharpness.

Use blue sutures in hairy areas to make removal easier.

Always use reverse cutting needles for skin except for elderly, friable skin then use taper needles.

The only deep sutures proven to work are PDS II, Monoplus, Monoslow. The only place to use them (as a rule) is on the back.

Use bipolar cautery for flap haemostasis to minimise tip necrosis.

Don't over-cauterise. Most bleeding is venous or arteriolar and settles with pressure, time and/or temporary clamping.

Put a locator suture or nick in before you fully excise the lesion (usually at 12 o'clock).

An assistant should watch you and anticipate.

'General anaesthesia was invented for the benefit of the surgeon'. A nervous, garrulous patient may have to be tolerated until they are reassured the operation doesn't hurt.

If a patient has a cold ask them to warn when they are about to cough or sneeze so as to secure the wound and untied sutures.

UNDERMINING

The cutaneous or subdermal vessels are the main blood supply to the skin. Located at the junction between the deep reticular dermis and subcutaneous fat, they are responsible for dermal bleeding from the edge of the skin flap and consist of both arterioles and capillaries that form the subdermal plexus with enough perfusion pressure to nourish random flaps. This plexus is situated in the superficial to mid-subcutaneous fat and this must be attached to the raised flap to ensure viability.

Undermining too superficially, as in the dermis, runs the considerable risk of cutting off this blood supply with subsequent necrosis of the flap.

Undermining 50–100% of the defect width [25] or to 2–4 cm [26] beyond the wound edge has been recommended to decrease the wound tension, but this should be taken as a guide only.

In vivo studies on pigs have shown that the force required to close a linear wound is reduced by 18.6–47.4% by simple undermining of the wound edges [27].

Benefits

Wounds heal optimally with good skin edge eversion and when sutured under minimal tension. Wounds repaired under tension are at greater risk for edge necrosis, tract marks, dehiscence, infection, scar inversion, scar spread and distortion.

- Undermining is the most useful technique to reduce wound closure tension.
- Undermining wound edges resulted in a significant decrease in force required to close wounds of up to 50% [29].
- Undermining in all directions, including the apices, distributes redundant tissue more evenly and minimises dog-ears.
- It also distributes the scar tissue and contraction over a larger area for better cosmesis and stability, forming a plate-like scar.
- Wide undermining of flaps is obviously needed to mobilise them but undermining of the recipient site also improves flap fit and reduces pin-cushioning.
- It allows a circular defect to align optimally as an ellipse.

Complications

Complications are usually the result of incorrect or poor technique:

- reduced skin edge perfusion
- nerve damage
- blood vessel damage and haematoma
- altered and poor cosmesis.

Technique

- Rhomboid/ellipses: the usual practical recommendation is to undermine an ellipse 25% either side, making 50% in toto.
- Flaps: it is necessary to undermine flaps so as to mobilise them to be repositioned. To do so, it is essential the subdermal plexus of blood vessels is not compromised. The skin, especially on the head and neck, varies and knowledge of this aids successful surgery. See Chapter 2, 'Essential anatomy for skin surgery'.

Undermining 2–4 cm [26] or 50–100% [25] of the defect diameter is recommended to decrease wound tension and minimise compromising blood supply (Figure 5.30).

- Test first: pull the edges together first as many wounds need no undermining.
- Mandatory:
  - good lights that illuminate both undermined edges as far as needed
  - good exposure – retraction by tissue forceps or skin hooks
  - thorough knowledge of the anatomy
  - correct plane of dissection, usually the fat layer, so as to leave a layer on the raised skin to provide the subdermal plexus with nourishing vessels (see below)
- Sharp:
  - A scalpel is arguably mostly used. The incised edge is gently grasped and elevated with toothed forceps, the correct plane identified and the area undermined with arc-like incisions parallel to the skin surface at right angles to the incision.
  - Open straight scissors are introduced in the wound edge parallel to the incision and the tips palpated with the free fingers of the hand holding the forceps or skin hook.
- Blunt: closed scissors are introduced at right angles to the incision and advanced cautiously then opened to provide shearing, rather than a cutting, and hence less risk of damaging vessels or nerves. This is mostly used on the dorsum of the hands and feet and the subgaleal scalp. Wens can also be blunt dissected out this way using the needle holder (inserted between the cyst wall and surrounding tissue and then just opening their jaws).

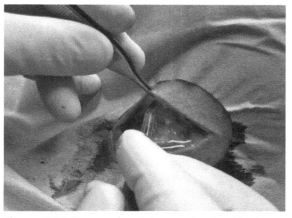

Figure 5.30 Here undermining on the shoulder is done in the mid-fat layer using the scalpel

Planes of dissection/undermining

In essence all undermining should be in the mid-fat layer except in the four danger zones of the face, where it should be in the superficial fat layer, and on the scalp, where it is subgaleal.

- Danger zones of the face (zygomatic arch where the temporal branch of the facial nerve crosses, mandible just in front of the masseter muscle where the facial artery crosses, temporal area where the superficial temporal artery lies above the fascia, inner canthus): while superficial, these lie deep to the subcutaneous fat and can be avoided by meticulous adherence to the superficial layer of the subcutaneous fat.
- Forehead: subcutaneous fat above the frontalis fascia; subgaleal (large defects).
- Temple/zygoma: superficial subcutaneous fat above the temporal branch of the facial nerve.
- Mandible: superficial subcutaneous fat above the mandibular branch of the facial nerve.
- Face: superficial subcutaneous fat.
- Nose: directly above the perichondrium/ostium.
- Scalp: under the fat layer of the scalp, in which the blood vessels run, the superficial and deep fascia that envelops the frontalis and occipital muscles becomes one dense fibrous sheath, the galea. Under this fascia, the subgaleal space is bloodless and blunt dissection is easy. The galea can be recognised because it is so dense and mobile whereas the underlying periostium, if cut, reveals bone. The difference becomes more difficult with the elderly. Ensure all undermining is done below the level of the hair follicles and that the incision is oblique and not vertical so that it is parallel to the oblique hair

shafts. This minimises cutting across hair follicles and a scar without hair growth.
- Hair areas: deep to the hair papillae – deeper fat layer.
- Neck danger zone (accessory nerve – Erb's point): superficial subcutaneous fat above the accessory nerve.
- Trunk: above the muscle fascia or mid fat.
- Hands and feet: subdermal.

The superficial subcutaneous fat is always safest. Just leave a layer of fat on the flap to provide nourishment.

Take care

Know the anatomy. Ensure a dry field with good vision. Even the apparently simplest lesion in a safe site can have a significant aberrant blood vessel running more superficially than expected (see Figure 5.31). The forearm and the lower leg, especially in patients with varicose veins, often present such problems.

Orientation location

Mark one edge so as to orientate the excised lesion. Do this before the lesion is completely excised, while still attached, so as to obviate mistakes if distracted. Marking may be by a small nick or a stitch but ensure they do not pass through the tumour. Note the location on the pathology request form as a clock face. 12 o'clock is usually taken as the default mark unless otherwise noted. This allows the surgeon to identify where the lesion is incompletely excised if this occurs.

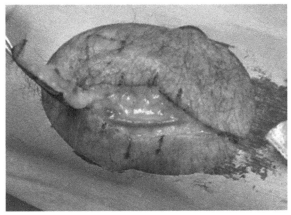

Figure 5.31 In the forearm there is invariably a large superficial vein as here

With varicose veins in the leg meticulous dissection to avoid nicking them will be rewarded as the time taken to do this is far less than finding and ligating any that may be cut.

DOG-EARS

Definitions

Dog-ear or **cone**: an excess of tissue formed by compression of the skin with closure of wounds. This is usually caused by the wound being too round or one side longer than the other or when movement of a flap pushes adjacent skin up.

Note: some authors also refer to the triangular excised ends of an ellipse where the central circle has been excised as dog-ears too.

Standing cone: perpendicular to the skin and occurs when symmetrical wounds are closed. These are repaired by symmetric procedures such as a fusiform excision.

Lying cone: half a cone that lies on the skin surface and is formed on the longer side of an asymmetric wound. These are repaired by asymmetric procedures such as a triangular excision.

Inverted cone: a depression at the apex of the wound and occurs in thick, rigid skin such as the back or acral when inadequately undermined. Repair involves undermining and mobilising the depressed cone and converting it into a standing cone.

Causes and prevention

- Tissue type: skin is elastic and accommodating but this alters with age, exposure and site. The back and acral skin are thick and unforgiving. Extensive undermining helps prevent dog-ears.
- Tension: wounds closed under excessive tension depress the centre of the wound and lift the ends/apices provoking a potential dog-ear.
- Flaps: dog-ears are prone to form:
  - Advancement flaps: at the base
  - Rotation flaps: opposite the point of rotation
  - Transposition flaps: at the base where the rotation element occurs
- Apical angles: the classic recommendation is for the apical angles of an ellipse/fusiform wound to be <30°. This is best achieved when the length-to-width ratio is >3:1 to 4:1. It is obvious that the sides of an ellipse are longer than the central axis. Therefore, closing to this shorter central axis causes tissue displacement and compression. Closing by the 'rule of halves' allows the skin to accommodate this if the apical angle is <30°. However, all wounds should be closed from alternate ends toward the centre. This

way dog-ears do not form. Excess tissue at the centre usually accommodates, given time, or can be more easily excised.

- Skin contour: convex surfaces are more prone to dog-ear formation, especially across the jaw and chin. Scar contraction can also depress the centre of the scar and exaggerate the apical rise.
- Excision technique:
  - Scalpel angle/wedging: the correct 90° vertical scalpel blade incision angle must be maintained right to the apices of the ellipse. Any altering of this angle with consequent bevelling of the side or wedging/shallowing of the apical wound base causes excess tissue at these apices and a greater likelihood of a dog-ear (Figure 5.32). These are less likely to resolve due to this excess wedge of tissue.
  - Undermining: the apices, especially, should be undermined in the subcutaneous plane as tissue is pushed out from the centre towards the apices and undermined apices better accommodate this push.
  - Creeping Charlie: the traditional advice is to make a central suture, halving the wound, and then go out both sides. Although this is sound for lacerations it is not sound for skin cancer deficit where, for any wound, whether it is of equal or unequal length, closure is begun at the ends of the defect to avoid unnecessary dog-ears. Any redundancies can be dealt with in the middle of the wound during closure. Irregularities or pleats in the middle of the wound generally resolve in time. Remember, skin stretches and accommodates.
  - Unequal sides: dog-ears can be prevented by still using the rule of halves, especially with the creeping Charlie technique, so dog ears can be sutured out by starting at the end and then scalloping of the longer side stretches and takes up.
  - Stretching: immediate prevention may be accomplished by stretching the wound

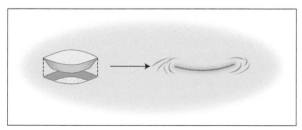

Figure 5.32 Wedging or shallowing of the apical wound base

longitudinally at both ends before any suturing. This is good for short excisions with apical angles >30°. The practitioner may be able to use the index finger and thumb of the non-dominant hand but the whole wound needs to be stretched at its apices. Then non-dog-eared stretched ends can be secured at either end. Optimally, or for longer wounds, an assistant is needed.

Dog-ear treatment and repair

Observation

Although several methods have been developed to prevent or correct dog-ears, most result in prolonged scars and operating times. Observe dog-ears without correction to examine regression with time.

One study found that, if the height of a dog-ear is ≤8 mm, observation rather than immediate surgical removal is recommended [30]. Many practitioners underestimate the skin's ability to redistribute tissue under tension and compression during the healing process. Although it is not always possible to predict which dog-ears will self-resolve, experience plays a significant role. A 2008 report followed 43 dog-ears after excisions in 26 patients and quantified dog-ear regression. Dog-ears regressed at least partially in all 43 and resolved completely in 19 (within a mean time of 132 days). Younger women were most likely to have self-resolving dog-ears [30].

Suturing techniques

Various suturing techniques have been reported to assist in dog-ear repair or avoidance. After a round lesion is removed, a horizontal square buried suture (HSBS) is deeply placed parallel to the longitudinal direction of the defect. The defect then becomes fusiform. A second HSBS is then placed parallel to the longitudinal direction of the defect but in more superficial fascia and using smaller horizontal buried loops than those of the first deep suture. The wound then becomes almost completely closed without dog-ears. Percutaneous sutures can then be placed to complete the closure. A small circular or oval defect on the face ≤1 cm in diameter could be closed in this way without any additional excision of the skin and without creating dog-ears. If the defect is >1 cm in diameter, minor corrections of dog-ears are probably required. Even in such a situation, the resultant scar is much shorter than that of conventional fusiform excision [31].

Defect ratios of 1.5 : 1 without resultant dog-ear formation were obtained using a horizontal oblique dermal suture to approximate the tissue, creating minimal wound edge tension. Additionally, the apex cutaneous suture can repair most dog-ear defects [32].

Shorter scars were also achieved by using subcutaneous and percutaneous figure-of-eight sutures. These can equally distribute the excess tissue along the scar and

alleviate dog-ears. In 65 cases a significant reduction of the length-to-width ratio was reported and achieved excellent long-term cosmetic outcomes while preserving healthy skin with shorter scars [33].

Repair

Various methods have been described:

1 Extension: the aim is to extend the original incision in the same line so that it is not noticed. There are three methods:

   A Use a skin hook to pull the dog-ear up by its apex (centre), then pull it to one side. Now extend the original incision in its straight line. Now pull this cut piece across to the other side and again extend the original incision cut. This results in a triangle of excised skin that is discarded and the wound sewn up continuing the straight line of the original incision (Figure 5.33a).

   B A simple new ellipse is made around the redundant cone with the same result as in (a) (Figure 5.33b).

   C In a variation of (a), the cone is raised by its central apex to form a tent of two triangles and then cut from this apex straight, in line with the original incision, to the tethered skin/wound end. This frees these two triangles, which are removed and then sewn up (Figure 5.34).

2 Hockey stick: incision and excising of the dog-ear is done at right angles to the main incision.

3 Right angle/crescent: incision and excising of the dog-ear is done at right angles to the main incision.

4 M-plasty

5 Lazy S-plasty

6 Curvilinear excision

7 Rule of halves

8 Staged elliptical excision and crescent excision with purse string sutures

9 Subdermal diathermy: a probe is inserted to dissolve the subcutaneous fat below the dog-ear to flatten it.

Methods 4–8 are covered elsewhere or are self-explanatory.

HEALING

Refer to Chapter 12, 'Postoperative care'.

FOLLOW-UP

Inform patients that it takes at least 6 months for scar maturation. Remove sutures ASAP but take care! Do not be in a hurry if there is any tension/threatened dehiscence. Apply tape-strips to facial wounds or those under tension at ROS. Patients can open wounds by dragging their face across the pillow while sleeping.

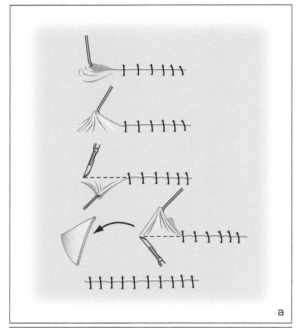

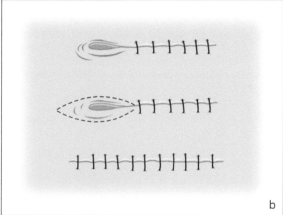

Figure 5.33 Repair of dog-ear deformity by **(a)** pulling excess tissue to each side of the incision line and removing a single triangular piece of excess tissue or **(b)** making a simple elliptical excision around the redundant cone

Adapted from Roenigk R, Roenigk H (eds). Dermatologic Surgery, 2nd edn. New York: Marcel Dekker Inc, 1989.

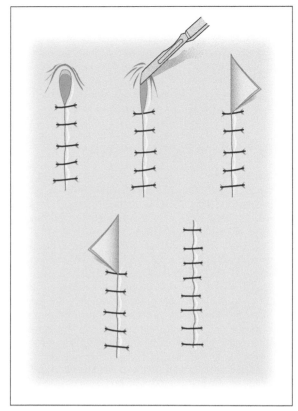

Figure 5.34 Correction of dog-ear deformity by division of the dog-ear in half and excision of two small triangular pieces of tissue

Adapted from Roenigk R, Roenigk H (eds). Dermatologic Surgery, 2nd edn. New York: Marcel Dekker Inc, 1989.

For at least 6 months, do not perform aggressive scar revision to allow for normal scar maturity. Earlier scar revision intervention is indicated if facial function will be compromised or distorted from contraction.

Camouflage make-up can be helpful for obvious scars.

If an incision appears to be developing into a hypertrophic scar, consider using injectable triamcinolone acetate and topical silicone-gel sheeting. A sign that excessive scar formation could be developing is a persistently non-tender, erythematous, raised-skin surface present after several weeks.

REFERENCES

[1] Madan R, Chen S. The so-called dysplastic nevus is not dysplastic at all. Dermatol Pract Conc 2013;3(1):1. Available: <http://dx.doi.org/10.5826/dpc.0301a01>; [accessed 2 Mar 2013].

[2] AJCC/UICC TNM Classification of malignant tumours, 7th ed. 2009.

[3] Rigel DS. Cancer of the Skin. Philadelphia: Elsevier Saunders; 2005. p. 119.

[4] Wolf DJ, Zitelli JA. Surgical margins for basal cell carcinoma. Arch Derm 1987;123:340–4.

[5] Kerns MJ, Darst MA, Olsen TG, et al. Shrinkage of cutaneous specimens: formalin or other factors involved? J Cutan Pathol 2008;35:1093–6.

[6] Sussman LA, Liggins DF. Incompletely excised basal cell carcinoma: a management dilemma? Aust N Z J Surg 1996;66:276–8.

[7] Griffiths RW. Audit of histologically incompletely excised basal cell carcinomas: recommendations for management by re–excision. Br J Plast Surg 1999;52:24–8.

[8] Schreuder F, Powell BW. Incomplete excision of basal cell carcinomas: an audit. Clin Perform Qual Health Care 1999;7:119–20.

[9] Kumar P, Orton CI, McWilliam LJ, et al. Incidence of incomplete excision in surgically treated basal cell carcinoma: a retrospective clinical audit. Br J Plast Surg 2000;53:563–6.

[10] Fleischer AB Jr, Feldman SR, Barlow JO, et al. The specialty of the treating physician affects the likelihood of tumor-free resection margins for basal cell carcinoma: results from a multi-institutional retrospective study. J Am Acad Dermatol 2001;44:224–30.

[11] Hallock GG, Lutz DA. A prospective study of the accuracy of the surgeon's diagnosis and significance of positive margins in nonmelanoma skin cancers. Plast Reconstr Surg 2001;107:942–7.

[12] Bisson MA, Dunkin CS, Suvarna SK, et al. Do plastic surgeons resect basal cell carcinomas too widely? A prospective study comparing surgical and histological margins. Br J Plast Surg 2002;55:293–7.

[13] Dieu T, Macleod AM. Incomplete excision of basal cell carcinomas: a retrospective audit. ANZ J Surg 2002;72:219–21.

[14] Hussain M, Earley MJ. The incidence of incomplete excision in surgically treated basal cell carcinoma: a retrospective clinical audit. Ir Med J 2003;96:18–20.

[15] Bogdanov-Berezovsky A, Cohen AD, Glesinger R, et al. Risk factors for incomplete excision of basal cell carcinomas. Acta Derm Venereol 2004;84:44–7.

[16] Wilson AW, Howsam G, Santhanam V, et al. Surgical management of incompletely excised basal cell carcinomas of the head and neck. Br J Oral Maxillofac Surg 2004;42:311–14.

[17] Richmond JD, Davie RM. The significance of incomplete excision in patients with basal cell carcinoma. Br J Plast Surg 1987;40:63–7.

[18] Nagore E, Grau C, Molinero J, et al. Positive margins in basal cell carcinoma: relationship to clinical features and recurrence risk. A retrospective study of 248 patients. J Eur Acad Dermatol Venereol 2003;17:167–70.

[19] Seretis K, Thomaidis V, Karpouzis A, et al. Epidemiology of surgical treatment of nonmelanoma skin cancer of the head and neck in Greece. Derm Surg 2010;36(1):15–22.

[20] Lask GP, Moy RL. Principles and techniques of cutaneous surgery. USA: McGraw-Hill; 1996. p. 165–70.

[21] Goldberg LH, Alam M. Elliptical excisions: variations and the eccentric parallelogram. Arch Dermatol 2004;140:176–80.

[22] Burton C, Rennie R, Turnbull L, et al. Can skin marker pens, used pre-operatively to mark surgical sites, transfer bacteria? ICAAC-IDSA Annual Meeting. Washington, DC, October 25–28, Abstract K-583, 2008.

[23] Wilhelmi BJ, Blackwell SJ, Phillips LG. Langer's lines: to use or not to use. Plast Reconstr Surg 1999;104(1):208–14.

[24] Larrabee WF Jr, Holloway GA Jr, Sutton D. Wound tension and blood flow in skin flaps. Ann Otol Rhinol Laryngol 1984;93(2 Pt 1):112–15.

[25] Boyer JD, Zitelli JA, Brodland DG, et al. Undermining in cutaneous surgery. Derm Surg 2001;27(1):75–8.

[26] Leach J. Proper handling of soft tissue in the acute phase. Facial Plast Surg 2001;17:227–38.

[27] McGuire MF. Studies of the excisional wound: I. Biomechanical effects of undermining and wound orientation on closing tension and work. Plast Reconst Surg 1980;66:419–27.

[28] Larrabee WF, Holloway GA, Sutton D. Variation of skin stress-strain curves with undermining. Surg Forum 1981;32:553–5.

[29] Mackay DR, Saggers GC, Kotwal N, et al. Stretching skin: undermining is more important than intraoperative expansion. Plast Reconstr Surg 1990;86:722–30.

[30] Lee KS, Kim NG, Jang PY, et al. Statistical analysis of surgical dog-ear regression. Dermatol Surg 2008;34(8):1070–6.

[31] Matsunaga J, Aiba S. Horizontal square buried sutures in a two-layered fashion enable direct primary closure for small circular wounds without dog-ears on the face. Dermatol Surg 2005;31:574–6.

[32] Stewart JB Jr. Tissue sparing repair. A new approach to shorten excisional lines. J Dermatol Surg Oncol 1992;18:822–6.

[33] Tilleman TR. Direct closure of round skin defects: a four-step technique with multiple subcutaneous and cutaneous 'figure-of-8' sutures alleviating dog-ears. Plast Reconstr Surg 2004;114:1761–7.

[34] Kunishige JH, Brodland DG, Zitelli JA. Surgical margins for melanoma in situ. J Am Acad Dermatol 2012;66:438–44.

[35] Kelly JW, Henderson MA, Thursfield VJ, et al. The management of primary cutaneous melanoma in Victoria in 1996 and 2000. Med J Aust 2007;187(9):511–14.

Suturing, knots and closures

I don't know who is the best for that operation as I never operate with or see other surgeons. The theatre sister is the one to ask.

A surgeon's reply

SUTURING TECHNIQUES

Basic, good suturing technique and good equipment are mandatory.

First the margins

As will be repeated in Chapter 8 'Flaps', the essential fact in skin cancer surgery is to excise all the cancer with the correct, evidenced margins.

Closure

The aims of closure are:

- obliteration of dead space
- even distribution of tension along deep suture lines
- maintenance of tensile strength across the wound until tissue tensile strength is adequate
- approximation and eversion of the epithelial portion of the closure
- cosmesis.

The defect must be closed in the best possible manner. No longer are 'rope' sutures leaving 'train lines' or 'snake bites' acceptable. Today, many scars can be hidden or minimised to just a fine white line if the surgeon understands tissue movement, incision placement and good technique and uses the best and most appropriate materials. Remember to use the minimum number of sutures to approximate the everted wound edges to allow the skin to heal itself. Too many sutures increase the chances of wound infection, necrosis and poor cosmesis. Skin/wound tension also needs to be minimised. Every time tissue is handled by instruments, cells are killed, so minimise handling and be gentle. Sharp dissection is generally less traumatic than blunt dissection. Skin cancer surgery, however, has a unique disadvantage in that a surface lesion has been excised leaving a large deficit and the wound edges are far apart when compared with most other surgery or injuries. A simple ellipse heals better and a curve is less noticeable than a straight line.

Anyone can do it

With a modicum of effort, understanding and technique the incidence of ugly scars for the simplest (and even the most difficult) excisions can be minimised. Despite best efforts some scars will spread and some will show suture marks, but it is now possible to learn how to minimise and hopefully prevent this (see Figure 6.1).

HINTS AND TIPS

- Instruments (forceps) kill cells when tissue is picked up. Minimise handling and be gentle.
- Use the minimum number of sutures to appose and evert edges.
- Approximation is all that is needed, at all tissue levels.
- Minimise tension.
- Do not pull sutures too tight.
- Ensure knot security.
- Epidermal shallow sutures leave marks/scars.
- Sharp dissection is less traumatic than blunt.
- Use the best sutures the patient can afford.
- Know the tissue reactivity potential of sutures and minimise.
- Consider subcuticular sutures for cosmesis.
- Arm needle holder correctly each and every time.
- Do not pull the needle by its tip (causes blunting).
- Do not pull or handle the needle with fingers (needle stick).
- Draw nylon between gloved fingers to minimise memory.

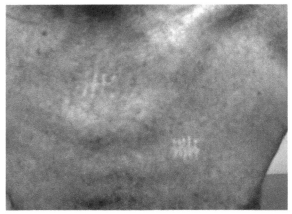

Figure 6.1 Between the two rather horrific, horizontal 'train line' white scars (done for benign lesions) on this man's chest, an elegant oblique reddish line can be seen where a 12-mm cancer was excised with 4-mm margins. Most excisions can be done elegantly and correctly. The patient stated that the first two 'hurt and pulled' but that the final one 'gave no trouble'. This was because the incision was placed in the 'action' lines, with the patient lifting his arms above his shoulders, and because the incision was long enough with sufficient undermining to reduce tension, using the smallest sutures possible (5/0), everting the edges and using a waterproof dressing, which the patient left on until removal of sutures. This redness will fade and the scar will be virtually invisible.

FUNDAMENTALS AND ESSENTIALS FOR SKIN SURGERY AND WOUND REPAIR

Careful matching of layers

No matter what suture is used it is essential to match each layer with the corresponding layer on the other side of the wound. If this is not done the scar will dip and rise, reflecting the light differently with a poor cosmetic result or even ugly and unsatisfactory inversion of the edges.

Knowing and recognising the various tissue layers (epidermis, dermis, fat, deep fascia and muscle) is essential (see Figure 6.2a). Matching may often best be achieved, especially on the back but also where the wound is very wide, by placing deep sutures to draw the dermis together (Figure 6.2b–d). This has the added benefit of provoking eversion (Figure 6.2e, f), if done correctly, and also reducing the tension on the skin sutures.

Often one 'side' of the wound may be lower than the other. This is frequently encountered in lower forearm flaps where the higher side then needs a shallow suture while the lower side needs a deeper suture to draw it up and level. This sounds simple but is sometimes difficult to achieve. Just remember to go as shallow as you can on the high side (high, high) and as deep as necessary on the

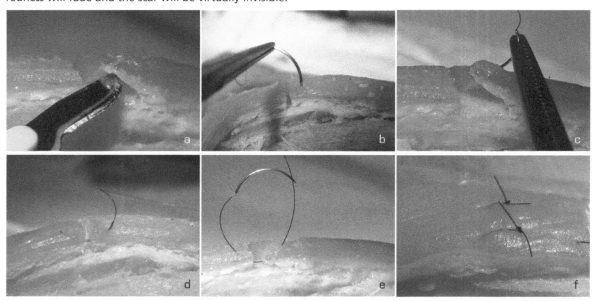

Figure 6.2 A pig model illustrates the layers of the skin and suture technique

a The epidermis or skin surface is the glistening top layer whereas, directly inferior, is the slightly thicker darker dermis below which is the white fat and then the pink muscle. Undermining is being done in the upper fat layer. **b** The needle is inserted vertically and rotated slightly out and away from the incision so the base is wider than the point of entry. **c** It is then allowed to prescribe the natural arc of its curve through the dermis, which is the toughest tissue, and into the fat if there is a small dead space to close. Large dead spaces are best closed with deep sutures. **d** The vertical needle, outward rotation and natural arc make the base of the suture flask-shaped. **e** When this is pulled together the wider base everts the wound edges. **f** This humps up the epidermis to meet in eversion. The knots are tied to the side of the incision further promoting the desired eversion and, as can be seen, the layers perfectly matched.

low side (low, low) (Figure 6.3), and more than one is often needed. Simple interrupted sutures are used. There are two methods:

1 Enter the higher side first and take a shallow bite, then a deeper bite on the lower side to bring it up.
2 Some prefer entering the lower side first and pulling it so the skin surfaces are coplanar, which allows assessment as to where the more superficial suture on the other side should go.

Eversion of sutured wound edges

The correct technique for superficial or skin sutures should ensure eversion (Figure 6.2e, f). Deep sutures may enhance this.

There cannot be too much eversion if the apposition is epidermis to epidermis (Figure 6.4a). However, there will be too much eversion if the wound edges are drawn up so that the apposition is dermis to epidermis, or dermis to dermis (Figure 6.4b), which results in a wide scar.

Lack of tension

Closing the deficit in skin cancer surgery creates **skin under tension**. In a wound under tension, the blood supply is compressed and restricted, which leads to poor healing, suture marks and bad scars. While 'no tension' may be recommended this is impossible to achieve. The aim is therefore to control, distribute and minimise the tension. Assessing how the skin moves and where it is lax allows placement of the incision so as to maximise this movement and minimise tension. The easiest way to assess this is by simply pinching the patient's skin between thumb and index finger in all directions. The incision is then placed longitudinally between the thumb and index finger where they can grasp the most skin. The usual illustrations of Langer's lines and the relaxed skin tension lines (RSTLs) are not always a good guide. It is far better and more logical to get the patient to grimace or raise the arms so as to see where the face, chest or back 'action' lines actually are. If the RSTLs were to be used on the extremities where they are mostly horizontal, they would not only result in much more tension on the wound, especially with bending the limb, but also be more dangerous as such an incision would cut straight across nerves and vessels.

Good blood supply

A good blood supply is essential for flap surgery to avoid necrosis. Most skin flaps depend on small, unnamed vessels or the subdermal plexus of blood vessels, which are classified as 'random'. The random plexus runs in the subdermal fat layer and so it is absolutely essential that a layer of fat stays attached to the skin flap as it is moved. The base of the flap must also be wide enough so the plexus can supply the whole length of the flap. A width (base)-to-length ratio of 1:1 means the base is as wide as the flap is long and ensures adequate supply. Usually the widths of flaps are shorter than their lengths, but when the ratio reaches 1:3 the blood supply is compromised. It is best not to exceed a length of 1.5 relative to a base width of 1. For further details, refer to Chapter 8, 'Flaps'.

Simplest procedure

Always use the simplest procedure that will do the job. A straight line (an ellipse) heals better than a flap, with fewer complications. Always consider a longer ellipse.

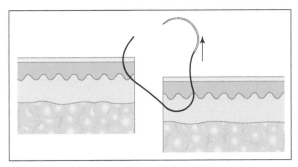

Figure 6.3 Layer adjustment: step down or adjustment sutures

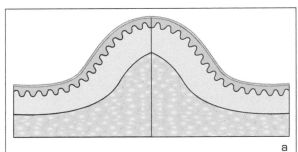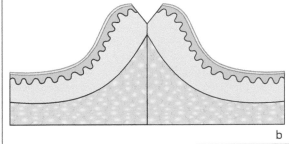

Figure 6.4 Eversion of wound edges
a Correct: epidermis to epidermis. **b** Incorrect: dermis to dermis; too much eversion.

Basic gems

1 A straight line (ellipse) heals better than a flap. Always do the simplest procedure.

2 Ensure the length of the excision is at least three times its width (3:1). In areas of high tension don't hesitate to make the incision longer; 4:1 is optimum.

3 Measure and mark margins. Line-up lines may also help if the wound is wide.

4 Cut outside marks in any event.

5 Hold skin-to-go (i.e. the lesion) but not the good remaining skin with toothed forceps.

6 Incise and undermine lesion.

7 Determine the level to excise and go across on the same level/plane, working from one pole to the other.

8 Assess mobility of the wound to draw close, especially in the middle, to ascertain if further undermining is needed.

9 Undermine as necessary proportional to need and circumstances (~25% don't need undermining).

10 Skin stretches and wounds that are initially too wide to place the first stitch in the centre may well come together if sutured from the ends ('creeping Charlie' technique). Alternate sutures from end to end.

11 Scars can contract up to 30% in length over time.

12 Consider S-plasty or O-S flaps where scars have to stretch over joints.

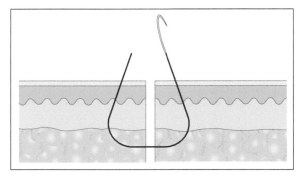

Figure 6.5 Flask or pear suture

DIFFERENT SUTURES AND THEIR USES

Interrupted sutures

Simple interrupted sutures

Interrupted sutures have the advantage of 'modelling' the wound by halves so potential problems and excessive tension can be recognised early and dealt with. Alternate sutures can also be removed if a wound infection develops, which maintains the integrity but helps treat the infection.

Flask or pear sutures

If the needle goes further out at the bases than at the entry and exit points, the needle holes will be closer together at the skin surface than at the wound base, resulting in eversion (Figure 6.5). These are referred to as flask or pear sutures – narrower at the top and broader at the bottom.

Most instructions state the needle should go in vertically; however, here this makes a flask shape more difficult. Instead, angle the needle away from the incision into either the dermis or subcutaneous fat by pronating the hand, and then make an equal bite on the opposite side, at the same level, to return closer and exit at the same distance from the incision as the entry (Figures 6.6, 6.7). This technique results in eversion of the incision edges. By tying the knots at the side, rather than on top, the skin is further pushed up and everted (Figure 6.8). This is the desirable objective.

Mattress sutures

Mattress sutures also evert the edges and provide greater support and less wound tension than simple sutures. They also close dead space better.

Vertical mattress suture

A pear or flask suture is not needed here as eversion is effected by the return suture. The needle this time is directed vertically into the dermis and/or subcutaneous tissue (Figure 6.9). The longer or wider the defect or wound, the further away the first points of entry and mirror image exit should be. This usually varies from 5 to 10 mm. The needle is then reversed to make a second stitch much shallower and at the same level either side into the epidermis and some dermis but closer to the incision edge some 2–3 mm away. Then this is tied off. A vertical mattress suture is sometimes used as the central stitch to gain eversion and make this easier to maintain by subsequent interrupted stitches.

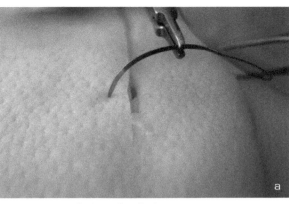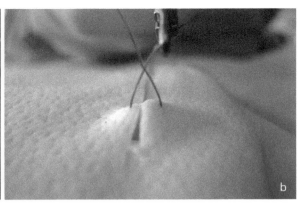

Figure 6.6 Technique for flask or pear sutures

a The needle is inserted vertically or angled out and away such that the base will be wider than the entrance. **b** The flask- or pear-shaped bottom naturally everts the epidermal edges.

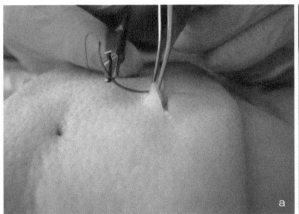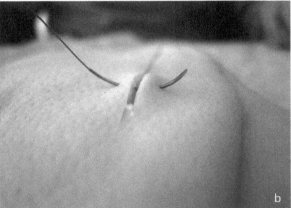

Figure 6.7 Second eversion technique

a Another way to achieve eversion is to evert both the epidermal edges with the forceps. **b** Then pass the needle through.

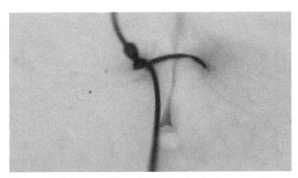

Figure 6.8 Tying off at the side also helps eversion

Horizontal mattress suture

These are most useful for reducing wound tension (Figure 6.10). Note that other sutures can be placed in between. The technique starts the same as for the vertical mattress but, when the first stitch exits, instead of returning across the wound the needle is taken parallel to the wound on the same side some 3–5 mm along and then across to the original side (Figure 6.11).

Do not use this stitch in areas or wounds with a compromised blood supply as it is more likely to tie off vessels. Take care not to pull too tight and strangulate tissue.

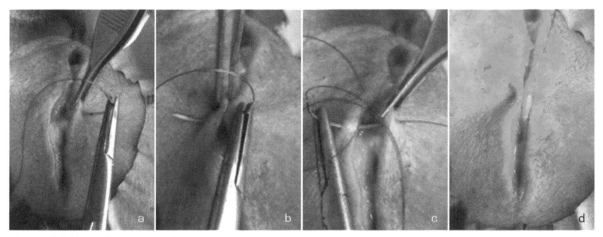

Figure 6.9 Vertical mattress suture

a The wound edge is everted and the needle inserted further away from the edge than for a normal interrupted suture. **b** It is passed to the other side, duplicating the same level and distance from the wound edge. **c** The needle is reversed to return and enter the skin but now closer to the wound and again exits duplicating the other side in depth and distance from the wound edge. **d** Both ends of the suture are drawn tight so that the epidermal wound edges 'kiss' and tied off leaving a perfectly sutured everted wound edge.

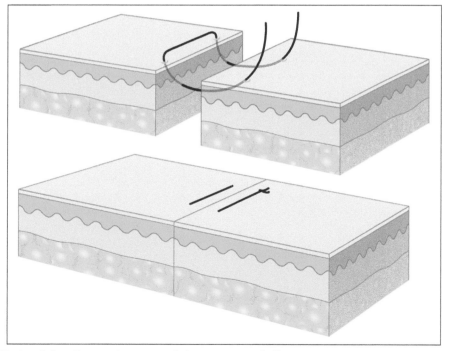

Figure 6.10 Horizontal mattress suture, one of the strongest of all sutures

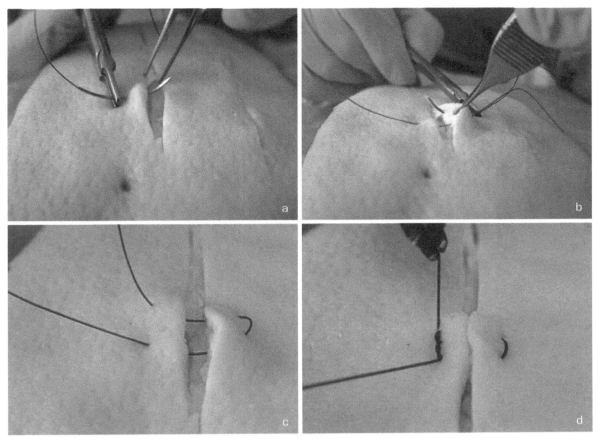

Figure 6.11 Horizontal mattress suture technique

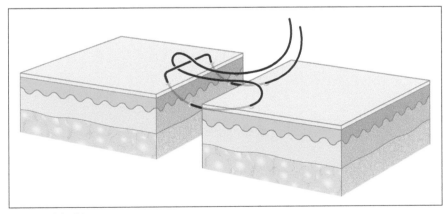

Figure 6.12 Horizontal locking mattress suture

Horizontal locking mattress suture

The horizontal locking mattress suture (Figure 6.12) provides haemostasis and edge eversion. Its main disadvantage is that with healing the suture tends to become buried and is difficult to remove. The locking horizontal mattress technique (Figure 6.13) facilitates suture removal and provides more control over wound edge placement while providing haemostasis, tensile strength and eversion and allows easier, faster suture removal with less patient discomfort.

This suture is useful for surgical and traumatic wounds of the hand, closing wounds of the scalp as they

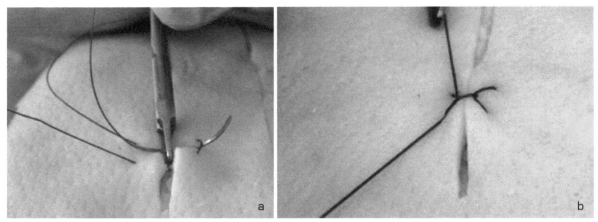

Figure 6.13 Horizontal locking mattress suture technique
Rather than tying off, (**a**) the needle is passed back under the horizontal first suture and (**b**) then tied off.

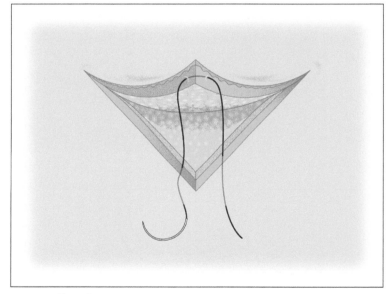

Figure 6.14 Gilles, corner or tip suture

frequently bleed freely and are fairly inelastic, and other wounds with thicker skin such as the back and thighs. It is not recommended for thinner, more fragile tissue and wound edges less able to tolerate some ischaemia from compression. Avoid over-tightening this suture to prevent tissue strangulation [1].

Gilles, tip, corner or half-buried horizontal mattress suture

This stitch is credited to Gilles, a New Zealand World War II surgeon who pioneered plastic surgery on burnt or battered Battle of Britain air crew. It is used to suture the triangle tip of a flap (Figure 6.14) but mostly to pull two 'A' flaps together to join the 'T' (Figure 6.15).

When an A-T flap is cut, the T skin base remains fixed while the A flap arms are undermined and raised. Suture entry is made into the dermis from the secure fixed skin of the horizontal T arm base slightly to the right of midline to exit into the wound (Figure 6.16a). Then, always at the same dermal level, the needle passes into the horizontal bottom of the pointed tip of the right A flap end (Figure 6.16b). It then curves parallel to the horizontal base to exit into the wound and

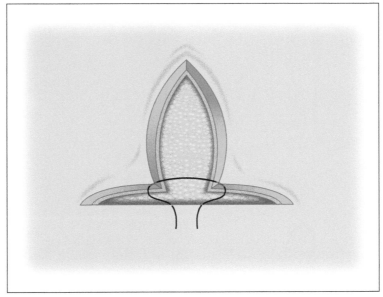

Figure 6.15 This Gilles or corner suture is mostly used for A-T flaps to secure the free ends of the raised A flaps and draw them together and bed into the base

duplicate this across at the other left flap tip (Figure 6.16c), then back to the base to exit just left of the midline (Figure 6.16d).

It is important that the sutures are all placed at the same level in the dermis.

The completed excision is shown in Figure 6.17.

Running or continuous sutures

Simple running suture

A running or continuous suture traverses the whole wound without any knots (Figure 6.18). It is much faster than interrupted sutures but not as strong and, if pulled tight, can cause strangulation of the blood supply. The problem of wound infection also arises because individual or alternate sutures cannot be removed. It is a fast 'emergency' suture.

Start as for an interrupted suture but don't cut the stitch. Then stitch on the diagonal to where the next suture is to be and go horizontally as for an interrupted suture but again don't cut it. Continual tension is needed as the surgeon pulls the wound closed, keeping the stitch end of the suture taut but not strangulating. Continue along the wound horizontal surface, diagonally in the dermis.

Locked or blanket suture

This blanket stitch is used to control postoperative bleeding where each of the running stitches is locked by passing the needle through the loop formed by the last suture (Figure 6.19). This places consistent pressure on the wound edges providing haemostasis. It is most often used on scalp wounds.

Subcuticular running suture

This suture gives the best 'scarless' cosmetic result but there are some hints and tricks not usually documented (Figure 6.20).

Many surgeons bend the sutures back slightly rather than going straight across.

When the wound is long or there is so much tension that it pulls apart, exit the wound, tie off and start again.

Techniques for tying off are illustrated in Figures 6.21 and 6.22.

> **NOTE**
> Subcuticular sutures work best when there is no tension. Unfortunately, most skin cancer surgery involves closing a large defect and hence there is tension with scar spread often at the point of maximum tension. Deep sutures may help as will a couple of 6/0 surface securing sutures, which some colleagues call 'sleepers' – because they allow them to sleep at nights.

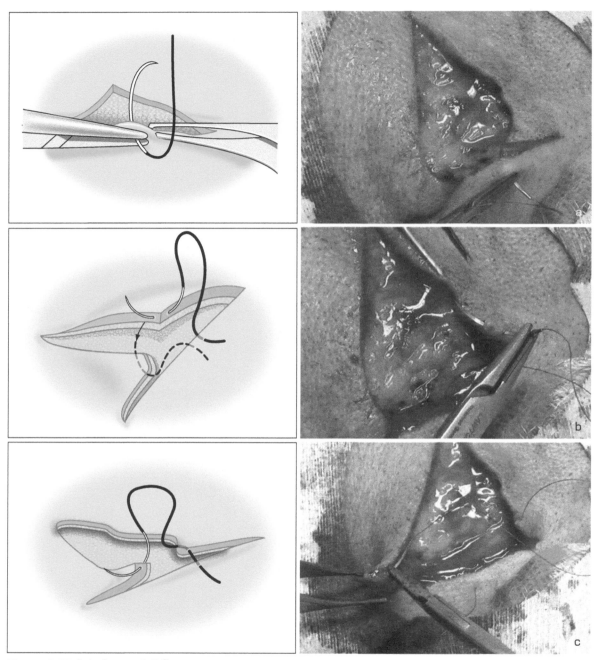

Figure 6.16 Suturing an A-T flap

a The apex of the A is distal to the needle, which is being inserted through the dermis at the right of the middle of the non-undermined T-axis base while the two lateral A flaps have been well undermined to facilitate their being pulled together. **b** The needle is inserted through the dermis of the right A flap. It goes in at the base, on the T side of the flap, and out exiting to the centre of the wound to head towards the same point on the left flap (all at the same dermal level). **c** The bottom of the left A flap is secured by the forceps to facilitate the needle passing through to duplicate the other side and exit facing the base (the T).

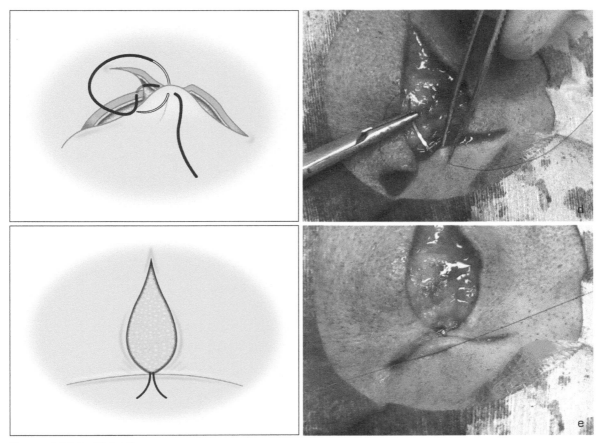

Figure 6.16 continued

d The needle now is passed to copy the original entry but slightly to the left of the midline. **e** Normally the A has been sutured together to minimise tension of the Gilles corner stitch tips but here, for demonstration, the tips have been pulled together first.

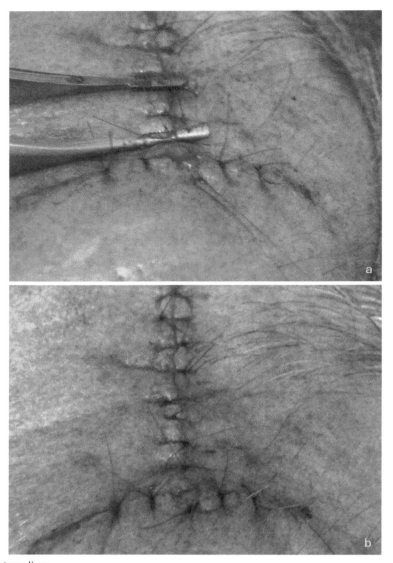

Figure 6.17 A-T suture lines

a The forceps are used to push the distal suture line down so as to show the eversion of the Gilles suture by revealing the distal wound edge. **b** The finished operation. This was a micronodular BCC and wider margins and Mohs pathology were done. Just as well – there was perineural invasion but margins were clear.

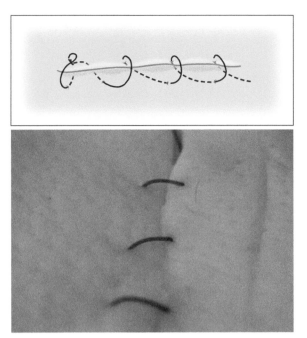

Figure 6.18 Simple running suture

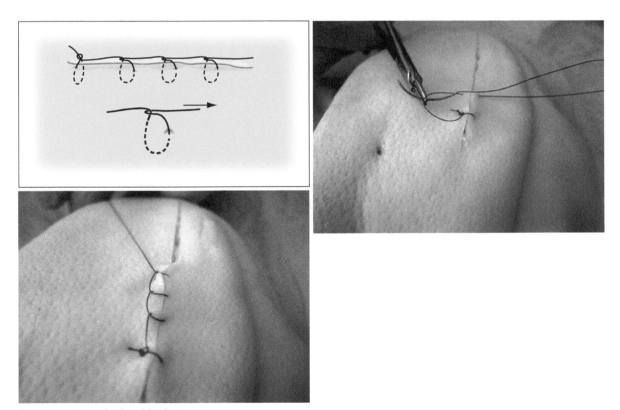

Figure 6.19 Locked or blanket suture

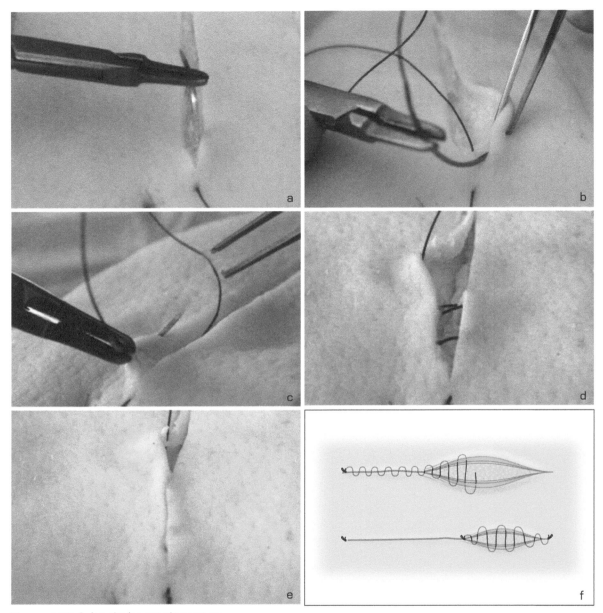

Figure 6.20 Subcuticular running suture

a Usually the suture enters 5 mm or so from the wound and comes out at the apex of its proximal base. **b** The edge of the wound is everted and the needle prescribes a semicircle through the dermis. **c** The needle now traverses the wound base to enter the opposite dermis at the same level. Most text books show this going straight across but many surgeons go back up higher. **d** These subcuticular (dermal) sutures now criss-cross the wound. **e** If the suture is pulled tight, the everted edges appose without any surface marks. **f** Schematic diagram of the subcuticular running suture.

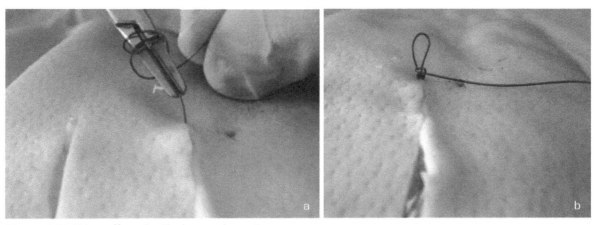

Figure 6.21 Tying off a subcuticular running suture

a Grasp the free suture that is either the start or finish end and wind it twice around the needle holder, then use the needle holder to grab the suture where it disappears into the wound. **b** This is effectively an instrument tie. Do two or three reversed throws.

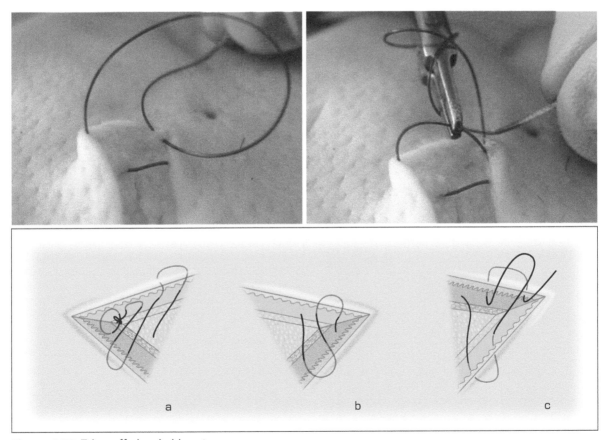

Figure 6.22 Tying off absorbable sutures

a If using absorbable sutures it is possible to bury both the start and the finish. Don't leave the wound at either end but take a small dermal bite while leaving the next or previous suture loose enough to provide a loop to grab. **b** Wind the needle end of the suture around the needle holder as for an instrument tie and now grab the last subcuticular dermal loop lying in the wound and do an instrument tie. This buries the knot in the wound. **c** Schematic diagram.

HINTS AND TIPS

1 Use a slippery, low friction suture such as polypropylene.

2 Do not use stretching sutures or those with some elasticity (polybutester).

3 Ensure sutures are placed exactly at the same levels on each side.

4 Rather than going straight across go somewhat proximal nearer to the previous suture on that side.

5 Pull the suture at regular intervals to ensure the wound closes.

6 Exit to the surface regularly, at a maximum of 3 cm, so as to be able to pull them out.

7 If the suture does break on removal, this is usually not a problem if the suture is biologically inert.

8 Absorbable sutures such as poliglecaprone (Monocryl) can be used and either pulled out or, if difficult, cut the ends and leave the middle in situ to absorb (do not leave exposed as then will not absorb).

9 Start and finish knots can also be buried in the wound.

10 Secure wound with strips.

11 Consider a central interrupted suture for added security.

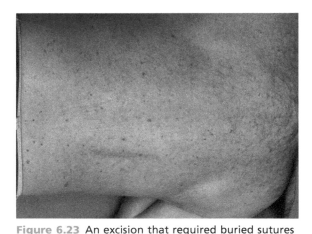

Figure 6.23 An excision that required buried sutures
A long simple ellipse for a large melanoma that required 10-mm(+) margins (i.e. >30-mm deficit). Deep Monoslow/PDS II sutures were used and interrupted nylon to close. Healing was uneventful with no scar spread 5 years later despite the patient's continued manual work and sailing. Despite all these best efforts and techniques, scar spread can still occur spontaneously on the back. The point is to nevertheless do the best possible to attempt to prevent this (i.e. deep slow absorbing sutures and minimal skin tension). Correct level of placement is most important: if too high in the dermis close to the epidermis/skin surface they may later extrude or 'spit'. Uneven/different levels result in a step-down deformity.

Buried sutures

Buried sutures take the tension off the skin edges of the wound by approximating the wound's deep tissues. In doing so, they eliminate the dead space, redistribute wound tension and allow for better skin closure. There is then less chance of dehiscence and scar spread, especially on the back, if sutures with a long absorption time are used (Figure 6.23).

Scar spread prevention

Dermal support for 3 weeks may reduce scar spread by 16% and for 6 months by 38% [2].

In effect, this means PDS II, MonoSlow or Monoplus deep sutures for back wounds.

They also provide wound edge approximation, which allows for subcuticular suturing to be done without tension and potential separation. Monosyn or equivalent is best used here.

An absorbable deep suture may be used for skin closure so as to minimise waste and opening another suture pack. However, absorbable sutures are degraded and absorbed by hydrolysis; when exposed, they do not degrade and have to be removed like nylon sutures.

Normal buried suture

The essential key to buried sutures is that the stitch starts at the base of the wound and goes upwards (Figure 6.24), which is the reverse of the normal skin suture. Preferably the wound should be undermined and the stitch commenced in the subcutaneous tissue up into the reticular dermis to exit and go across to the other side at the level of the mid-dermis then down and out mirroring the other side to emerge at the base of the wound. The suture is then tied with the knot now at the bottom of the wound to minimise reaction (Figure 6.25) as is cutting the suture 'on the knot'. The same level of exit and entry is important to obviate step-down deformities. A three-throw locking knot is invariably needed or a one-handed tie keeping the tension on and drawing the wound closed.

Absorbable deep sutures are almost mandatory for back excisions but also for any long and wide excisions or where there would be undesirable tension on the skin sutures, such as some facial wounds. PDS II/

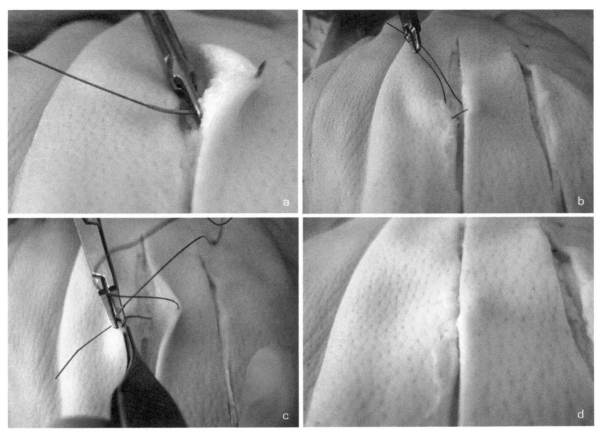

Figure 6.24 Normal buried sutures

a The needle enters from the base of the wound and exits upwards through the dermis. **b** It then traverses to the other side to enter the dermis and go down and out in the wound base. **c** These sutures are pulling the wound together and there is a lot of tension. **d** The pulled together wound allows for no-tension skin suturing.

Monoslow, which last for 180 days, are used but nylon sutures dissolve after 14 years or so and have been used successfully by the author (with no spread and no irritation after 4 years).

Vertical mattress buried suture

The vertical mattress buried suture is just the same as the normal one except the initial curve is wider and turns down in the dermis to exit lower in the wound edge. It then mimics this, entering the far wound edge to prescribe a higher arc before turning down to exit in the fat layer.

Buried butterfly suture

The buried butterfly is an exaggeration of the vertical mattress suture wherein the initial arc turns down to exit in the fat layer to be mimicked in the opposite wound edge (Figure 6.26). The wound needs to therefore be undermined but the result is even greater wound edge eversion.

Purse string suture

The purse string suture consists of small horizontal bites scalloping around the circumference in the mid-dermis of a usually circular wound (Figure 6.27). When the circle is complete and the two ends meet, they are drawn, pulled or tightened as in an old-fashioned purse. It is seldom a wound can be so closed but what the purse string suture does is reduce the radius of the deficit and allow faster healing. As can be seen in Chapter 9, 'Ear, nose and lip', it can be used not only for speeding up but also for modelling secondary intention healing.

Some techniques alternately exit the suture to the surface.

Layered purse string sutures can be used to close dead space.

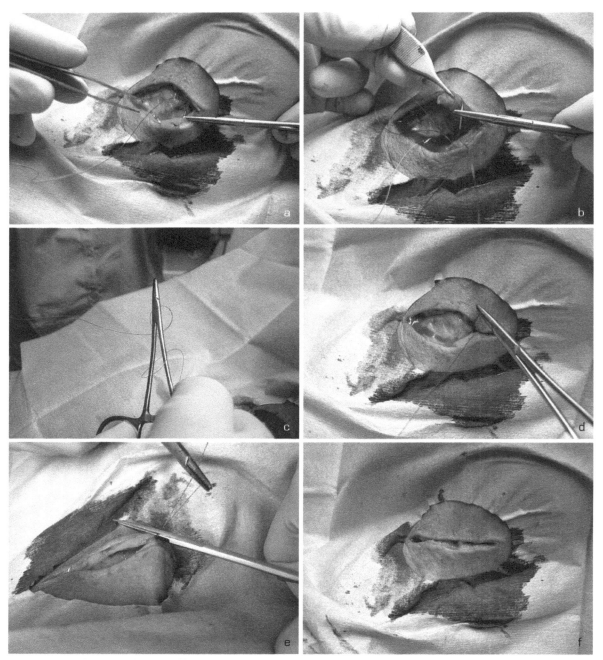

Figure 6.25 Placing and tying off normal buried sutures

a The needle is inserted from the base of the wound to exit in the dermis. **b** It then prescribes an arc to enter the opposing dermis and exit out into the bottom of the wound. **c** Wind the suture around the needle holder _three_ times (two shown here – do one more so it holds). **d** It is important to keep both free and needle end of the suture on their same sides and not crossed. This will allow the three loops to lie along the suture and easily be drawn tight. If crossed, a cinch will be formed. If there is difficulty tightening these first three throws, try sawing both suture ends back and forth and/or holding one and pulling the other (rather than the usual pulling both equally). **e** Cut on the knot. **f** Comparison of the end result of four deep sutures with the initial wide defect in **b** shows how the deep sutures have closed the defect and obliterated any dead space and that there will be no tension on the skin sutures.

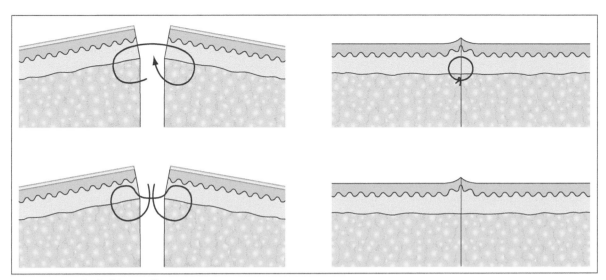

Figure 6.26 Buried butterfly suture

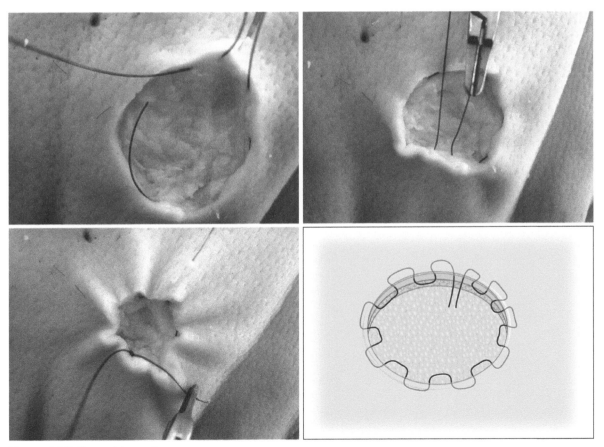

Figure 6.27 Purse string suture

Running subdermal suture

Running subdermal sutures are the same as a running skin stitch but start in the fat layer to exit mid-dermis and to run down the wound. The disadvantage is, as for skin sutures, if there is a break or infection the whole lot goes whereas interrupted sutures give individual control. They are not good where there is high or even moderate tension.

Wide wounds – high tension sutures

Closure of wide wounds under tension poses considerable problems [3]. It can lead to suture marks, dehiscence, infection and skin slough [4].

Techniques for closure of wide wounds under tension include the following:

- Deep sutures – layered closure.
- Pulley or far-near-near-far sutures [5]: each pulley delivers 50% more pull (Figure 6.28). One or even two pulleys can be used but there is arguably too much tension if this is needed. They may, however, initially pull the hole together allowing other sutures to then distribute the strain and tension. The pulley, far-near-near-far technique

causes concern for cosmesis because of tension on the epidermis [5].

- Undermining widely.
- Creeping Charlie: despite the usual advice to start the first suture in the middle of the wound and go out in halves, starting at the ends and working in, more often than not, closes the hole by creeping up on it.
- Big, temporary and gliding sutures: a thicker, often braided or even silk suture (yes, they still exist) can be used to pull the wound together. Suturing and stretching then allows approximation and this big suture is removed.
- Towel clips [6]: these are frequently used to pull the wound edges together. Their disadvantage is that it takes time for the skin to stretch and the patient under local anaesthetic gets restless. Towel clips can also cause substantial trauma to the skin by focusing the tension on four discrete points. For this reason, a towel clip should not be used on thin skin including the face, since it may tear.

A modification of the method more equally distributes tension along the wound to produce nearly immediate tissue expansion (Figure 6.29).

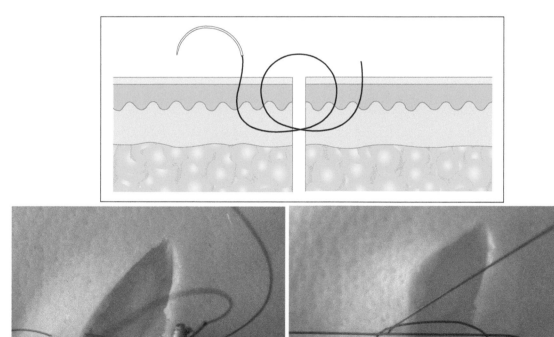

Figure 6.28 Pulley or far-near-near-far suture

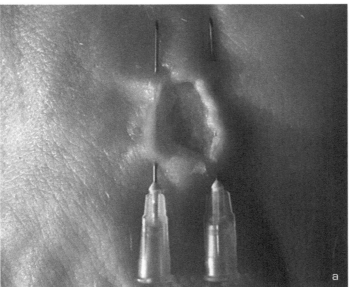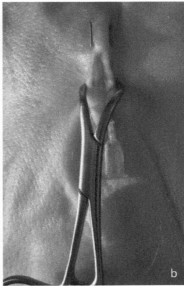

Figure 6.29 Modified towel clip method

a Two needles are placed intradermally approximately 1 cm from the wound edges. **b** A towel clip is placed across the wound and over the two buried needles. The clip is pulled together to reapproximate the wound edges in a quick and relatively atraumatic manner.

The wound edges should not be undermined because that may compromise the vascular integrity of the stretched skin. To further protect vascular integrity, the towel clip may be closed tightly but should not blanch or tear the skin. The towel clip may be further tightened after 5–10 minutes have elapsed and some initial elasticity has been gained if additional area is required. Leaving the towel clip in place for 10–15 minutes is often sufficient to adequately stretch the skin. An additional towel clip is usually required for every 3 cm of wound length. The stretching method of reapproximating wounds is particularly useful on the scalp, back and extremities [7].

- Assistant to push the wound edges together.
- Horizontal mattress sutures [8]: offer more if not the most strength but can compromise the blood supply. For this reason, bolsters are sometimes used if the horizontal mattress suture is to be left in for additional support [8].
- Multiple relaxing skin incisions: cause trauma to the surrounding skin with possible scarring [4].

Suspension periosteum (plexing/tacking) sutures

These are buried sutures used to secure unwanted slack or deformity, such as a ptosis, or to prevent a free margin distortion. Start with a stitch into the dermis of the wound margin (not through the skin) that needs securing, is causing distortion or is under tension. As it will take significant strain it should be a good bite of some 2–3 mm of actual dermis and in >5 mm from the wound edge. Ensure it does not dimple the skin surface. Continue this stitch down into the mid-wound floor where wound closure is desired. Direct the needle down to the bone (Figure 6.30) to then turn up and exit taking up the periosteum and then up through the floor of the wound and tie down.

CONSIDERATIONS TO REPAIR AND CLOSE A DEFECT

Firstly, the size of the defect has to be known: the hole, not the tumour size, is what is important.

Think of all the closures successfully done before or seen done before in that area and select the one you think will work best. Always have a plan B. Some surgeons advise considering up to four options or possibilities (but this often includes side-by-side and secondary intention).

Closure options

If possible, perform primary closure under minimal tension. Layered closure of the wound helps decrease tension at the skin level. Absorbable buried sutures can be used to approximate deeper layers to avoid

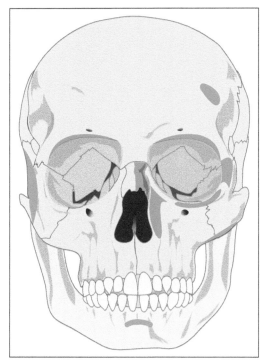

Figure 6.30 Bone anchoring points for suspension sutures

Adapted from Robinson JK, Hanke WC, Sengelmann R et al (eds). Surgery of the skin. Philadelphia: Mosby, 2005; Fig 19.12.

excessive tension on the skin. Nonabsorbable or absorbable sutures can be used on the skin surface with gentle eversion of skin edges. Generally, use 5/0 to 3/0 absorbable sutures for deeper layers and 6/0 to 5/0 sutures (permanent or absorbable) for skin. Perform undermining within the same depth of plane on each side of the wound to allow for correct re-approximation of the corresponding tissue layers. Differential (one-sided) undermining in the subcutaneous plane may be needed to advance only the undermined side of the wound so that the non-undermined side will not be as mobile, thereby preventing distortion of nearby structures.

A 'trapdoor' deformity resulting from a bevelled wound edge can be prevented by conservatively excising the excess skin tangentially to the wound surface to create a more vertical skin edge. Also excise the opposite skin edge to match it.

If the defect cannot be closed primarily, additional surgical planning is required. Reconstructive choices include: 1) healing by secondary intention, 2) skin grafts (full-thickness or split-thickness), 3) local flaps (random or axial), 4) regional flaps and 5) free flaps. Defects >3 cm need flaps.

Secondary intention healing

Healing by secondary intention is a treatment option for superficial wounds. This process occurs when the wound is left open, allowing it to spontaneously contract and epithelialise on its own. Healing by secondary intention is inappropriate for complex defects where multiple tissue layers are missing and structural support is needed.

Cosmetic results of a defect healing by secondary intention depend upon the facial region involved. Concave facial surfaces (e.g. medial canthus, temple, nasofacial crease, nasomalar grooves, auricle) heal with good results. Convex facial surfaces located on the nose, cheek, chin, lips and helix do not heal as well by secondary intention. At these regions, depressed and hypertrophic scars frequently occur.

Disadvantages of healing by secondary intention include: 1) a longer period of healing; 2) often, increased hypopigmentation of re-epithelialised scars; and 3) added contraction of surrounding soft tissue, which causes drifting of neighbouring structures.

Pig carts
How to move the skin:
Primary
Intention (secondary intention)
Graft
Flap:
Complex (combined)
Advance
Rotate
Transpose
Subcutaneous island pedicle and myocutaneous

Deep suture sites

- Back
- Trunk
- Large face deficits
- Not on arms (usually)

Suture lines

Place suture lines in boundaries of cosmetic units where and when possible and in functioning or relaxed skin tension lines (whichever dominates).

WOUND CLOSURE

The rule of halves versus 'creeping Charlie'

The traditional advice to close a wound is to make a central suture and then go out both sides, halving the wound. Although this is sound for lacerations it is often not the best technique for skin cancer excisions. A 12-mm lesion requires a minimum of 4-mm margins, creating a defect width of 20 mm. To avoid dog-ears and achieve the optimum 30° end angles, the 4:1 ratio requires the incision to be 80 mm. If a central suture is put across a 20-mm central defect, there is very little chance of closing it as the tension will be too great.

With the creeping Charlie technique the wound is closed progressively and equally from both apices, 'creeping' towards the centre. This recruits the surrounding end skin such that, as the centre is approached, the defect is no longer 20 mm but far smaller so that it can invariably be closed without difficulty. Any redundancies can be dealt with in the middle of the wound during closure. Irregularities or pleats in the mid portion of the wound generally resolve over time. Remember, skin stretches and accommodates.

In addition, many wounds that initially are too wide to close across their widest point (e.g. the widest part of an A-T flap) can be closed by this 'creeping Charlie' technique with the narrowest part closed first.

Match-up lines

Although experienced surgeons may eschew drawing across an intended excision so as to provide orientation match-up lines, tissues move when the excision is made, and may even fall apart, and correct matching and alignment can be difficult. Lines (see Figure 6.31) are simple enough and provide extra security and fewer hassles, so why not use them? They also provide unexpected help in areas such as the middle of the T in an A-T flap, showing where the corner stitch goes, as tissue movement frequently displaces this previously obvious central point.

This excision of a scalp sebaceous carcinoma (Figure 6.32) healed without a trace no doubt helped by matching using the lines.

If the sides are of uneven length, matching the lines will invariably allow the skin to stretch and even out with no deformity or crenation.

HINTS AND TIPS

Don't forget a locator suture or nick at 12 o'clock while the lesion is still partly attached. This is best done as soon as possible, so undermine the 12 o'clock end first if possible so it can be nicked.

'X' sutures: closing small circular excisions

- Skin: good for small circular defects such as punch biopsies >6 mm. The X goes across the centre, making the circle an ellipse (Figure 6.33).

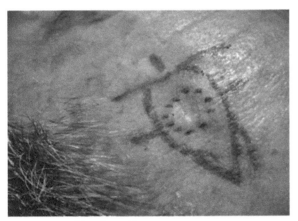

Figure 6.31 Match-up lines

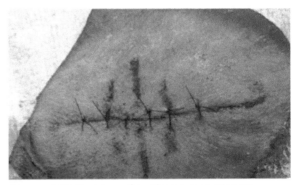

Figure 6.32 Excision of a sebaceous carcinoma

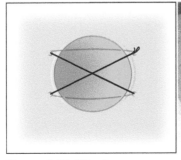
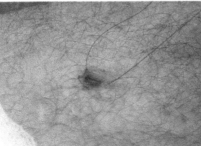
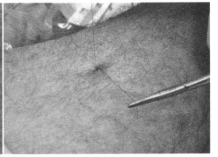

Figure 6.33 'X' suture

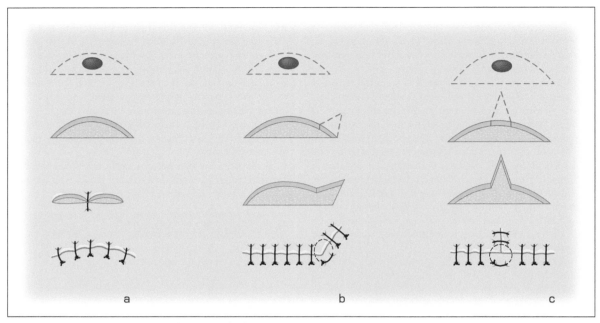

Figure 6.34 Closing wounds with unequal edges
a Closure using the rule of halves. **b** Closure using a Burow's triangle. **c** Placement of the Burow's triangle at any position on the long side.
Adapted from Roenigk RK, Roenigk HH Jr (eds). *Dermatologic surgery,* 2nd edn. New York: Marcel Dekker, 1989; (Fig 1).

- Subcuticular: same suture but buried in subcuticular tissue (i.e. interrupted deep X sutures with buried knots). Used to approximate wide wounds to reduce tension on skin sutures and reduce or prevent wound spread. Mostly used on backs.

S-plasty

This excision allows for a better result over convex surfaces or over joints where the scar will have to stretch. Scars can contract by 30% of their length over time so excisions over joints need scars that can stretch. The S shape that S-plasty and an O-S flap provide allows for the scar to stretch. The elongation of a scar with an S also minimises the result of any contraction.

Closing wounds with unequal edge lengths

The simplest method for closing wounds with unequal edge lengths is the rule of halves (Figure 6.34a). Start in the middle and keep halving the long side to the short. Although this may result in some initial puckering the

skin will stretch and adapt. Obviously, gross puckering such that edge anastomosis is impossible precludes this technique.

A Burow's triangle (named after the German surgeon Karl von Burow) is a triangle or wedge of skin cut so as to shorten the length of the longer side of a wound (Figure 6.34b). One or more can be cut to make the length of the long side equal to that of the short side. The Burow's triangle can be placed anywhere on the long side and thus may be able to be well hidden in a crease (Figure 6.34c).

Alternatively, the shorter side can be lengthened/enlarged by extending the excision out on that side.

Closure of serial excisions

Large lesions such as congenital naevi or even a BCC can be excised in stages. Excise as much of the lesion as possible without tension through its centre. Do not take the edge/side or any normal skin. Suture and wait 3 months or so, which allows the skin to stretch. Then excise the remnant taking normal skin on either side, thus removing the whole lesion with a smaller scar.

Summary:
Fundamentals of wound closure

1 Plan: have options, know the anatomy.

2 Handle tissues gently.

3 For any wound, whether its edges are of equal or unequal length, begin closure at the ends of the defect to avoid unnecessary dog-ears. Deal with any redundancies in the middle of the wound during closure. Irregularities or pleats in the mid portion of the wound generally resolve over time.

4 Eliminate tension at the wound edges.

5 Evert the wound edges, epidermis to epidermis.

6 Use the finest sutures possible and remove as early as possible.

7 Use the most non-reactive suture material.

8 Use reverse cutting needles.

9 Absorb excess wound exudate to prevent maceration of the surrounding skin.

10 Divert any salivary drainage away from the wound to minimise bacterial contamination.

11 Maintain a moist wound environment with occlusive dressings.

12 Protect the wound from trauma.

13 In wounds with potential for infection, institute appropriate oral and topical antibiotics for 7–10 days.

14 To avoid cellular damage and delay healing, do not apply skin cleansers (e.g. hydrogen peroxide, Betadine®, Hibiclens®) to a wound.

15 Apply tape-strips to the face or any wounds with potential tension at removal of sutures (ROS).

16 Cover the scar with paper tape at ROS for 2–4 weeks.

17 Massage thereafter with moisteurisers.

18 Allow time for scars to mature before repeat intervention.

KNOTS

The aim of any wound closure is to provide the minimum support (sutures) to allow the wound to heal. The tension created across a wound with closure is critical and must be minimised to prevent dehiscence, a widened scar and even breakdown. The use of deep sutures, understanding tissue and skin movement, the placement of the final skin sutures and the suture material used all contribute to a good result.

Knot security is obviously paramount. Nylon and the other synthetic suture materials slip and can present a major problem to the novice surgeon.

Instrument tied knots are invariably used in skin surgery. Using instruments means the surgeon should never touch the needle with his or her fingers. The one-handed knot is sometimes used to secure deep suture knots where slipping is a problem.

Surgeon's knot

The fundamental knot is the square or surgeon's knot (Figure 6.35), which is a modification of the reef knot (Figure 6.36). It adds an extra twist (or more) when tying the first throw, forming a double overhand knot, thus adding friction that makes the knot more secure. This knot is also used by fishermen to tie hooks, lures and flies and in other situations where the thread is slippery and security is needed, such as jewellery. Like the reef knot, the surgeon's knot capsizes and fails easily if one of the working ends is pulled away from the standing end closest to it.

The reef knot is fundamentally two loops that pull against each other with the ends of each loop exiting through the neck of the other loop on the same side. This is accomplished by tying the first throw one way and then reversing it.

If the throws go the same way, it makes a granny knot, which slips and is hence very dangerous for surgery. The reef knot is taught as *left over right,* then *right over left.* The granny knot is the first step repeated twice, *left over right and repeat.* This is a very common mistake made by people learning to tie a reef knot. In a granny knot the thread goes under then over the loops (pink under then over green and vice versa; Figure 6.37). When a granny knot slips, the wound will open.

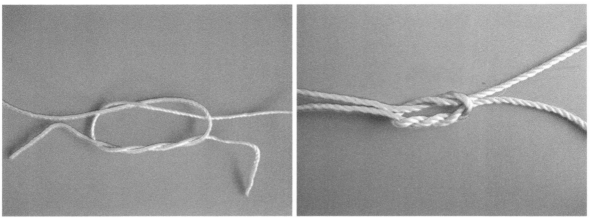

Figure 6.35 Surgeon's knot has two (or more) initial throws but the ends exit the loops on the same sides

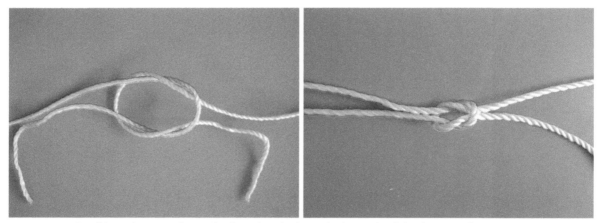

Figure 6.36 Reef knot has one throw; both ends exit through the neck of the loop on the same side – both green over pink, both pink under green

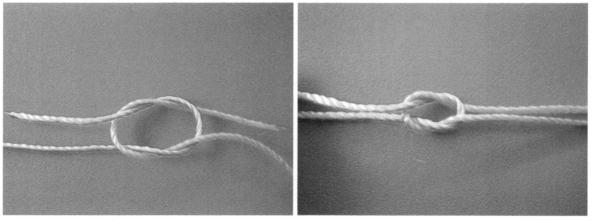

Figure 6.37 Granny knot

The instrument tie

With the instrument tie the needle is passed through both sides of the wound and the suture pulled through leaving a short length on the non-needle side and a long length below the needle (Figure 6.38). The needle holder is then wound around this long length a number of times below the needle and then picks up the short end to pull it through creating a knot. The number of winds determines knot security and prevents slipping but also can cause so much friction that it can't be pulled closed. The classic surgeon's knot uses just two initial throws. However, with nylon and skin surgery, where a significant gap has to be closed and the wound wants to pull apart, the usual technique is for three initial clockwise winds to prevent slipping, then two anti-clockwise, then two clockwise again. If the first winding is clockwise around the needle holder, the second 'throw', after pulling the first throw tight and then releasing the short end, is then wound anti-clockwise.

It's a cinch

A cinch is where the two ends of the suture are pulled to the same side, thus locking the length likely to slip (Figure 6.39). Alternatively, the suture ends go back against the run of the knot to do the same. This can, at times, be a valuable help but at others it impairs tightening the knot.

HINTS AND TIPS

Look at the knot to ensure the suture ends are pulling it in a linear alignment and not cinching it by pulling back against the run.

For deep sutures reverse the order (i.e. anticlockwise – clockwise – anticlockwise), which 'automatically' prevents cinching.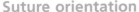

Suture orientation

Suture ends should open across the sutured wound and not along its length (Figure 6.40). If they are wrongly oriented to lie along the wound, they will invariably insert into the wound allowing the skin to grow over it, increase the chances of inflammation and infection and worsen cosmesis (Figure 6.41). Making the knot and suture ends open or lie across the wound is simple; it all depends on the direction the first throw is pulled. Pull both ends away from the incision (90° and 270°).

Handling long lengths of sutures

Sutures usually come in 45-cm and 75-cm lengths and the latter can literally be 'a hand-full'. Initially, when pulling the first pass through, it is so long, almost the span of the surgeon, that any close lights may be inadvertently touched. This can best be avoided by ensuring no low lights and by gathering up the long length and gaining control.

Problems with knots

- Reduced suture strength – a knotted suture has one-third the strength of an unknotted one. The more throws, the less the strength. Nylon and most synthetics need a minimum of three initial throws and two thereafter.

  Knots are where most sutures fail since local stress weakens the suture fibre. The US Pharmacopeia (USP) has thus specified minimum knot-pull tensile strength requirements for sutures.
- Knot untying and/or breaking – knots can become untied and fail if the suture material is slippery. In addition, knots can split or break if tied improperly or if damaged by surgical instruments. Breakage of barbed sutures has been verified in non-industry funded research.
- Suture extrusion – spitting – suture knots may erupt through the wound if left below the skin. This is due to the bulk size of suture knots and could cause patient discomfort, infection and inflammation. The rate of occurrence of spitting may be as high as 5%.
- Infection – spaces between the filaments of a braided suture and the interstices within a suture knot have been shown to harbour bacteria.
- Rupture, or splitting open, of a surgical wound – closure failure at the site of tightly approximated wounds is primarily caused by tissue pull-through. Up to 88% of suture loops in disrupted wounds may be found intact at the time of disruption.
- Exacerbated inflammation – wound closure strength can be reduced up to 77% due to excessive tension. Wounds that are closed under strong tension have been shown to exhibit an inflammatory response, releasing neutrophilic cell infiltrates and increasing tissue myeloperoxidase activity.
- Ischaemia and scarring – sutures that are overly taut can produce pressure necrosis. Microangiographic examinations have shown that tightly tied sutures caused avascularity within the tissue and the area surrounding the suture loops. The resulting microinfarction leads to increased scarring in addition to compromising the wound closure strength.

Themes, variations and tricks

The first throws can be as many as needed according to the tension on the knot and the slipperiness of the suture. The only prohibition to the number of throws is if the suture material is 'sticky' and won't allow the loops to slide. This can pose a problem with PDS II/Monoslow deep sutures where there is significant tension as they are being used to close the dead space.

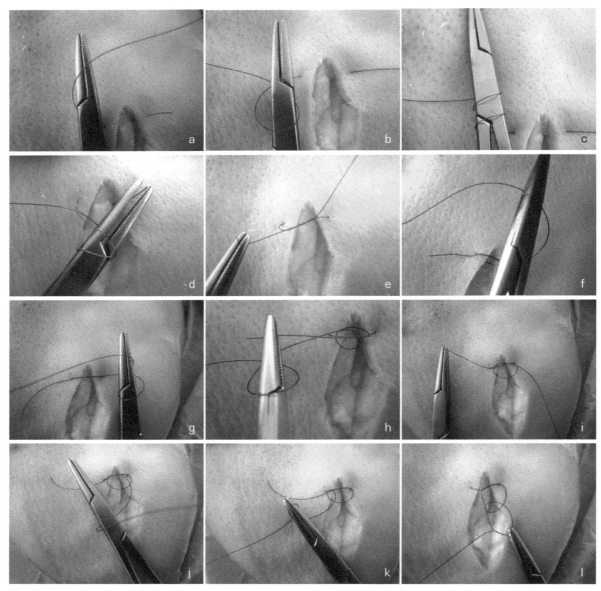

Figure 6.38 Instrument tie

a The needle having passed through the excision, the suture has a short free end and a long needle end. The needle holder is moved against the inside loop of the long suture end. **b** Using the other hand the needle-end suture is wound clockwise around the needle holder, at least twice for a surgeon's knot, but may need three or even four or more throws to stop it slipping. This 'winding' is done by combining spiralling the needle holder and holding the needle end of the suture secure or by helping to wind them on. **c** Two loops have been wrapped around the needle holder. **d** The needle holder now grasps the free end of the suture. **e** Hands cross to align the knot and pull. **f** Releasing the suture, the needle holder now reverses its path pushing into the long needle end but this time throwing the loop counter-clockwise. **g** The long needle-end suture is wound counter-clockwise once around the needle holder. **h** The free end of the suture is grasped. **i** The second throw of the knot can be tightened. **j** Finally, the last clockwise throw is made. **k** The free end of the suture is grasped and pulled through. **l** An 'exploded' view of the surgeon's knot: the first double throw on the skin surface, the second single counter-clockwise throw and loop and the third single clockwise throw and loop.

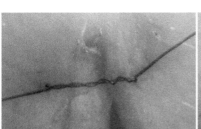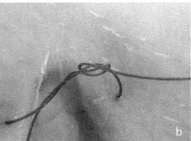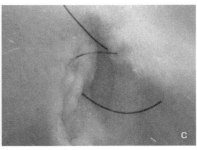

Figure 6.39 Avoiding a cinch

a Ensure the throws align along the suture. **b** A cinch is formed when the loose end of a suture is pulled the wrong way, back on itself as on the right. **c** With blood and the reduced working space, it is easy to exit a deep suture so that both ends are not on the same side, as here. Make sure they are on the same side or a cinch will form, making closure inadequate.

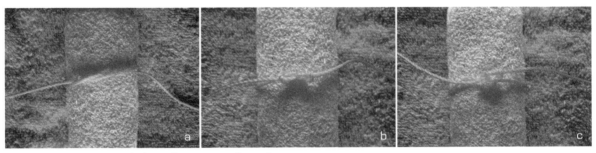

Figure 6.40 Correct technique for suture orientation

a The suture ends are pulled laterally, either side, across the 'wound'. This first throw is all important: it dictates the direction of the suture ends. **b** The second double surgeon's knot is still made to lie as per the first throw orientation. **c** Even the third throw does not alter this desired orientation where the suture ends go across the wound and not lengthways.

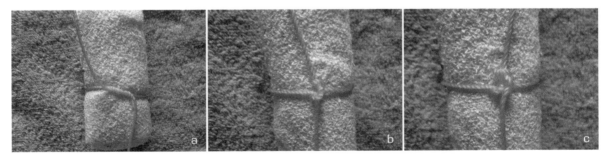

Figure 6.41 Incorrect technique for suture orientation

a The first throw is made lengthways. This is easy to do, especially with an instrument tie and fine sutures wherein the needle holder is pushed away rather than deliberately pulling it laterally across the incision. **b** The second throw just reinforces this mistake. **c** The third throw also cannot alter the direction of the free ends, which now run along and then in the wound incision so that the skin may grow over.

Tricks:

1 Ensure the loops of the first throws (three or more) are aligned along the drawn ends. Often, in the 'heat of battle', an inadvertent cinch is formed by the suture ends exiting on different sides of the main suture loop itself.

2 The surgeon may cross hands the wrong way. Look and ensure the loops are running along in the same direction.

3 If there is trouble sliding the knot because it grabs, try see-sawing both ends or even fix one end and just pull the other.

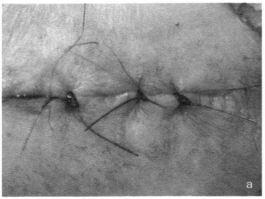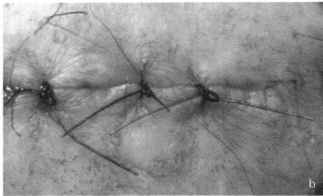

Figure 6.42 What is wrong with this photo?
a The right end suture lies along the incision and its internal end is already buried in the wound because the first throw was not made across the incision. **b** It has been dug out so that the skin will now heal over it. (The gaps were also closed and the epidermal edges heaped up to optimise healing.)

4 If a loose but secure knot is desired, as when there may be no tension and the epidermal edges are easily and satisfactorily apposed, just tie the first throw gently or loosely but tie the second and third throws securely.

OTHER CLOSURES

Tape skin closures
Tape closures are made by several different companies in various sizes. The excised deficit in skin cancer surgery is too large to be closed by tape closures. In this context they have three main uses:
1 Extra support where there is unavoidable wound tension. This may be just psychological (for the practitioner as well as the patient) but may help spread the focus of tensions.
2 At removal of sutures to provide on-going support. All wounds are at their weakest at ROS and these may well help.
3 Wound protection. This is their main help. ROS for wounds on the face is usually done on the sixth postoperative day. If the patient then rolls over in their sleep and drags the wound across the pillow, it may well rip open. It is recommended that all face or similarly vulnerable wounds be taped to prevent these shearing forces.

The correct technique is all-important. Most tapes are in sterile envelopes to be used during operations. Postoperatively, however, if the wound has healed and sealed, non-sterile continuous tape (such as Fixomull or Hyperpaque) can be cut into strips. First, never touch the tapes with hand or glove. Use forceps only. Extra adhesion is obtained by painting the under-tape skin area with tincture of benzoin compound (Tinct Benz Co or Friar's Balsam) or Skin-prep and applying the tapes when it is tacky – nearly dry but not wet. The proprietary tapes are usually on a backing board that breaks towards the ends. Individual tapes can be lifted off with forceps and applied or the free ends placed on one side of the wound and secured by fingers while the board is bent and pushed across the wound dispensing the remainder of the tape across the wound. This, if and when mastered, gives the even spread as per the packaged product and looks reassuringly professional.

Refer to the 'Dressings' section in Chapter 12, 'Postoperative care' for more detail.

Staples and glue
In practice, skin cancer excisions result in such a significant deficit that staples and glue are not usually used.

REFERENCES
[1] Hanasono MM, Hotchkiss RN. Locking horizontal mattress suture. Derm Surg 2005;31(5):572–3.
[2] Elliot D, Mahaffey PJ. The stretched scar: the benefit of prolonged dermal support. Br J Plast Surg 1989;42(1):74–8.
[3] Stough DB, Spencer DM, Schauder CS. New devices for scalp reduction. Intraoperative and prolonged scalp extension. Dermatol Surg 1995;21:777–80.
[4] DiStasio AJ 2nd, Dugdale TW, Deafenbaugh MK. Multiple relaxing skin incisions in orthopaedic lower extremity trauma. J Orthop Trauma 1993;7:270–4.
[5] Giandoni MB, Grabski WJ. 1994 Surgical pearl: the dermal buried pulley suture. J Am Acad Dermatol 1994;30:1012–13.
[6] Liu CM, McKenna J, Griess A. Surgical pearl: the use of towel clamps to reapproximate wound edges under tension. J Am Acad Dermatol 2004;50:273–4.
[7] Perlis CS, Dufresne RG Jr. Immediate skin stretching with towel clips and needles. Derm Surg 2005;31(6):697–8.
[8] Coldiron BM. Closure of wounds under tension. The horizontal mattress suture. Arch Dermatol 1989;125:1189–90.

Operating

Preoperative preparation

To be prepared is half the victory.

Miguel de Cervantes

DIAGNOSIS

Some clinicians may be confident enough to excise a lesion on their clinical judgement; a nodular basal cell carcinoma (BCC) or a squamous cell carcinoma (SCC) may appear to be an easy diagnosis. However, many BCCs are mixed and what appears to be a nodular BCC may, in fact, be micronodular wherein wider margins or even slow Mohs would be preferable. An SCC may be undifferentiated, suggesting the same, whereas a thin melanoma may have actually penetrated the basement membrane, thus also increasing the recommended margins. A lesion reported as a solar keratosis or even a seborrhoeic keratosis may actually be an SCC. A punch biopsy only allows some 1% of the lesion to be examined. If in doubt, take 3- or 4-mm punch biopsies from different areas of the lesion or shave the whole lesion off co-planar to the skin.

In other words, the clinician is well advised to gather all available information about the lesion by punch, shave or excisional (preferably) biopsy. The necessary and most appropriate procedure can then be best planned. Not all skin cancers need to be excised. An intraepidermal carcinoma (IEC)/Bowen's disease and superficial BCCs can

---

NOTE

Solar/actinic and seborrhoeic keratoses can mimic SCCs and result in false negative pathology reports.

Take larger samples from large, raised suspicious lesions that do not exhibit the classic diagnostic features of a seborrhoeic keratosis (crypts and cysts).

---

be treated by other methods according to the surgeon's preference and experience.

Skin cancer priorities

There are different priorities for the various cancers, based on seriousness and urgency, which determine preferred excision times:

- Priority 1: life-threatening (melanomas) – excise as soon as possible, preferably within 2 weeks.
- Priority 2: serious and potentially life-endangering (SCCs; rare dangerous [Merkel cell, sebaceous cell]) – excise within 2 months if possible.
- Priority 3: non-life threatening but malignant (BCCs, IECs, Bowen's disease) – excise as soon as possible.
- Priority 4: cosmetic – no urgency.

Ensure you are across all possible options and able to give the patient the evidence for each treatment.

Curettage in experienced hands with cautery or repeat cycle cryosurgery is arguably the treatment of choice for superficial BCCs and Bowen's. Although MALA and imiquimod have been approved for some BCCs, the recurrence rate is higher than that of correct margin excisions. They are viable options, however, to try for the nose and face as, if successful, there is usually no scar.

Excise all other BCCs, SCCs and melanomas with the correct, evidenced margins.

A competent clinician who is confident of performing the operation can discuss the options: simple side-by-side diamonds, flaps (including what type), a graft or even secondary intention. Slow Mohs is now regarded as the best option for difficult-to-demarcate melanomas and other skin cancers.

INFORMING THE PATIENT

It is very good advice never to give results over the phone. These are fraught with potential misinterpretations and mistakes. If a biopsy is worth doing, the patient should pick up the hard copy results at the clinic and be seen if pathological. If the patient gets the hard copy, there can be no argument that it was received and what the lesion was.

If pathological, the implications of the lesion, as to its seriousness, its metastatic potential and the need for an operation, can be best explained to the patient by the responsible doctor. The medical practitioner is advised to present the diagnosis and the alternative treatments, if any, as well as the fee for any operation but not to impose upon, persuade or 'sell' the patient.

HINTS AND TIPS

Don't rush the patient. Although you may try and do them a favour by postponing a BCC so as to do their melanoma immediately, the patient most often perceives this as being rushed and possibly coercion. If you have a trained assistant, they can inform the patient often more fully than the doctor and, without you being present, the patient doesn't feel any pressure. A good assistant will know the Medicare rebates and give the pros and cons of doing the operation.

Costs and fees

The immediate next step, seldom, if ever, discussed in texts, is to discuss the fee. Most doctors are abysmally ignorant of the costs involved but, to survive and do the best job, these costs need to be addressed. It is recommended that the AMA recommended fees (which are indexed), as a minimum, be charged. However, there are certain operations where the AMA recommended fee may not cover the time and skill needed and the individual practitioner must put his or her own value on these. For example, the author has been 'caught short' with large melanomas on the back (done by a long side-by-side excision and necessitating numerous deep sutures) and by bi- and tri-lobed flaps on noses and wedge resections of ears, all of which require more time than is covered by the suggested fee.

On receiving bad news, patients are usually confused and worried. It is best to issue a written 'quote' that covers both the simplest and the most complex procedures. For example, initially it may be felt that an operation around an eye can be done with a simple ellipse, but 'on the table' it may be found a flap is necessary. The fee for the latter will come as a nasty shock to the patient unless previously covered and quoted.

PATIENT ASSESSMENT

Fast pre-op screen

There is no point discussing an operation if the patient is medically unsuitable or a risk. A fast history can be taken when you deliver the results to assess their suitability.

Six-point fast procedure screen (3M3P)

1. Medical
   a. Diabetes/BPH/frequency
   b. CVS problems – pacemaker – TIAs
   c. Hep C/HIV
   d. Epilepsy
   e. Coughs and sneezes*
2. Medications
   a. Anticoagulants (+ antibiotics)
   b. Steroids
   c. Beta-blockers
   d. Diuretics
3. Musculoskeletal
   a. Operation position
   b. Can they lie down in the best position for the allocated time?
4. Pathology, plan and position
   a. Check and re-check results/diagnosis for margin needs
5. Personal
   a. Urgency (BPH, diabetes, diuretics)
   b. Ability to walk/drive afterwards – ? transport
   c. If they live alone – monitor or change dressings
   d. Idiosyncrasies (vaso-vagal, needle phobia etc)
6. Personality
   a. Very anxious/needle phobic – ? anxiolytics

*Beware coughs and sneezes as such violent 'explosions' can burst unsecured sutures or the patients sudden movement cause surgical damage.

Complete the pre-op exam

The following preoperative assessment is only a suggestion and too long to be practical. It is designed to be adapted and covers most contingencies, many of which can be assessed by staff.

If done each and every time, the assessment not only protects the medical practitioner medico-legally by revealing potential and avoidable problems but, most importantly, allows the best arrangements for the best result for the patient. The disciplined progression through a systematic assessment will avoid mishaps and need not take as much time as it might appear, as the experienced clinician will rapidly assess the remainder of their skin, their flexibility, suitability and such. It is false economy and not worth the risk for the solo or private medical practitioner not to spend the same time following the same protocol as that which the hospitals allocate and insist upon for a preoperative assessment.

Preoperative assessment

PATIENT NAME _____

1 DIAGNOSIS: _____

2 SITE: _____

3 SIZE: _____ mm

4 PHOTO:

5 TREATMENT OPTIONS:

Non-surgical (to be offered if appropriate)   **Surgical**

☐ Salicylic acid   ☐ Punch excision
☐ Cryosurgery   ☐ Shave excision
☐ 5-Fluorouracil   ☐ Simple ellipse
☐ Imiquimod   ☐ Flaps – possibilities and alternatives
☐ Diclofenac   ☐ Deep sutures (back)
☐ IPL   ☐ Subcuticular sutures (cosmesis)
☐ PDT   ☐ Graft

6 DURATION: _____ min

7 ALLERGIES: _____ Local anaesthetics / Iodine / Antibiotics / Wound dressings

8 MEDICATIONS: _____ Anticoagulants – Aspirin / Clopidogrel / Warfarin
Any new or recent changes (e.g. pacemaker)

9 LOCAL ANAESTHETIC:

☐ Drugs interacting with adrenaline: beta-blockers, tricyclic antidepressants, phenothiazines, butyrophenones
☐ Contraindications to adrenaline use: recent AMI / unstable angina, severe HTN, uncontrolled diabetes, uncontrolled hyperthyrodism
☐ Drugs interacting with lignocaine: amiodarone, beta blockers, cimetidine, disopyramide
☐ Recent CABG / refractory arrhythmia
☐ Conditions predisposing to lignocaine toxicity: HF, renal / liver failure
WARNING: Older patients are often on older medications (e.g. propranolol). Check.

10 PAST MEDICAL HISTORY (PMH)

i	CVS problems	a Bleeding diathesis d Angina	b Pacemaker e CCF	c SBE / heart valve prophylaxis
ii	RS	a Smoker	b Asthma	c Orthopnoea
iii	Musculoskeletal	a Can they lie in a fixed position for duration?	b Arthritis/spine problems	
iv	CNS	a Ménière's/vertigo (preventing lying down) c TIAs	b Tremors d Epilepsy	e Anxiety / personality
v	Endocrine	a Diabetes	b Thyroid	
vi	Renal / liver impairment	a Lignocaine toxicity		
vii	Transmissable conditions (double-gloving)	a Hepatitis	b HIV	c HSV

Preoperative assessment continued

11 CURRENT MEDICATIONS

   i Anticoagulants including fish oil, ginkgo, vitamin E

   ii Steroids

   iii Alternative medications / supplements

   iv Interaction with local anaesthetic – as above

12 PAST SURGICAL HISTORY (PSH)

   i Other skin cancers   ii Hypertrophic scarring/keloid prone   iii Other

13 LOCAL FACTORS / HYGIENE   Pre-treat skin infection(s)

14 PROCEDURE PLANNING

   Margin requirements: _____ mm

   Anaesthesia: Local infiltration   Nerve block   Item No. _____

   Important underlying structures / danger: 1 Zygomatic arch   2 Temporal   3 Anterior masseter

   Problems:

   ☐ Lower calf   ☐ Friable skin (steroids)

   ☐ Venous stasis   ☐ Tight skin – no harvest areas

   ☐ Peripheral vascular D   ☐ 11% complications below knee

   ☐ Varicose veins   ☐ Lips and lids

   ☐ Smoker

   Functional effects:

   ☐ Forehead – raised eyebrows, eye – ectropion, face – contractures, mediastinum – keloid

   ☐ Wound closure plan: primary / flap / graft

15 TRIAL POSITIONING: _____

16 DURABILITY (hold position for required time): Urgency (diabetes, BPH), M/S, CNS, Psych

17 RULES OF ENGAGEMENT:
Explain that, to ensure the best result, the patient may have to maintain an uncomfortable position for some time and, especially if the excision is on the face, not talk and not move. If these can be presented as conditions that are all and only for their benefit, it helps obviate or minimise problems during the operation. This is best done preoperatively and (gently) reinforced, if necessary, during the operation.

18 POST-OP OBLIGATIONS:

   Immediate: a Driving   b Driven   c Public transport / walking

   (Specific questioning needed) Healing: a Social   b Work   c Sport   d Travel

19 WORK:

   Patient can resume work   a Immediately   b Needs light duties   c Time off (certificates)

20 HOME SITUATION:

   a Partner   b Support   c Solitary   d Help

Preoperative assessment continued

21 **SUTURES:** Nylon interrupted, deep – absorbable, subcuticular

22 **DRESSING:** Waterproof, non-stick / Fixomull, other, conforming / pressure bandage

23 **DEPILATORY CREAM / TRIM**

24 **PREOP HANDOUT GIVEN**

25 **PHONE NUMBERS:**   Home _____   Mobile _____   Work _____

26 **ITEM NUMBER:**   1 _____   2 _____   3 _____

27 **FEE:**   1 _____   2 _____   3 _____

28 **CONCESSION:** _____

29 **DEPOSIT or GUARANTEE CONFIRMATION:** _____

30 **CONSENT FORM SIGNED:** _____

Examination

If this has been recently done, just salient re-checks are necessary, especially with respect to:

- CVS:
  - BP – if high, gain control
  - Pulse (regular) ? bradycardia/beta-blockers
  - Anti-coagulation – only prescribing doctor to cease
- Respiratory: cough, hay fever/sneezing
- Skin: furunculosis, infections/cold sores, undiagnosed rashes close to operation site
- Psychiatric assessment:
  - Stable enough to endure 1 hour under local anaesthetic; unreal expectations
  - Vexatious or potential litigants – angry and disturbed – odd or strange. ? Ability (and circumstances) to cope. Cognisant or relative with power of attorney needed.
- Social: home situation (live alone – ability to care for wound – especially if on back). Hygiene. Specifically ask about postoperative obligations.

PRE-PLANNING THE OPERATION

Type of operation
- Simple diamond (ellipse)
- Flap – possible types
- Wedge resection

Seeing the patient as close to the operation date as possible allows for better final planning and greater efficiency. It has been said that the most valuable consultation for skin surgery is seeing the patient the day before.

Sketches
A pathology/lab report often provides a useful sketch pad for the preliminary plan as well as confirming the preoperative diagnosis. Drawing the operation on the patient may affirm the proposed plan or may reveal a problem. Showing the patient is both a courtesy and reassuring to them. Any plan may have to be altered on the day.

Sketch pads for computers are now available that allow a digital photo to be taken of the lesion and the proposed operation to be drawn on the computer screen (Figure 7.1).

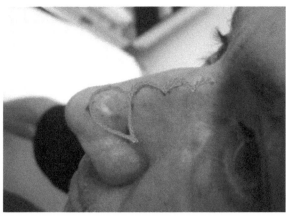

Figure 7.1 This preoperative plan was drawn on a tablet/pad with the aid of graphics software

Suture selection

Note special sutures or techniques (deep, subcuticular).

Duration estimate and optimal timing

- Duration: allocating the appropriate duration is tricky. Many surgeons boast how an op 'only takes 20 minutes'. That may be so from the first incision to the last suture in an uncomplicated case, but it seldom takes into consideration the preparation, positioning and anaesthetising of the patient or the dressing and postoperative advice and operation notes. There are some 50 steps to even the simplest operation. Leaving time between patients is less stressful. A practical tip is to add 15 minutes between patients and ensure the person making the appointments allocates this time.
- Timing: decide what time of day best suits you to operate and try to arrange this theatre slot. Block booking is most efficient. Doing the simplest operation first allows for any bugs in the system to be ironed out and the surgeon to 'warm-up' to maximum efficiency. Leave the most difficult operation until last with no following appointments in case of over-run.

NOTE

Only 50% of the surgeon's time in the theatre is actually spent operating, and this has been documented in hospitals with all the clerical, support staff, wardies, scrub nurse, theatre sister, lights operator and gophers (and probably an assistant to write up the notes ... let alone look up the item numbers and record them).

Operation planning

Factors to consider:

1. Lesion
2. Size and location
3. Danger areas
4. Type of operation (simple ellipse S/E, flap)
5. Duration estimate
6. Appointment time
7. Margins
8. Cosmetic problems (ectropion, eyebrow lift)
9. Anaesthesia: local infiltration/nerve block
10. Antibiotic cover (diabetes, sites)
11. Treatment of intercurrent problems: open sores, resolution respiratory infections – coughing
12. Item numbers/fee
13. Complications warnings
14. Booking and informed consent
15. Patient phone numbers (home, work, mobile) for confirmation and emergency alterations
16. Preparation of operation list
17. Special dressings (waterproof, form-fit/crepe pressure bandages)
18. Depilatory cream for hairy areas with instructions
19. Reduce smoking/use nicotine substitutes 2 weeks before and 1 week after

Heavy smokers who consume more than one pack per day have an increased risk of complications (wound dehiscences, necroses), especially with flaps and grafts. It is recommended to explain this to them and ask them to reduce their consumption, as it is not realistic to ask them to stop completely, at least 2 weeks before the operation and for 1 week after. They can use nicotine substitutes. Tobacco consumption increases skin ageing (wrinkles), but is probably not a risk factor of skin cancer [1].

INFORMED CONSENT

If and when the patient wants their cancer excised they must be acquainted with the potential risks and complications. Then an informed consent form is signed by them and the doctor with a witness. There are two legal standards that can be applied as to what risks should be disclosed in the informed consent:

1. the 'reasonable practitioner' standard
2. the 'reasonable patient' standard.

In the first, those risks must be disclosed that would be disclosed by a *reasonable practitioner* in the relevant specialty. In the second and tougher standard, those material risks that a *reasonable patient* would need to know to make an informed decision must be disclosed. To adhere to such standards, a good guide is to select those risks that could be 'material' to the patient's decision-making. The relevant question is: 'What potential results would a person need to know to make an informed decision to consent or refuse consent?' Material risks include those that have a *high severity* or a *high frequency*. For the less serious risks, a rough rule of thumb could be if the risk event occurs in 3% of cases. For the more serious risks, 1% would be sufficient to be a material risk. Examples of high severity would be death, paralysis or brain damage. Obviously, the risks differ for the excision of a BCC on the back of a healthy person on no medication versus a melanoma or SCC over the zygoma on a patient who has had a heart attack, is on anticoagulants and has diabetes. Although the patient may appear reasonable and very anxious for the operation to be done, any complication may translate to a litigious situation. Although it may be the natural inclination to downplay any serious potential problems to allay the patient's fears, it is a wise precaution to point out any potential problems and to document this in your notes. Specifically address the dangerous areas of the face, scarring, anticoagulation and inter-current medical risks, as warranted.

Figure 7.2 contains a standard informed consent form. Specific risks can be added and initialled by the patient.

SCHEDULING

Allocate priorities, as above: 1) melanoma, 2) SCC, 3) rare and dangerous, 4) BCC. Scheduling then depends on workload, theatre time (if sharing a theatre) and patient availability/cooperation. Each doctor will have a time frame for the duration of their operations and needs to communicate this clearly to the surgical coordinator who sets the appointments and allocates the time. There are various scheduling methods but a dedicated chit (Figure 7.3) would seem the safest. The doctor fills these out and gives them to the surgical coordinator who schedules the patient's appointment. The operation list can then be changed to suit the surgeon. Inform patients that the exact time is to be confirmed and hence the need for their phone numbers.

This allows the staff to book Mrs Doe in as the last operation, which will last an hour or more, and to add up her total fee with an estimate of her Medicare rebate (in brackets). The second item number is where the fee is 'coned' or halved as for the actual excision 31270, whereas the flap 45203 is full fee. Here the supraorbital nerve block has been charged at rebate only.

If the surgical coordinator will assist at the operation, it is most desirable to have them present when you do the pre-op history and examination so as to be completely familiar with the procedure and able to provide a friendly face and link for the patient.

WARNING

The most overlooked item in booking the patient is obtaining their phone numbers to confirm or alter their operation appointment. This will minimise the inconvenience of sitting around for an hour because a patient has forgotten his appointment or having to bump a BCC to another day because a melanoma result has come in.

LISTS

Lists allow the surgeon to see the timetable (see Table 7.1). They should be available the day before and checked then as well as confirming appointment times for operations with patients.

Patient privacy considerations prevent operation lists being displayed where others can see them. Discrete print-outs above the sink where the surgeons scrub up is usually a safe place to access them.

Operation times in Table 7.1 allow 15–20 minutes between operations to clean up and prepare for the next operation and compensate for running late with complex operations. The 'nerve blocks' are not detailed for the nose as both a maxillary and an external nasal may be needed and can only be assessed after being performed.

TABLE 7.1 Suggested wall list operation schedule

Time	Name	Age	Lesion	Site	Size	Op	Min	Item No. /Fee*
8.00 am	SMITH John	66	NBCC	R Deltoid	>10	S/E	30	31285/515
8.45 am	JAMES Ann	72	NCBCC	Supraorbital	<10	A-T	60	45200, 31265,18236 (BB)
10.00 am	DOE John	45	NBCC	Nose	<10	Bilobe	90	45206/965, 31255/267 + nerve block(s)
11.15 am	Doe Jane	43	SCC undiff	L Maxilla	>10	A-T	60+	45203/1020, 31270/312, 18234 /122.50

*Note: Item numbers and fees as at 2012.

Consent for Surgical Procedure

I,_____, of_____

_____

hereby consent to undergo

or

hereby consent to_____ **undergoing the**

operation / treatment of _____

the nature and purpose of which have been explained to me by Dr._____.

I also consent to such further or alternative measures or treatment as may be found necessary during the course of the operation or treatment and to the administration of local anaesthetic for these purposes.

I understand that skin surgery may result in complications including but not limited to the following.

• Scarring [including pronounced hypertrophic or keloid scars]

• Bleeding / Bruising

• Wound infection

• Wound dehiscence [stitches failing to hold wound edges together]

• Loss of function including numbness and altered appearance of nearby anatomical structures

• Incomplete skin cancer removal requiring further surgery or future recurrence

• Allergic drug reactions to medications used to perform the procedure

• Miscellaneous reactions such as fainting or seizures

• Risks specific to this operation

I also understand that during the post-operative period I may be required to

• Take analgesic drugs for pain

• Restrict my activities to ensure good wound healing

• Change my wound dressing at regular intervals and to return to the practice for removal of stitches as advised by the doctor performing the procedure

I am also aware that I am to notify the doctor as soon as possible if any of the abovementioned complications occur or if I have any other concerns regarding the aftercare / progress of my surgical wound.

Signature _____   **Date**_____
              [Patient / parent / guardian]

I confirm that I have explained the nature and purpose of this operation/treatment to the person[s] who signed the above form of consent.

Signature _____   **Date**_____
              [Medical Practitioner]

Figure 7.2 Sample informed consent form

'I have considered my options, reflected on my own values and preferences, and would now like you to proceed with surgery' is the wording that should appear on the consent forms of the future, according to an article in the Journal of the Royal Society of Medicine (2013, doi:10.1177/0141076813490686).

Source: Royal College of Medicine

Operation booking form

NAME: *Jane DOE*

LESION: *SCC – undifferentiated*

SIZE mm: *>10*

SITE: *Forehead*

OP: SHEX: S/E: FLAP: *A-T*

ITEM No(s).   *45203, 31270*

NERVE BLOCK: Supraorbital   ITEM No(s): *18236*

SUTURES: *Subcuticular prolene*

DRESSING: *Waterproof / Conforming wrap*

FEE: *45203/999 (332), 31270/619/2=310 (211/2=105), 18236/51.15*

DURATION mins: *60 +*

TIME: *Last*

PHONES: HOME _____

                          WORK: _____

                          MOBILE: _____

PREOP HANDOUT:

INFORMED CONSENT:

Figure 7.3 Suggested operation booking form

The operation

If you can keep your head when all around you are
losing theirs and blaming you …

Rudyard Kipling, IF

Be still and know that I am God.

*Psalm 46:10 (and a patient's response at being asked
to 'be still')*

Skin cancer surgery that is performed in a clinic can
best be equated to a hospital emergency room scenario.
As the peritoneum is not being cut, full aseptic technique and stripping the patient completely are not
necessary. Only the excision site needs to be exposed,
isolated and prepped and a sterile field established.
Scrubs, sterile gowns, caps and masks are not necessary
other than to protect the operator's clothes. Full scrubbing up with 4% chlorhexidine for a full 2 minutes
and sterile gloves and sterile technique, however, are
mandatory.

It is the firm recommendation that no twilight
sleep or general anaesthesia be contemplated. Most
lesions can be excised under local anaesthesia, which
is safer. For those with a needle phobia or great anxiety,
some diazepam oral or IV can be considered. Antibiotic
cover for diabetics or the unkempt may also be
necessary.

CALM, PEACE AND QUIET, TIME TO GATHER ONE'S WITS

The golden rule is that practitioners who operate must
be in total control and arrange everything to suit themselves for the benefit of their patients. This, in essence,
means:

- arranging lists to suit (time of day, duration, order)
- ensuring all instruments are in first class order and ready
- ensuring the patient is there 15 minutes before time
- trialling and checking to optimise patient positioning
- assistance as needed
- no interruptions.

These are the real jobs of a practice manager, and to
provide a smooth, calm environment in which 'case irrelevant chatter' is kept to a minimum. Sudden, unexpected
noise when operating over a critical or difficult site area
is, to say the least, very dangerous. Good medicine and
good surgery can best be practised if the doctor's conditions are optimised.

Sleep deprivation is an issue that can affect practising doctors. A recent study indicated that lack of
sleep can result in higher rates of surgical complications if the surgeon had less than 6 hours of sleep
the preceding night [2]. Select a day and a time of
day that best suits you to operate and ensure a good
night's sleep prior.

In a study of 300 operations in which surgeons were
ranked for their behaviour, a correlation between civility
in the operating room and fewer postoperative deaths
and complications was noted. When team leaders act
rudely, the stress response is activated, blood pressure
increases and the body's immune system is weakened.
Studies show that incivility in the surgical workplace is
associated with increased staff sick days and decreased
nursing retention, both of which are associated with
increased medication errors [3].

On operating days, arrive early and prepare those
things that only you can do – e.g. drawing up the
anaesthetic(s), checking the list and pathology reports,
going over your operation plans (those items which otherwise cause a geometric progression of delays).

ON PATIENT ARRIVAL

Preliminaries

On arrival, the staff confirm the identity of the patient,
the operation, the fee and payment to avoid any confusion or mutual embarrassment.

Once the paperwork has been done, the staff may
'instruct' the patient that, 'Doctor won't be long – if
you'd like to use the toilet there's enough time'. Diabetes,
diuretics and prostatomegaly cause urgency. Diuretics
should have been ceased prior to any operation. Encourage all diabetics and nervous patients to void immediately before their operation. Triple micturition is often
needed for diabetics.

All patients are apprehensive. Imparting reassurance
and confidence with a smile from the doctor goes a long
way towards relaxing them. For those with morbid
anxiety, 10 mg diazepam 2 hours prior is helpful. Nevertheless, there are those patients who insist on general
anaesthesia and the surgeon is best not to try and operate
on them under local.

Patient clothing and cleanliness

The patient can usually leave their clothes on other than
around the operation site. In fact, it has been found that
patients in street clothes disperse the same amount of
bacteria as those in a clean cotton gown [4] and that
infection rates for same-day surgery are not significantly
affected when patients remain fully dressed [5]. There is
little, if any, evidence that street clothes and shoes increase

infection risk for skin cancer surgery. There is no reason or evidence in the literature to remove patients' rings or other jewellery unless they are in the operative or anaesthetic field and in the absence of specific infection evidence.

As the patients' skin is a major source of bacterial contamination, in clean wound operations it was traditional to ask the patient to bathe or shower before elective surgical procedures. However, there is no evidence to suggest this influences infection rates in small area skin surgery, although a preoperative shower with chlorhexidine or povidone–iodine has been shown to decrease wound infection rates [6,7]. Skin excisions are seldom, if ever, an emergency and preoperative advice to shower beforehand and wear freshly washed, clean clothes makes it more pleasant for the medical staff and reinforces to the patient their own obligation to look after themselves.

OT dress code

Skin surgery is performed on ambulatory patients and equates more to emergency department outpatient or ambulatory day-case minor procedures. The potential wound is, or should be, clean and relatively superficial, and most ambulatory patients are in reasonable health with good resistance to infection. Thus, major hospital operating theatre codes can be modified.

- Wear approved theatre clothes, either scrubs or a non-sterile gown. These confer no benefit other than patient reassurance and protection of one's own clothes.
- No wristwatches or jewellery of any kind including wedding or dress rings, bangles and earrings.
- No nail polish or artificial nails.
- Masks are a debatable benefit as are caps. No need.
- Long shirt-sleeves and ties were forbidden but this too is now disputed. Obviously, arms should be scrubbed to the elbows and ties not allowed to dangle, so rolled or short sleeves and no ties are easiest.
- Wearing theatre clothes outside theatre/change room is prohibited.
- Plastic 'Crocs' or similar open sandals have resulted in injuries from dropped sharp instruments.

Site exposure

It is advisable not to compromise in exposing the surgical site. Clothing that has been pulled away, rather than taken off, can creep back into the area and blood can spill and stain the clothing. Hair is always a problem. Trim the site so none intrudes.

SITE IDENTIFICATION AND ASSESSMENT

Time-out protocols

Important: Time-out protocols

Everyone is busy preparing for the operation. The staff and the patient are asking questions or injecting white-noise chatter. These are potentially dangerous interferences to the surgeon's concentration and how mistakes happen.

Allocate time when previous relevant notes can be read. Obtain the biopsy/pathology report. Find a quiet area and check and re-check what the operation is and why it is being done. Re-confirm the margins necessary. Then ensure the correct site. Even with photographs, sites can heal and lesions regress.

- Confirm the patient's identity.
- Verify the procedure.
- Verify the site.
- Confirm the lesion.
- Check the pathology.

Time taken to read the patient notes, check the pathology report and quietly consider the possible options again at the operating table will be well rewarded as different operation options present: e.g. what may have been a complex flap may be able to be done as a less difficult, less time-consuming and less dangerous simple ellipse.

Preventing wrong-site surgery

Identifying a well-healed biopsy site can be difficult; preoperative photography can help. Wrong-site surgery was responsible for 14% of professional liability cases against Mohs surgeons [8]. The potential for wrong-site skin cancer surgery is considerable. Patients cannot reliably identify lesions accurately and often prefer not to take responsibility for knowing the biopsy site or tumour location. Photography at the time of biopsy seems by far the most reliable method for reducing the risk of wrong-site Mohs surgery. However, lesion identification by patients should remain part of the preoperative evaluation because it includes patients in decision making and facilitates their acceptance of responsibility for their care [8]. Some doctors actually get the patient to touch the site, thus transferring ink from the purple marker pen to their finger as 'the purple finger sign' [9].

Suggested procedure for dubious/healed sites

- Get patients to identify the site, in a mirror if necessary, with family/caregiver input.
- Mark the site after verification.
- Digitally photograph the marked site.
- Have a documented pre-surgery time-out.

When patients and escorts are unsure of the site:

- Loupe examination and skin abrasion are performed to identify the site with local anaesthetic infiltrate.

If uncertainty remains:

- Do another biopsy. If this biopsy does not show tumour, follow the patient/site every 3 months for 2 years.

HINTS AND TIPS

If the biopsy site can't be identified, infiltrate the suspected site with local anaesthetic in the dermis. The previous biopsy site may form a blister due to the separation of the epidermis from the dermis [8].

Tangential and/or reduced light also often helps identify the site.

Marking out the site

An alcohol-based 'permanent' marker is preferred over advertised surgical pens. Studies have confirmed the alcohol provides sterility and insurance against cross-infection. Cutting outside the marks ensures no pigment is left on the patient (although it does wipe off completely).

Skin preparation solutions have varying effects on the visibility of surgical site markings. One study showed chlorhexidine erased significantly more markings than iodine when a black permanent marker was used to mark the skin [10]. The author has experimented with different colours, but the only recommendation is to let the marking dry for as long as possible before prepping.

LOCAL ANAESTHETIC

Use adrenaline in the anaesthetic to provide vasoconstriction and minimise blood ooze. Although anaesthesia is almost immediate vasoconstriction takes a good 10–15 minutes to work. Don't panic if a digit is inadvertently anaesthetised with adrenaline – there would seem to be no hard documentation of alleged 'tip necrosis' and adrenaline is progressively being considered safe to use. 1% lignocaine and 1:200,000 adrenaline provide optimum available anaesthesia and vasoconstriction.

HINTS AND TIPS

Pre-fill the syringe and needle with local anaesthetic and bicarbonate and hide them so the patient doesn't see them. Inject this local anaesthetic first thing, then get the rest of the operation ready. Delay the incision for 15 minutes as this maximises the vasoconstrictive effect of adrenaline.

Contraindications to adrenaline and lignocaine are listed in Chapter 3, 'Local anaesthesia'.

The greatest drawback of local anaesthetic is that the patient can talk and, the more nervous they are, the more they talk. It is when they ask questions that the surgeon's concentration can be broken and smooth theatre procedures interrupted. Having an assistant present who can chat to distract them and answer their questions is invaluable.

It is not a very pleasant experience to have chunks of one's skin, nose or ears removed and some kindness, reassurance, good humour and distraction by the surgeon and staff go a long way to allaying the patient's most reasonable fears and concerns. Reassure the patient that they will not feel any pain and that, if they even feel a twinge, more local anaesthetic is available. Most patients seem most impressed and grateful (and surprised) that they 'didn't feel a thing'.

POSITIONING THE PATIENT

Position the patient to allow the best presentation and access to the operation site. This not only provides and allows the best techniques and thus achieves the best operation outcome for the patient but it is also beneficial for the long-term musculoskeletal health of the surgeon. Abnormal positioning, craning, stretching or being in the leastways uncomfortable compromises the operation and leads to fatigue and long-term sequelae for the surgeon.

It may be some time since the patient has been seen and the lesion may also have grown, mandating a different approach or technique. A day-before consultation to re-assess everything is arguably the most valuable consultation the surgeon can undertake.

Shoulder lesions are particularly problematical as they can cross three planes from posterior to superior to anterior. Try asking the patient to lie on their side.

The face

Explain to patients not to talk during the operation as this causes the site to move and to warn of any impending coughing or sneezing.

Scalp hair

Ask patients to tie up long hair for any head and neck operations. Long 'ibis bill' hair clips are handy. Paper tape often won't stick unless bare skin can be found. For the scalp, a stretch net-gauze can be a great help.

Ensure all hair is secured or trimmed. Hair will re-grow but wisps interfering with the operation, especially on the temple, can be off-putting.

MUSIC

Music is now an evidence-based treatment for depression, anxiety and general functioning, admittedly after 3 months [11], but it may also have an immediate calming effect. An age-appropriate music selection may help to calm the patient during surgery. Some surgeries make available i-Pods so the patient can self-select music that makes them relaxed. On the other hand, music the surgeon likes can be a definite help (to the surgeon).

STERILE SURFACES

Sage packs or the equivalent are folded such that exposed corner edges can be pulled out from what will be the non-sterile underneath side (Figure 7.4). Surgical instruments, sutures and other swabs and equipment can then be dispensed onto this surface on the tray. For minor or small sterile areas, some clinics use the inside of the sterilised instrument or glove pack.

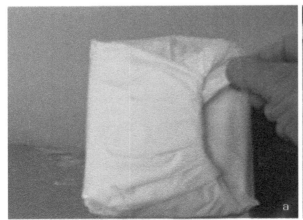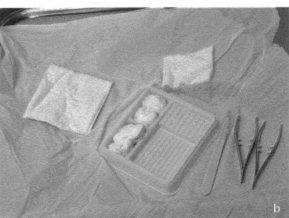

Figure 7.4 Commercial sterile skin lesion packs
a The protruding loose corner is pulled to display the whole square of inner sterile contents. Then the bottom side of the plastic sheet is pulled at each corner. The top sterile side is never touched. **b** The complete pack has a plastic container with various wells, a sterile paper towel that can be cut for a drape, some gauze swabs, sterile swab forceps and a disposable scalpel – either an 11 or a 15.

TRAY SET-UP

The sage pack opens with its plastic container inconveniently in the centre (Figure 7.5). The top disposable (yellow) forceps can be picked up using a sterile, no-touch technique and the superfluous 'superstructure' (plastic drape, napkin, disposable scalpel) removed, if so desired. The tray can then be moved to the corner furthest away from the surgeon so as to allow instrument set-up.

Arrange all necessities so they can be seen and are in a logical order, viz: the scalpel blade nearest the surgeon, and not covered, with the instruments next to it; swabs close and to one side; sutures near and able to be seen (Figure 7.6). The sterile drape can be further away as it will be taken off. Some surgeons also include a sterile cotton bud and dental rolls.

On the non-sterile, bare tray are:

- the site prep (here BD Persist)
- the open, labelled pathology jar
- sterile water for cleaning the wound.

PHOTO DOCUMENTATION

Rebates depend on the size and site of the lesion. It is strongly recommended that all lesions greater than 10 mm be photographed as documented proof. The first of the top five Medicare offences is the inappropriate use of MBS procedural items with up-coding of skin cancer removal items (e.g. claiming >10 mm when it was not). There is no point in recording a lesion under 10 mm for Medicare purposes unless it is to confirm the site warranted flaps and show the operation plan drawn on the patient. However, it may be valuable as a practice record for the doctor's own reference. Use an appropriate digital camera; computer digital dermoscopy units also have a macro feature. Incorporate a post-it note with the patient's name and date and outline the lesion (Figure 7.7). A transparent circle ruler readily obtainable from pathology laboratories can be used to quantify its size.

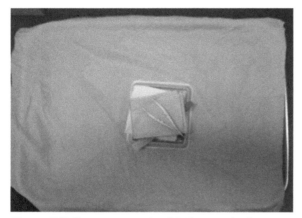

Figure 7.5 Open sage pack with the tray in the centre

SCRUBBING UP: PREOPERATIVE HAND WASHING

It is important for the surgeon to wash his/her hands prior to operating. Preoperative surgical hand washing will remove or destroy transient microorganisms and significantly reduce detachable resident microorganisms and helps prevent intraoperative infections.

Surgical scrubs

Chlorhexidine gluconate has good activity against Gram-positive bacteria, somewhat less activity against Gram-negative bacteria and fungi and only minimal activity against tubercle bacilli. It has in vitro activity against enveloped viruses (e.g. herpes simplex virus, HIV, cytomegalovirus, influenza and RSV) but substantially less activity against nonenveloped viruses (e.g. rotavirus, adenovirus and enteroviruses). Preparations with 2% chlorhexidine gluconate are slightly less effective than those containing 4% chlorhexidine.

Take care to avoid contact with the eyes when using preparations with ≥1% chlorhexidine because the agent can cause conjunctivitis and severe corneal damage.

Chlorhexidine gluconate 2% soap solution (green) is normally used in clinical areas and can be used in all indications for hand hygiene. It provides substantial residual activity but can cause dryness and skin irritation.

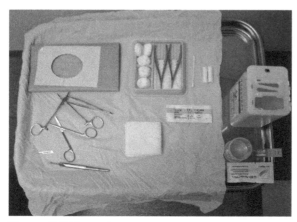

Figure 7.6 Tray set-up

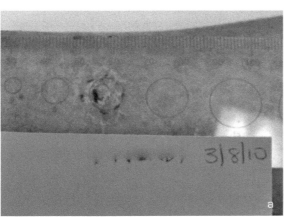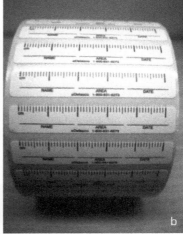

Figure 7.7 Photographic record of a lesion

a Simple method of including patient's name, date and size. **b** These labels can also be used. One seemingly insurmountable problem is parallax error. A lesion >10 mm can appear to be <10 mm because the ruler is closer to the camera or because the lesion is slightly curved over a convex surface.

Chlorhexidine gluconate 4% soap solution (pink) is normally used in theatre or when surgical procedures are performed. It has a slower antimicrobial activity than alcohol-based hand rub (ABHR).

Chlorhexidine allergy

Alternative antimicrobial hand hygiene products include triclosan (clinical setting) and povidone–iodine (surgery and multi-resistant organisms).

Triclosan has been incorporated into soaps for use by health care workers. Concentrations of 0.2–2% have antimicrobial activity. Triclosan has a broad range of anti-microbial activity, like chlorhexidine, and has persistent activity on the skin. The majority of formulations containing <2% triclosan are well-tolerated and seldom cause allergic reactions. Triclosan is also impregnated into 'bacteriocidal' sutures.

> **NOTE**
>
> Studies have demonstrated that formulations containing 60–95% alcohol alone, or 50–95% when combined with limited amounts of a quaternary ammonium compound, hexachlorophene or chlorhexidine gluconate, lower bacterial counts on the skin immediately post-scrub more effectively than do other agents. The next most active agents (in order of decreasing activity) are chlorhexidine gluconate 4%, iodophors, triclosan and plain soap.

Preoperative hand washing technique

Australia currently recommends a conservative approach to surgical hand hygiene, such as scrubbing for 5 minutes, whereas the WHO and Centers for Disease Control (CDC) in the USA recommend less time or alcohol-based hand rubs as alternatives.

A review of the literature regarding the duration of washing, the use of a brush and the reagents used found that:

- Preoperative hand washing for 10 minutes is not recommended; 2–5 minutes is adequate.
- There is no evidence supporting the use of a brush.
- Alcohol-based hand rubs (ABHR) are equally effective as conventional reagents such as chlorhexidine gluconate and povidone–iodine in preventing SSI.
- ABHR have the advantage of better user compliance and causing fewer occupational hazards.
- A 1-minute non-antiseptic hand wash, followed by thorough rubbing with ABHR until dry and without brushing, is a safe and effective alternative to the conventional scrubbing technique [12].

Although it is a legal requirement for practitioners to surgically scrub before all invasive surgery, skin cancer surgery is not invasive and an initial surgical scrub with 4% chlorhexidine for at least 2 minutes and, thereafter, the use of ABHR can be recommended. If the practitioner wants to be doubly sure, use the ABHR, three squirts, twice.

Preoperative hand-washing technique

- Antiseptic detergent solutions are required for this level of hand hygiene (e.g. 4% chlorhexidine, povidone–iodine). Rapid growth of bacteria can occur if hands are washed with a non-antimicrobial soap.
- Mechanically remove gross dirt and oil from hands with ordinary soap first.
- Aims:
  - reduction of transient microorganism count as close to zero as possible
  - prolonged depressant effect on the resident microflora of the hands and forearms.
- 10-minute scrub is not necessary.
- Scrubbing is not recommended. It damages the skin and increases the microorganisms colonising it.

Scrub according to the manufacturer's guidelines/instructions (normally 2–6 minutes):

1 Wet hands and forearms under gently running water. Always keep hands higher than elbows: as the water runs from the hands down to the elbow, this avoids re-contaminating hands.
2 Apply antiseptic detergent to the hands and forearms to the elbows for 2 minutes.
3 A sterile nailbrush may be used at the start of a list to clean under nails if needed. Nail brushes are not otherwise recommended as they may cause micro-abrasions. Drop it in the sink after use and do not touch it again.
4 Rinse, using the elbows to adjust the flow of water. Do not touch tap with hands to prevent recontamination.
5 Using the surgical scrub solution, wash again from hands to just above the elbows.
6 Then, beginning with the little finger, rub each side in straight strokes and continue on to the next finger until all are rubbed. Using circular motions, work your way to your palm and then the back of your hand.
7 Repeat with the other hand.
8 Maintain a lather at all times, adding more water and soap if needed (using elbows).
9 Holding the hands above the elbows, rinse both hands and allow excess water to drip off.
10 Repeat the procedure with the hands and arms but do not include the elbows.
11 Rinse thoroughly under running water.

How to dry hands after a surgical scrub:

1 Pick up a corner of a sterile towel and allow it to unravel, being careful not to touch any other surface with the towel or your hands. Try not to shake out the towel to avoid accidental contamination.
2 Use your imagination to split the towel into four sections.
3 Holding the towel in your right hand, dry your left hand with the first quarter, front and back and all fingers.
4 With the second quarter, dry the left forearm to the elbow.
5 Now take the fourth quarter with the left hand, drape it over your right hand and dry the fingers and palm.
6 Finally, dry the right forearm to the elbow with the third quarter.

Note: Use of an alcohol handrub/gel between operations is recommended, but not yet approved. If the hands are physically clean, this method can be used between cases. Ensure that the alcohol handrub/gel purchased is suitable for preoperative hand disinfection. Two separate applications of alcohol handrub/gel are rubbed onto hands and forearms until dry. Consult the manufacturer's recommendations, but usually if the hands are dry before 15 seconds not enough ABHR has been used.

OTHER HYGIENE MEASURES

Gloves

Gloves play a dual role:

1 as a barrier for personal protection from patients' blood and exudates
2 to prevent bacteria from the surgeon's hands entering the surgical site.

All examination and surgical gloves must conform to national standards. Scrub team members should wear sterile gloves, donned after the sterile gown (if worn). Change to a fresh pair of sterile gloves for each procedure. Change gloves promptly if punctured or if they touch an unsterile object.

Perforations

Protection of the surgeon is the main indication for preoperative change of damaged gloves (especially against human immunodeficiency virus [HIV] and hepatitis B virus [HBV] and C [HCV]). Perforations were found in 12.7% of gloves and occurred in 34.5% of operations. No increase in bacterial contamination of the surgeon's hands or the outside of the surgical gloves in operations where gloves were shown to be punctured could be demonstrated and no association between glove perforation and postoperative wound infection could be found [13].

Double-gloving

Exposure to bloodborne pathogens is a serious occupational risk for health care workers. The bloodborne pathogens most commonly involved in needlestick and sharps injuries are HBV, HCV and HIV, even though the transmission of at least 20 different pathogens has been reported [14]. Randomised studies within various surgical specialities have shown that wearing two pairs of gloves decreases leaks by 3–9-fold in water permeability tests, when compared with wearing one pair of gloves.

Double-gloving may be uncomfortable and reduce manual dexterity and tactile sensitivity but it provides increased protection from penetration of needlestick injuries. It also reduced the percentage of hand contamination. It is estimated that as many as 87% of surgeons will experience a percutaneous injury at some point in their career [15]. The average risk of infection after percutaneous injury with a contaminated sharp instrument is 0.3% for HIV, 6–30% for HBV and 4–10% for HCV [14, 16]. These three viral infections are not rare in Australia. An estimated 260,000 plus people are currently infected with HCV (as at 2007), the majority of whom do not present signs or symptoms of the disease. The number of people living with chronic HCV and advanced liver disease is projected to increase by around 38% by 2015 [17]. This poses a risk to anyone performing surgery since people suffering from HIV or hepatitis have an increased risk for developing a medical problem requiring surgery and, therefore, the prevalence of these infections may be higher in general surgical patients than in the general population [15]. Skin surgery patients also have their share of viral illnesses.

The use of double-gloving in surgical procedures is regarded as the major risk management factor in the control of disease transmission in the clinical setting, as it provides an additional level of protection against bloodborne infections and greatly reduces the hazards of glove penetration. Double-gloving is the recommended practice of numerous professional organisations [18–20].

Double-gloving decreases the risk of blood exposure by as much as 87% when the outer glove is punctured [21]. Furthermore, in the event of a percutaneous injury, the blood on a solid suture needle is reduced as much as 95% when passing through two glove layers [21]. Double-gloving significantly reduces the perforation rates of the glove in contact with the skin, helps to cut down the number of potential exposures and reduces the risk of surgical cross-infection, as the greatest risk for transmission of infectious agents occurs when a glove is torn or punctured during procedures [18]. This is extremely important when considering that chronic HBV infection among surgeons is three times greater than that of the general population [22] and that every year more than 200 health care workers die from bloodborne hepatitis infections [23].

Recommendations:

- It is a personal decision whether to operate on a patient with known HBV, HBC or HIV. The hospitals are better equipped to do so and you have an obligation to your family and staff as well as the patient when such other avenues of treatment are available to them.
- The majority of patients with chronic HCV do not present signs or symptoms of the disease, so use extreme caution on patients with tattoos or a history of drug abuse.
- Wearing double gloves at surgical procedures helps to protect the wearer from viral transmission. The addition of a second pair of surgical gloves significantly reduces perforations to innermost gloves.

Gloving technique: gloving up

It is essential that the bare hand never touches the outside of the sterile gloves. Hence, the first glove is pulled on by its inside turned-over internal edge (Figure 7.8). Then, *the key to the whole procedure* is hooking or extending the gloved thumb up to hold the margin of this glove as it is pulled on. This is 'the key' because this prevents the first glove from rolling into a band at the wrist that will then be impossible to lift. Pushing the thumb up and away from the palm allows the second gloved hand later access between the first glove's thumb and the palm.

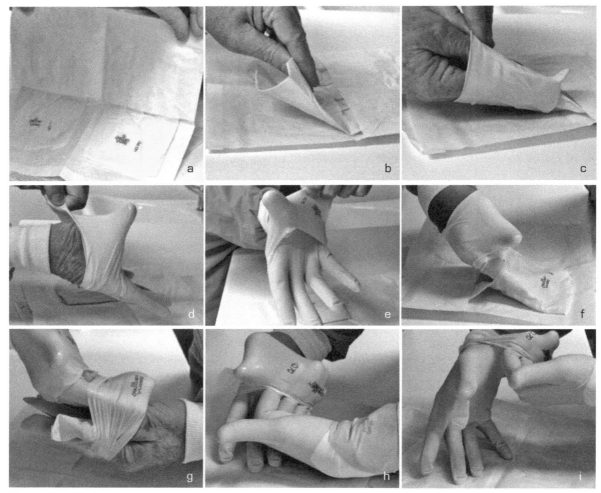

Figure 7.8 Gloving up

a Holding the inner glove envelope at the top allows the gloves' open ends to flop down ready for sterile hand insertion. Where this envelope has been grasped is now not sterile and should be avoided. **b** After scrubbing up the left thumb is inserted into the right glove and its mouth grasped and opened to facilitate insertion of the right hand. Ensure that the fingers only touch the reflected inner surface of the glove. **c** The right thumb and fingers are inserted until they are correctly located at the base of the appropriate glove finger, but do not push them in any further. Instead, elevate the thumb to indent and secure this reflected part of the glove as shown. **d** Another view of how the thumb secures this reflected part of the glove. **e** The glove can now be pulled down towards the wrist maintaining the thumb elevating the reflected glove while the rest of the fingers can be pushed home. **f** With the thumb of the right hand still elevating the reflected glove, its fingers are now used to slide under the sterile outer surface of the left glove. **g** It is then pulled up along the (left) forearm. **h** The fitted left glove is used to insert under the gap made by the elevated thumb on the right glove (i.e. the whole purpose of this thumb is to provide easier access to the right glove by the left hand). **i** The sterile left glove is only touching the external sterile part of the right glove, which can now be pulled up. It only remains to pull the caught thumb part of the glove out so it can rebound over the thumb correctly and pull down all fingertips so there is a close fit.

Face masks

Facemasks were introduced in 1897 as one layer of gauze and became routine in 1920. Their design improved but their effectiveness mostly went unchallenged. A review of all the relevant literature found many studies poorly designed or irrelevant and concluded that the Tunevall study of 1991 [24] was 'the only trial in the literature that shows respectable results according to which there is no difference in the incidence of postoperative wound infection in masked and unmasked groups' [25]. The controlled, prospective study by Tunevall recorded incidence of wound infection in 3088 patients over a 2-year period in acute and general surgery (Table 7.2). The study design randomised patients into weeks during which staff were 'masked' or 'unmasked', and the results were statistically insignificant. The 1537 'masked'

TABLE 7.2 Results of the Tunevall study

	With face mask			No face mask		
	Infections	Operations	% wound infection	Infections	Operations	% wound infection
Acute operations	21	350	6.0	17	349	5.4*
Elective clean operations	11	688	1.6	9	707	1.3*
Elective non-clean operations	41	499	8.2	27	500	5.4*
Total	73	1537	4.7	55	1551	3.5*

*$p < 0.05$ (statistics according to 2-tailed chi square test).
Adapted from Tunevall TJ (1991)[24].

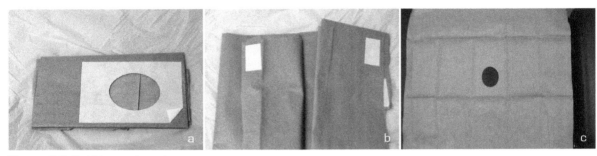

Figure 7.9 Fluid-impervious drapes
a The under (skin) side of a fluid-impervious drape. The paper is peeled off leaving a sticky surface that adheres to the skin, with a fenestrated central hole that is placed over the lesion to be excised. Remove this last. **b** Sticky peel-off tabs at all corners prevent the drape from slipping. Remove these first. **c** A whole drape is 60 × 60 cm with a 7.5 × 6.5 fenestrated hole. If enlarging the hole is necessary, do this before the sticky cover is removed. Don't put the sticky part on hairs as it will painfully rip them out when removed.

operations had an infection rate of 4.7% compared with 1551 'unmasked' operations with an infection rate of 3.5% [24].

There is still no clear evidence that face masks benefit or harm the patient by preventing postoperative wound infection in clean surgery [26]. However, the pendulum has now swung to protecting the surgeon: the rate of blood contact during surgical cases was found to be 10.2% with surgeons twice as likely to be affected as other health care individuals [27]. Masks not only provide a barrier for airborne organisms but also protection for the wearer against blood and body fluid splashes. Most studies were also for major operations (invasion of the peritoneum or joint spaces) and most hospitals still insist on face masks. Skin surgery does not usually involve such potential problems but have masks, caps and protective gear available; assess each individual case.

In one small study, plates for culturing bacteria were placed where an ophthalmologist's patient's head would be. When doctors talked while wearing a mask or stood in silence, hardly any bacteria grew on the plates. But when they didn't wear a face mask, while either facing the patient or turned away, most plates sprouted bacterial colonies. And when patients talked, about half of the plates grew bacteria [28].

Recommendation: masks are not necessary for skin surgery but don't cough, sneeze or talk loudly; otherwise, wear a mask.

Drapes

The simplest drape is a lint-free, strong paper towel that is sterilised; the surgeon can cut a hole in the centre of the appropriate dimensions. Plastic sheets, as in Sage packs, move and are troublesome. Fenestrated fluid-impervious drapes with adhesive surrounds and corner adhesive tabs are now available and are recommended (Figure 7.9). Their sole defect is that blood runs over them quickly and can reach the edge and drop onto gowns or the floor unless immediately soaked up.

Smoke plume

There is a need for staff to be protected from inhalation of surgical smoke and laser plumes. The definitive evidence for the potential danger from smoke plume is provided by the National Institute for Occupational Safety and Health (NIOSH) of the CDC, USA [29]: 'Research studies have confirmed that ... smoke plume can contain toxic gases and vapors ...' The consensus-based recommendations of the American Sleep Disorders Association (1994) [30] also recognise the potential hazard of smoke plume during laser surgery [31]. Since prospective trials involving humans to evaluate the health risks of smoke plume would not be ethical, most of the studies assessing the risk of smoke plume are based on *in vitro* or animal experiments. In general, these studies have found smoke plume from laser/electric surgery to contain pathogens. A prospective *in vitro* study [32] compared bacterial and viral cultures from operating room air filters prior to (control culture) and during laser resurfacing surgery (two cultures taken at different time periods). Although no pathogens were grown in samples collected from control filters, bacterial cultures were grown in samples collected during surgeries of five of 13 patients (38%).

Hygiene, sterility and below the table

Assume anything below the operating table is non-sterile. Whereas some hospitals used to insist on overshoes, this now seems to have lapsed. As noted, skin surgery does not penetrate the peritoneum and may be best compared with emergency room procedures. Absolute sterility of the whole theatre cannot be achieved but every effort can be made to ensure the operation site and 'above the table' are sterilised and everywhere else is as clean as possible. To that end, it would seem reasonable to minimise risk by insisting patients wash before their operation and leave their shoes outside. OT staff may have a pair of dedicated OT shoes with the soles immersed in antiseptic wash.

WOUND INFECTION PREVENTION – SURGICAL SITE INFECTION (SSI)

Clean vs sterile

For all surgery relevant to this text, the wounds would be classified as class 1: clean wounds (meticulous observance of aseptic techniques; uninfected operative site; no entry to respiratory, GI or GU tracts). In this case the expected infection rate is 1–4% (<5%).

Much of the received dogma regarding operating room sterility for dermatological surgery is unsupported by clinical studies. For dermatological surgical procedures, clean rather than sterile technique (e.g. gloves) may be sufficient.

In a recent review on surgical garb, the evidence regarding the effectiveness of specific protective measures to minimise patient infection was systematically evaluated. Among the findings were:

- No randomised, controlled trials of the utility of sterile gloves are available. Clean gloves may be as protective as sterile gloves. Moreover, many studies showed undetected microperforations in gloves; when sterile gloves are appropriate, double gloving may be preferable.
- Masks and head coverings do not appear to reduce surgical site infections; surgical personnel with scalp *Staphylococcus* colonisation can cause widespread infection in patients despite use of head coverings.
- Gown materials and construction vary. Conclusions for protective benefits, if any, are difficult to establish.

- Street shoes have been shown to harbour and transfer more bacteria than OR-only shoes, but studies showing that this increased colonisation results in patient infection are lacking. Shoe covers are not particularly helpful and may increase hand contamination [33].

Although sterility may not be crucial for some dermatological procedures and clean operating rooms with use-once gloves may be acceptable, in private practice it may well be circumspect to ensure totally sterile conditions. If infections or more serious complications occur, the records will attest that everything possible has been done correctly.

Preoperative cleansing of the patient's skin with chlorhexidine–alcohol is superior to cleansing with povidone–iodine for preventing SSI after clean-contaminated surgery [34].

Preventing SSIs in nasal carriers of *Staphylococcus aureus*

The number of surgical site *S. aureus* infections acquired in the hospital can be reduced by rapid screening and decolonising of nasal carriers of *S. aureus* by treatment with mupirocin nasal ointment and chlorhexidine soap, on admission [35]. Nostril instillation of chloramphenicol ointment is suggested for perinasal operations (but see section below, 'Nostril antibiotic ointment').

Behaviour and rituals in the operating theatre

There are many rituals in the operating theatre that have evolved under the pretext of preventing postoperative wound infection. Whilst there is little doubt that the degree of bacterial contamination of the operative wound is the major determinant of the incidence of post-operative infection, the virulence of the organisms contaminating the wound, the amount of tissue trauma, and the body's ability to resist that contamination are all-important factors. The skill of the surgeon undertaking the operation is reflected not only in the degree of trauma that he/she causes but also in his/her general conduct of the operation and awareness of what is, and what is not, important in reducing bacterial contamination of the wound. Maintenance of infection control discipline by all members of the team is important to the patient outcome [36].

Assess precautions for specific procedures in individual patients and institute. Skin cancer surgery, like cataract surgery, carries minimal operative site risks but the general health and hygiene of the patient is important, viz: impeded circulation/stasis, diabetes, anticoagulation, poor hygiene and inability to care for oneself. Undertake a full preoperative assessment including home status. Many old people live alone and cannot tend their wounds, let alone inspect their backs.

Sources of SSI

Infected cases
Delay procedures in patients with a serious infection or illness if possible.

Clean cases
The bacteria that cause postoperative surgical wound infection can arise from endogenous or exogenous sources.

Most SSIs are caused by contamination of an incision with microorganisms from the patient's own body during surgery [37]. The skin is colonised by various types of bacteria, but up to 50% of these are *Staphylococcus aureus* [38].

- Endogenous contamination: some 95% of postoperative wound infections are caused by endogenous bacterial contamination, which in skin surgery is invariably from the patient's own skin but other sites include the nares and perhaps bacterially colonised tracts of the body – gastrointestinal tract, genitourinary tract, bronchial tract, sinuses and antra of the skull and diseased biliary tract. In analyses of contamination rates after cholecystectomy, the main source of wound contamination was found to be the skin of the patient [39].
- Exogenous sources: arise from the environment in which the operation is conducted. Sources here include the instruments used to perform the operation or the hands of the surgeon and other health care workers involved in the procedure. However, the major exogenous source is transmission by air. Many minor procedures are performed with natural ventilation. Other sources of airborne bacteria are the skin and hair of the health care workers present in the OT being shed into the atmosphere and circulated into the wound.

The unkempt patient and the elderly who live alone present potential problems and the experienced clinician and staff can predict with some accuracy those whose wounds will become infected despite all preventive measures being taken. In such cases, topical chloramphenicol ointment and even systemic antibiotics may be considered.

Skin preparation
Skin preparation or 'prepping' is the process by which the skin is cleansed to reduce the number of transient (up to 50% of these are *Staphylococcus aureus*) [38] and resident (e.g. *Staphylococcus epidermis*) skin bacteria before incision. The aim is to reduce the potential of SSI; hence, prep close to the time of incision to ensure the best possible patient outcome. Based on epidemiological evidence most SSIs originate from the patient's own skin, mucous membranes or viscera. When mucous membranes or skin is incised, the exposed tissues are at risk of contamination mainly from endogenous flora. Alcohol is the 'gold standard' for prevention of SSIs because of its speed in 'killing' microorganisms. Among the other commonly used antiseptic agents are iodophors (e.g. povidone–iodine [Betadine®]), chlorhexidine gluconate in aqueous solutions or solutions of these in alcohol (termed tinctures). The use of a preoperative wash containing chlorhexidine decreases the bacterial count on skin by 80–90%, resulting in a decrease in preoperative wound contamination [40].

Selection of prepping agent
Studies have shown that 2% chlorhexidine with 70% alcohol is best [34]. Multicentre, randomised controlled trials concluded that 2% chlorhexidine gluconate and 70% isopropyl alcohol reduced total SSIs by 41% (from 16.1% to 9.5%), compared to the use of povidone–iodine solution. Povidone–iodine can be neutralised by blood and other organic matter, reducing its effectiveness and persistence. The efficacy and safety of 2% chlorhexidine gluconate and 70% isopropyl alcohol for skin antisepsis are supported by more than 35 clinical studies and recommendations by 18 internationally recognised organisations or guidelines. Isopropyl alcohol rapidly kills microorganisms and chlorhexidine maintains persistent antimicrobial activity. Further, gently scrubbing the skin helps the solution penetrate the first five layers of the epidermis, where 80% of microorganisms reside [34].

In Australia, the closest the author can find to such a product is BD Persist Plus, which is 1% chlorhexidine gluconate and 70% isopropyl alcohol in a swab stick in a sterile rip pack that leaves a green identifying transient stain.

Application of prepping agent
- Advise patients to shower on day of surgery to remove any obvious dirt.
- Remove gross contamination and meticulously clean the incision site.
- Assess the skin for breaks, rashes or infections.
- Check for any allergies or contraindications (e.g. iodine).
- Document all skin preparation.
- Dispense the solution so as not to compromise the sterile field (i.e. splashing).
- Swab the excision site with chlorhexidine 2% + alcohol 70%. Prepacked swab-sticks of 1% chlorhexidine with 75% ethanol (BD Persist Plus) are also available.

Technique:
- Proceed from clean to dirty (i.e. begin at the incision site and move towards the periphery in *concentric circles moving away from the proposed incision site to the periphery* allowing sufficient

prepared area to accommodate an extension to the location of the incision).

- The application and type of skin preparation may need to be modified according to the incision site (e.g. on the face, chlorhexidine is damaging to the cornea) or the condition of the skin (e.g. burns).
- Prepare heavily contaminated areas (e.g. axilla, perineum) last.
- Prep multiple incision sites separately, including graft or donor sites.
- When preparing an area where a stoma is present, cover the stoma with a sterile swab and prepare the surrounding area before removing the swab and cleaning the stoma.
- Take special measures and use alternative solutions when preparing the facial area (chlorhexidine is dangerous on the face if it gets into the eyes).
- Alcohol solutions are preferred to aqueous solutions for skin preparation but allow sufficient time for an alcohol-based skin preparation to dry thoroughly before commencing the procedure to ensure that all combustible ingredients have evaporated.
- Avoid solutions coming into contact with diathermy plates and other equipment.
- Avoid seepage or 'pooling' of solutions under the patient. Sterile towels may be used to absorb excess solution under the patient and removed as soon as possible to avoid irritation.

 CAUTION

Chlorhexidine is dangerous to the conjunctiva and tympanic membrane.

Electrocautery can ignite alcohol prep: allow it to dry completely.

Body wash

A preoperative body wash containing chlorhexidine decreases the bacterial count on skin by 80–90%, resulting in a decrease in preoperative wound contamination [40]. The effect on SSI incidence has, however, been more difficult to demonstrate and it is possible that prolonged washing releases organisms from deeper layers of the skin.

Hand washing

Correct hand washing technique for at least 2 minutes before surgery significantly reduces the bacterial count [41].

Safety

In 2000 in Florida, USA, in response to concerns about the dangers of office-based procedures, it was mandated that all adverse events that necessitated hospital admission or caused death be reported. Office-based procedures of mandatory reporting data for 7 years (1 March 2000–1 March 2007) were reviewed and showed that board-certified plastic surgeons were responsible for 58% of all deaths and 83% of cosmetic surgery deaths, and 52% of all hospital transfers and 83% of hospital transfers after cosmetic surgery. Eight of the 31 deaths occurred after liposuction performed by a plastic surgeon, the single most common cause of death. Of these 8 cases, 7 were performed under general anaesthesia, and the deaths were attributed to pulmonary emboli in 4 and unknown causes in 3 cases. There was 1 death after liposuction with intravenous sedation [42].

MRSA

Methicillin-resistant *Staphylococcus aureus* (MRSA) is thought to be more prevalent than most doctors realise in a clinical situation. Among patients shown to carry MRSA, more than half had colonisation at extranasal sites – most commonly in the oropharynx and the groin. HIV infection showed the strongest association with MRSA colonisation, with a nearly 14-fold increased risk.

The current practical advice is to put patients with known MRSA 'at the end of the list'. Obviously, if possible, all infection should be visually healed and consideration may be given to prepping extranasal sites.

Some of the populations at risk:

- compromised immune systems (immunosupressants/OTR (Organ Transplant), HIV/AIDS, lupus, cancer patients, steroid patients)
- diabetics [43]
- intravenous drug users [44]
- college students living in dormitories [44]
- people staying or working in a healthcare facility for an extended period of time [44]
- users of quinolone antibiotics [45]
- young children
- the elderly
- exposure to known MRSA contaminated water
- occupants of confined spaces: shelters, prison inmates, military recruits, athletes (change rooms/gyms)
- urban under-privileged
- indigenous populations, including Native Americans, Native Alaskans and Indigenous Australians [46]
- veterinarians.

Wound irrigation

Water, at least in first world conditions, is a safe and effective alternative to sterile normal saline for wound irrigation prior to suturing, as has been found in a prospective, double-blind, randomised, controlled clinical trial at Stanford University Medical Center Department of Emergency Medicine [47].

Hair removal

Removal is only necessary if hair will interfere with the incision site or there is a risk of wound contamination.

Shaving damages the skin and the risk of infection increases with the length of time between shaving and surgery [48]. In one study, if the patient had been shaved more than 2 hours before surgery the clean wound infection rate was found to be 2.3% [49]. However, if patients had not been shaved but their body hair had been clipped the rate was 1.7%, and if they had not been shaved or clipped the rate dropped to 0.9% [49]. If it is essential, shave as close to the time of surgery as possible. Depilatory creams the night before are now often used. Only remove hair from the incision area. The patient should consent to hair removal after explanation.

- Preoperatively, hair removal is best achieved by:
  - depilatory cream the day before surgery
  - with clippers in the anaesthetic room immediately before surgery; use electric or battery-operated clippers with a disposable head (reuseable heads need to be disinfected after each use)
- Do not use a razor or shaving brushes.
- Document the type and site of hair removal.
- For surgery on an already contaminated or infected wound, hair removal is not recommended.

Wound closure

The healing of closed surgical wounds depends on many factors, one of the most complex of which is the influence of technique and expertise [50].

Healing by primary intention

Surgical wounds may heal by primary intention, delayed primary intention or by secondary intention. Most heal by primary intention, where the wound edges are brought together (apposed) and then held in place by mechanical means, allowing the wound time to heal.

Healing by delayed primary intention occurs when non-viable tissue is removed and the wound is initially left open or when left open as with slow Mohs. Wound edges are refreshed and brought together at about 4–6 days before granulation tissue is visible [51]. This method is often used after traumatic injury or dirty surgery. Experimentally as well as clinically, it has been shown that a delay in wound closure of 4–5 days increases the tensile strength of the wound as well as resistance to infection. The overall rate of SSIs in traumatic war wounds using delayed principles was 3–4%, compared with more than 20% after primary closure [50]. In civilian practice, delayed healing has been used successfully in cases of severe incisional abscesses, mainly after laparotomy. Another benefit of delayed closure is the cosmetic result after healing. The appearance of a wound closed after a delay of 4–5 days is comparable to that of primary closure. A wider scar follows late closure (10–14 days), but this is cosmetically better than the result obtained after the healing of an open granulating wound.

Healing by secondary intention

Healing by secondary intention happens when the wound is left open, because of the presence of infection, excessive trauma, skin loss or dehiscence. The wound edges come together naturally by means of granulation and contraction [52].

Wound infection prevention measures

- Ask the patient to shower the day of the operation.
- The patient's own skin is the source of most infections. ? personal hygiene/antibiotic cover
- Do not shave the area. Use depilatory cream the night before or trim on the day if necessary.
- Draw margins using an alcohol-based 'permanent' marker.
- Prep the patient's skin meticulously with chlorhexidine 2% + 70% ethanol. As a second choice, prep the site with BD Persist Plus or alcohol–iodophore solution.
- Swab the area using enlarging concentric circles from the incision site.
- Wash hands >2 minutes with 4% chlorhexidine.
- Cut outside the marked lines.
- Ensure good technique (asepsis, no haematoma, no dead space, no wound tension or compromised blood supply).
- Employ air-conditioning, minimise stress (reduction of surgeon sweat).
- Use waterproof/occlusive dressings – undisturbed; pressure dressings lower limbs.
- Give the patient written postoperative instructions (no stretching, elevation of lower limbs).
- An open wound for 4 days heals well (slow Mohs).

POSTOPERATIVE INFECTION RATES

Most data regarding incidence and predictors of surgical site infection are based on hospital studies [48, 53, 54], and most studies looking at infection rates following minor dermatological surgery outside hospital have been conducted in specialist dermatology clinics [55–57]. In contrast, the quality of evidence regarding infection rates following minor surgery in general practice seems to be poor [58], and a comprehensive MEDLINE search revealed only one study that adequately recorded the incidence of infection following minor surgery in general practice [59]. However, a Queensland study by 19 GPs from four practices in the Mackay area assessed 857 patients for risk factors for wound infection after minor surgery in general practice, which is arguably the most relevant study to date with respect to skin surgery. Infection occurred in 74 of the 857 excisions (8.6%). Infection rates for the four centres were 2.9%, 7.8%, 10.0% and 10.2%. A similar general practice cohort infection rate was 1.9% [59] and that for a similar dermatology clinic cohort was 2% [57]. Mackay, however, is a tropical, sweaty area and facial excisions were excluded, plus, as they pointed out, it is difficult to compare the infection rates between different studies as different variables and methods were used [55].

Their results suggested that diabetes, excisions from the lower leg and foot or thigh and excisions of non-melanocytic skin cancer (SCC and BCC) are independent risk factors for infection after minor surgery. The latter finding is consistent with a study conducted in a specialist dermatology clinic, which suggested that oncological surgery (excision of skin cancer) is associated with a higher risk of infection [60]. Body extremities, with reduced blood supply, have also previously been associated with a higher incidence of infection [60, 61].

Australian prospective study of infection rates associated with skin surgery

- Non-diabetics = 2.0%
- Diabetics = 4.2%

Hence, diabetics have a 66% higher risk for infection.

- For both non-diabetics and diabetics:
  - Leg wounds = 4 times more likely to become infected
  - Flaps/grafts = 3.5 times more likely to develop wound infections
  - Other complications (bleeding, dehiscence, edge necrosis, contact dermatitis, wound depression/elevation, hypertrophic scar/keloid, granuloma, deep scar) = 1.8% [62]

ANTIBIOTIC PROPHYLAXIS

Systemic antibiotics

In general, antibiotic prophylaxis is not recommended and is no substitute for correct site preparation and aseptic technique. Antibiotic prophylaxis is probably prescribed excessively or inappropriately for dermatological surgery [53, 63] and is thought to be best reserved for high-risk patients [63, 64]. Recommendations from the Mayo Clinic, based on guidelines from the American Heart Association, American Dental Association and the American Academy of Orthopedic Surgeons, state that antibiotic prophylaxis in clean dermatological surgery that does not involve the oral mucosa or infected skin (even with endocarditis) is not warranted.

There are, however, exceptions to consider:

- poor patient hygiene (unkempt, lives alone)
- systemic illness (diabetes, compromised immune status, immunosuppressives, high WCC, age, obesity, malnutrition, renal failure)
- smoking (which some allege does not impede healing, but see Chapter 8, 'Flaps')
- dirty areas (lower limbs, groin, axilla, external genitalia)
- site – lower leg
- poor skin – lower leg, steroids – friable or tight skin
- poor circulation – lower leg, varicosities
- diabetics
- type of operation (graft/large flap).

Regimen if systemic antibiotics warranted
All 1 hour before operation: dicloxacillin 2 g or cephalexin 2 g or roxithromycin 300 mg.

Topical antibiotics

The use of topical antibiotics is a vexed and contentious issue. Most studies and trials have not found them necessary but many text books nevertheless recommend them in passing and experienced surgeons still use them, especially for grafts on the lower limb and for wounds left to heal by secondary intention. A survey of UK plastic surgeons reported that 66% used chloramphenicol eye ointment mainly as prophylaxis against infection [65].

Infection occurs after surgery in 1.5–20% of cases but good quality trials as to the effect of topical antibiotic prophylaxis are lacking [66]. It has been noted that most SSIs are caused by contamination of the incision from bacteria on the patient's own skin and that good preoperative antisepsis is probably more a function of the method rather than the agent used [67] and that removal of gross contamination and meticulous cleansing of the incision site reduce SSI [66].

One study compared the application of bacitracin and white soft paraffin (Vaseline) and found no significant difference [68]. Another prospective study of prophylactic antibiotics used in clean surgery showed only a modest reduction in SSI [57]. Three small studies found that a petrolatum-based ointment advanced wound healing as well as topical antibiotics [69–71]. A study in tropical Queensland (Mackay) found a statistically significant reduction (6.6%) in infection compared with the control group (11%) with the single use of topical chloramphenicol with clean dermatological surgery but not a clinically significant absolute reduction at 4.4% as the authors predetermined criterion was 5% [66]. However, for high-risk sutured wounds a single application of topical chloramphenicol reduced infection by 40%. For high-risk wounds, in addition to meticulous cleaning and technique, consideration may be given to chloramphenicol ointment as well. Another trial found that medical staff who sweat profusely are more likely to contaminate the surgical site than staff who do not [72]. Rates of SSI by practitioners experienced in dermatological surgery in specialist primary care settings, such as cancer clinics and dermatology clinics, are low [57, 73].

The conclusion of a *British Medical Journal* editorial was that: 'In clean minor surgery meticulous preoperative preparation and aseptic technique by appropriately trained practitioners with access to appropriate facilities will prevent most surgical site infections without antibiotic prophylaxis' [66].

A review of the literature carried out through searches of peer-reviewed publications in PubMed in the English language over a 30-year period between January 1980 and May 2010 found that, apart from the specific indications of joint arthroplasty, cataract surgery, possibly breast augmentation and abdominal surgery in obese patients, the evidence for use of topical antibiotics in surgery is lacking in conclusive randomised controlled trials [74].

Contamination-prone regions

A controlled prospective study of four groups of 2165 outpatients undergoing skin surgery evaluated the utility and the effects of several antibiotic schedules for prophylaxis of wound infections.

- Group A: 23 of 541 patients, given no antibiotics, had wound infections (4.25%).
- Group B: 8 of 542 patients, given systemic antibiotics from immediately after surgery until the third day, had wound infections (1.5%).
- Group C: 4 of 540 patients, treated only with local sterile antibiotic powder sprinkled into the wound during surgery, had wound infections develop (0.75%).
- Group D: only one infection occurred in the 542 patients given systemic antibiotics from 2 days before surgery until the second day after surgery (0.2%).

This last schedule was the best for prophylaxis of wound infections in contamination-prone regions. Local antibiotic administration is a simple method for prevention of infections in routine skin surgery [75].

Nostril antibiotic ointment

Decolonising of nasal carriers of *Staphylococcus aureus* by treatment with mupirocin nasal ointment and chlorhexidine soap reduces the risk of *S. aureus* infection [35]. Mupirocin was introduced into clinical practice in the UK in 1985 and was an extremely effective treatment of skin infections and for clearance of nasal *S. aureus* isolates including those resistant to methicillin. Unfortunately, resistance was described shortly after its initial use [76] and resistance keeps increasing [77]. Given this increasing resistance of *S. aureus* and the documented contamination of the nostrils, the author now coats the nares/nostrils with chloramphenicol ointment preoperatively for operations on the nose and perinasal areas. Below the knee and diabetics also have a higher postoperative infection rate, which may influence surgeons' decisions.

CLINIC EFFICIENCY

It has been estimated that in UK hospitals about 50% of available operating time is actually used for operating. Although this may not transfer to a small clinic, aim to be efficient:

- Understand the current processes for getting patients to theatre.
- Understand the flow through theatre and out of recovery.
- Identify and eliminate blocks to patient flow.
- Improve the patient experience.

In particular minimise issues in the preoperative pathway (e.g. patients arriving for surgery without specific tests having been undertaken or without informed consent) and also issues around the admission process on the day of surgery.

Assistance

A theatre assistant can enhance efficiency and productivity. Staff can also serve as surgical coordinator ensuring the clerical and business side of things run smoothly as well as setting up and coordinating post-op care. Train staff to do as many of these jobs as possible.

WORKING ALONE

It has been suggested that, like dentists, no doctor should work without assistance. That said, staff get sick, emergencies happen and it is often quicker to do a simple

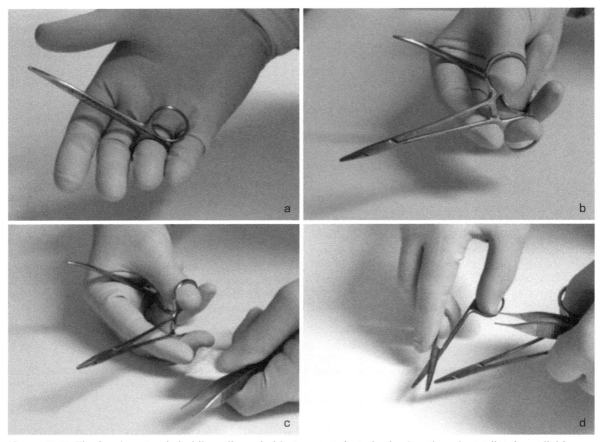

Figure 7.10 The key is not only holding all needed instruments but also having them immediately available and useable

a This begins with palming the scissors. After the lesion is excised the defect has to be sewn up. Rather than putting the needle holder down and picking up the scissors each time, they are palmed. **b** By placing one eye over the ring finger, this allows the middle finger and thumb to use the needle holder in the same hand. **c** The other hand uses the forceps for the wound edge and grasping the needle. Some operators also manage a cotton swab in the forceps hand. **d** When the sutures have to be cut, the needle holder is transferred to the forceps hand. Over time, it becomes automatic to maintain tension using the needle holder by pulling it up with fingers in its eyes while grasping both suture ends equally, holding them together, as it would be if you were holding them for an assistant to cut. The other hand now holds only scissors to facilitate cutting the sutures.

diamond/ellipse yourself. In such circumstances learning how to handle and hold all necessary instruments is a great help and simple to achieve so that it becomes automatic. This only becomes necessary when suturing and cutting the sutures (Figure 7.10).

HAND STABILISATION

Dentists are taught to brace and stabilise their hands to gain better control, but this is not a routine skill taught in medicine. Even bracing in mid-air gives better stability and control (Figure 7.11).

ERGONOMICS

All Mayo Clinic surgeons currently performing Mohs surgery and Mohs surgeons trained between 1990 and 2004 received a questionnaire survey between May 2003 and September 2004. Some respondents were videotaped during surgery. The main outcome measures were survey responses and an ergonomist's identification of potential causes of musculoskeletal disorders.

Results showed that the greatest risk for musculoskeletal disorders related to the surgeon's posture while performing surgery. Extreme or static postures assumed by various body parts during procedures may contribute

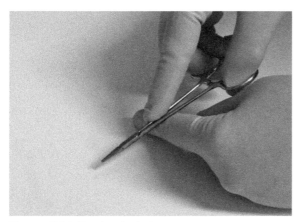

Figure 7.11 Bracing techniques

Here the needle holder (or whatever instrument) is braced across the other non-dominant hand's finger, which is in turn braced against a firm support. However, even the support of the other hand's index finger in mid-air will provide bracing and greater control.

immediately to the left (left handers may wish to reverse this). The hyfrecator/cauteriser can then be on the far side of the instruments with its sterile cable on the sterile instrument sheet. Locate foot switches to raise the table or trigger the cauteriser and check before scrubbing up.

 CAUTION

Locate the table up/down pedal outside the footprint of the table; otherwise, the surgeon's seated flexed thigh may be trapped and continue to depress the pedal. Fracturing femurs do not make a pleasant sound. (It may not necessarily be the femur that breaks, but there have been no offers of prospective trials.)

An assistant is best positioned directly opposite the surgeon, space permitting, otherwise to the surgeon's side affording best access.

---

greatly to development of work-related musculoskeletal disorders. Past studies have highlighted this risk in other jobs. Studying the relationship between posture and neck/shoulder musculoskeletal disorders, associations were found [78] between neck and neck/shoulder diagnoses with time spent in neck flexion, with critical angles greater than 15° and neck/shoulder diagnoses and time spent with upper arm abduction [78]. Similar associations due to imposed abnormal postures have also been reported [79–81]. After a review of more than 31 studies relating to posture-induced musculoskeletal disorders in various industries, the US Department of Health and Human Services [82] concluded that there is strong evidence of association between static and/or extreme postures and neck and neck/shoulder musculoskeletal disorders. Similar associations between static or extreme postures and musculoskeletal disorders were also reported for the shoulder and lower back.

Surgeons' symptoms

The 'arc'

It is not ergonometric sense for the surgeon to have to turn, twist, reach or contort for anything (instruments, equipment or to throw away swabs). Position the patient to allow best access, at the most comfortable height, with an excellent, shadowless light source. If possible, create a discrete arc of no more than 180° maximum (i.e. straight to the surgeon's sides), such that all equipment and waste bins are immediately handy and within reach. Instruments can be arranged on the right with the waste bin

TABLE 7.3 Summary of most common symptoms and proposed interventions

Symptom	Intervention
Neck-related symptoms	Angle patient or operating table to keep surgeon's gaze angle between 15° and 40° below horizontal Position patient closer to surgeon Short breaks during surgery to stretch and adjust position Stool with sternal support
Shoulder-related symptoms	Keep operative field at a 45° angle to the surgeon Position patient closer to the surgeon Stool with sternal support or a sit stand
Lower back pain	Stool with sternal support or a sit stand Frequent position changes Foot rest or foot rail
Eye fatigue and headaches	Decrease intensity of surgical lighting Goggles or glasses with antiglare film Brushed steel instruments instead of polished steel
Leg oedema	Compression stockings Foot rest or foot rail Antifatigue floor mats Gel insoles

Based on Esser, AC, Koshy, JG, Randle HW. Ergonomics in office-based surgery: a survey-guided observational study. Dermatol Surg 2007;33(11):1304–14.

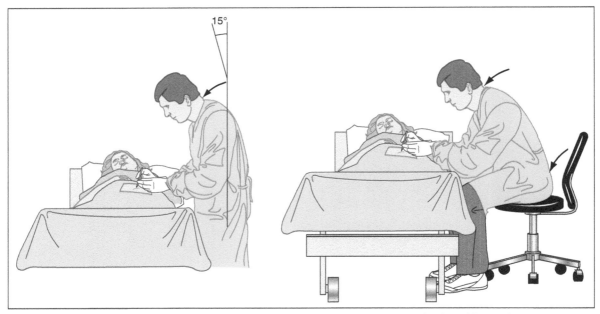

Figure 7.12 Flexing the neck more than 15° may lead to long-term cervical skeletal problems. The surgeon's head should not be dropped but aligned with the thoracic-lumbar spine at less than 15°

Tables should have minimal infrastructure to allow the surgeon's knees and legs to get underneath. Ensure both ends can be raised to best position the patient for face surgery without having to turn the bed around.

Train staff to *always* secure the surgeon's chair when he sits down as chairs have a tendency to roll away and, when scrubbed-up and sterile, there is little the surgeon can do.

Many surgeons suffer injuries from minimally invasive techniques

In a recent study, 87% of laparoscopic surgeons have experienced physical symptoms or discomfort [83]. This was especially true among those with high case volumes. Previous surveys had found only a 20–30% incidence of occupational injury among these surgeons. Sadly, it is easier for a surgeon to obtain an ergonomic assessment and direction to improve his golf swing than his posture or movement during surgery. Although laparoscopic surgery has problems peculiar to itself, this survey serves as a warning for any surgeon to ensure he is setting himself up in the most comfortable, ergonomic position possible.

The seven rules of surgery

Rule 1: 'The most important person in the operating theatre is the patient.' (Russel John Howard, *The Hip*)

Rule 2: Make the surgeon comfortable. That way the best job can be done for the patient.

Rule 3: Ensure a great light. Two sources eradicate most shadows.

Rule 4: Use the best equipment that you like and that you have selected.

Rule 5: Ensure the patient is positioned to allow the surgeon best access with minimal stretching.

Rule 6: Ensure the correct margins. Get it right the first time. The biggest factor leading to a high recurrence rate is inadequate margins. 'Measure twice, cut once'. First measure the correct margins, then work out if you can close the hole or not. If not, refer.

Rule 7: Don't rush. Check the patient notes, the pathology and the site. Confirm with the patient.

OPERATION NOTES

LESION: *NBCC*

SITE: *R Scapula*

SIZE: *>10 mm*

PHOTO: *Macro*

OPERATION:

Simple ellipse (S/E). *S/E*
Flap – determined as per PSR protocols and site Type:

L/A: *1% Xylocaine + adrenaline 1 : 200,000 × 10 mL*

INCISION: *Functional skin lines*

MARGINS: *4 mm*

HAEMOSTASIS: *Secured – bipolar*

CLOSURE: Deep sutures: *3 × 3/0 Monoslow*   Closure: *7 × 3/0 interrupted, central mattress nylon*

SUTURE No.: 7

DRESSING: *Opsite Postop*

RECOVERY: *Uneventful*

Figure 7.13 Sample template for operation notes

OPERATION NOTES

The surgeon is well advised to record good notes (see Figure 7.13) for personal recall, medicolegal and possible investigation insurances. With computer records a keystroke template is possible to ensure such complete records are filled in.

If the lesion is over 10 mm a photo is good proof. Measure lesions immediately preoperatively: although they may shrink during pathological processing, a preoperative photo with a measure scale is proof positive. The number of sutures is of interest to health departments as, perhaps reasonably, it would be hard to claim an operation as 'complex' if fewer than 10 sutures were necessary.

THE CHECKLIST

Checklists have proved to be a simple but dramatic improvement, especially in the ICU. In 2001, at John Hopkins Hospital, Dr Peter Pronovost constructed a simple 5-point checklist for doctors inserting an IV line: 1) wash hands, 2) clean patient's skin with chlorhexidine, 3) put sterile drapes over the entire patient, 4) wear a sterile mask and 5) put a sterile dressing over the catheter site when the line is in. This seemed unnecessary but observation found that, in more than a third of patients, at least one step was skipped. Adoption of the checklist resulted in the 10-day line infection rate falling from 11% to zero, and it was calculated that over 15 months the checklist had prevented 43 infections and 8 deaths and saved $2 million in costs. The introduction of checklists to other USA hospitals has afforded similar benefits, such as a decrease in Michigan's ICU infection rate by 66% in 3 months [84].

The checklist has two main functions:

1 to help memory recall, especially with routine, mundane steps easily overlooked with interruptions
2 to simplify and reinforce the importance of certain precautions.

In theatre
An operation can be divided into many parts but the most simplistic is:

1 setting up
2 excision
3 closure.

Each of these should be addressed as a separate entity. Take time to set up meticulously: prepare, prepare, prepare. Set up everything as *you* want and prefer so as to optimise your results. Some of the most valuable time the surgeon can spend is adjusting everything (HELP – height, exposure, light, position) to individual satisfaction. If anything goes wrong it is you and you alone who has to accept total responsibility.

The following steps and checks are an amalgam of various checklists as well as incorporating the experience of practising surgeons. It certainly is not meant to be didactic but rather to provide a list from which to extract what is needed.

Summary:
Steps necessary to perform an operation correctly

PRELIMINARY
1 Need for operation (biopsy report) – explain to patient
2 Options – surgical: punch/shave/ellipse/flap/deep sutures/subcuticular – plan most likely surgery
3 Fee
4 Booking and scheduling – completed booking form – duration of operation
5 Preoperative examination – complete check
6 Pre-op information sheet
7 Doctor's operation list (confidential)

COMPLETE OPERATION CHECKLIST

PRE-OP

Patient reception/receptionist
1 Confirm booking the day before
2 Ensure depilation done if necessary
3 Re-confirm phone numbers for Op day in case of delays etc
4 Arrive patient 15 min early for paperwork
5 Welcome patient and confirm ID on arrival
6 Confirm operation plan/photo
7 Confirm with patient (no prompting) (purple finger sign)
8 Confirm no recent health changes (pacemaker/medication/anticoagulants/skin infections)
9 Confirm fee and method of payment before operation (check item nos. with Dr)
10 Confirm consent
11 Get pathology request form signed
12 Open patient's records on Dr's computer

Patient preparation – assistant
1 Escort to change-room/theatre when Dr requests
2 Help patient remove all necessary clothes – 100-mm clearance from site

---

Summary:
Steps necessary to perform an operation correctly continued

3 Shoes – best left outside OT

4 Trim hair if necessary/get ibis pins/tape to hold back/tubi-gauze

OPERATING THEATRE

Assistant

1 Check OT clean and stocked

2 Pillow and blueys

3 Test and position equipment

4 Pathology request forms/jar(s), labelled

5 Air conditioning on – early

6 Music on

7 Ensure all necessary stock and spares

8 Test electrical equipment – switch on

9 Operating table – on, test, clean, position, adjust

10 Surgeon's operating chair – ensure in theatre

11 Lights – on, test

12 Pen, fine alcohol-based (+ spare)

13 Loupe

14 Gloves – non-sterile

Doctor

1 Patient's notes

2 Pathology results (biopsy reports)/operation plan/photos

3 Double-check: nodular or multinodular; undifferentiated or differentiated; Clark Lv 1 or Clark Lv 2 – these require different operations

4 Time out – gather wits – think it through – have a plan B

5 Call patient only after double-checking and 'time-out'

Patient to theatre – assistant

1 Bring patient when Dr specifically requests

2 Position patient to provide best access to lesion; check pre-op assessment

3 Clear the site – all clothes well away

4 Tape or pin back hair prn

5 HELP (height, expose, lights, position)

6 Camera/photo/ID (dedicated strips or post-its)

7 Alcohol swabs

8 Syringes and draw up needles (? prefill) – hide

9 25G 38-mm needles for L/A

10 Sodium bicarbonate

11 Lignocaine (xylocaine with adrenaline) 1% 1 : 200,000 optimum concentration

12 Lignocaine 2% plain for maxillary/nerve blocks

13 Mayo trolley or tray to right – the 'arc'

14 Yellow lined pathology/throw bin immediately to left (or vice versa)

15 Coagulation: (a) on & checked; (b) bipolar

16 Waterproof undersheet/bluey: (a) on pillow; (b) under operation site

Summary:
Steps necessary to perform an operation correctly continued

17 Foot switches outside table footprint – check if working

18 Catchers – place well away from lesion

19 Sterile hand towel

20 Gloves sterile

21 Pathology jar – open & labelled

22 Sharps bin

Doctor – operation
Use loupe and/or dermatoscope to meticulously define edges/margins

1 Measure – transparent plastic circles – and record in notes

2 Draw operation on site (alcohol-based pen) – ensure correct margins

3 Inject slowly and gently

4 Have a 'tea break' – adrenaline takes 15 minutes to act – the wait will repay you

5 Start your notes if impatient

6 Gown up – assistant to tie

7 Scrub: 2 min 4% chlorhexidine pink. Then ABHR × 2 and glove-up

8 Prep site – chlorhexidine 2% + 70% alcohol (BD Persist Plus closest)

9 Warn patient you are about to cut and to advise if any pain felt

10 Ensure orientated lesion before excised; put in jar immediately

Wall checklist

1 Sage pack

2 Alfoil

3 Drape(s) – sterile, fluid impervious

4 Operation kit: (a) scalpel handle; (b) needle holder; (c) tissue forceps; (d) scissors; (e) scalpel blade 15

5 Sutures (6/0 face → 3/0 back): absorbable and tie-off prn

6 Swabs gauze sterile

7 Chloramphenicol ointment

8 Dressing

9 Conforming/crepe bandage

10 Kidney tray – for used instruments

11 Dirty instruments to be cleaned statim → ultrasonic bath

Stand-by equipment

1 Artery/mosquito forceps

2 Plain Adson forceps

3 Skin hooks

4 4/0 dissolvable sutures

5 Cotton-tip long applicators

6 Dental rolls

7 Dressing scissors for nose/ear dressings – non-stick, gauze, Fixomull

8 Steri-strips, tincture benz. co/skin-prep

9 Waterproof dressings

10 Towel clips (to approximate wound edges)

11 Mirror

Summary:
Steps necessary to perform an operation correctly continued

POST-OP

Doctor
1 Sharps to sharps bin
2 Contaminants to pathology waste
3 Check pathology request, specimen and jar label
4 Post-op help, talk and assessment of patient
5 Notes

Receptionist
1 Recheck item nos. and fee (? altered operation needed)
2 Post-op instruction sheet – give to patient
3 ROS date (card)
4 Confirm ROS appointment & pathology form signed
5 Operation notes – check they are done

OTHER NECESSITIES FOR SURGERY/OPERATIONS

Stock (OT)
1 Surgical hand scrub
2 ABHR (alcohol-based hand rub)
3 Sterile drying towels
4 Gown/scrubs
5 Mask/cap optional
6 Non-sterile & sterile gloves
7 Local anaesthetics
8 Syringes and needles
9 Site prep: alcohol – chlorhexidine
10 Sterile water/normal saline (clean around eyes/ears)
11 Sterile surface sheet/Sage pack
12 Scalpel blade
13 Instruments (other sets + artery forceps, skin hooks, plain forceps)
14 Marker pens
15 Drape – sterile
16 Sutures – complete range including absorbable
17 Gauze squares, sterile & non-sterile
18 Dressings
19 Chloramphenicol ointment
20 Swab sticks/cotton buds
21 Kidney dishes for used instruments

Other OT equipment/necessities
1 Operating table
2 Lights
3 Coagulation unit bipolar
4 Topical haemostat solution
5 Sharps bin

Summary:
Steps necessary to perform an operation correctly continued

6 Waste bin(s)

7 Cleaning solutions – table, benches, floor

8 Cotton wool ball (external auditory meatus protection)

9 Hair clips/tape

10 Tubular mesh gauze, head size

11 Emergency light

12 Mirror

13 Conforming/crepe bandages

14 Spray dressing (scalp)

15 Reinforcing tapes/strips

16 Ultrasonic unit

17 Cleaning brush and instrument solutions

18 Lint-free cloths

19 Steriliser

20 Distilled water

21 Sterilising pouches

22 Indicators

23 Tracking items/log book

24 Pathology necessities (forms, jars, swabs)

MISCELLANEOUS

Sterile surfaces

Sterile surfaces can be provided by pre-packaged 'Sage' packs, which provide a sterile base towel, drape, disposable 15 scalpel, gauze squares and plastic forceps. Another alternative is to sterilise a lint-free tissue such as a Sontara®. In an emergency the inside of the instrument sterilising bag or glove packet can be used.

Instruments

Number packs to suit site (small needle holders for face etc).

'If you have the bi-polar connected, skin hooks and tie-off sutures you won't need them', or don't take the risk – have them out and ready.

The single most-forgotten item is the scalpel blade. Unless a checklist is used it is often assumed the blade is under the swabs, but by then everyone is gloved up. Place the scalpel blade in the same position every time where nothing is put on top of it.

Working alone/without an assistant

If working alone without an assistant it is most preferable to get everything right before scrubbing up. In the main this can be done, but there will be times when more sutures or swabs are needed. Although an assistant is obviously preferable, an emergency call-bell that can be pushed with an elbow can be installed and all staff trained in aseptic principles and techniques, how to open sterile packs and snap anaesthetic vials. If really caught out and alone, get the extra equipment you need while still gloved up and empty it onto your sterile area *then* open a new pack of sterile gloves, de-glove and then re-glove.

Bleeding

Never stop anticoagulants. Clopidogrel causes most severe complications. Thrombosis–embolus risk increases after 67 years of age.

Cleaning the patient

This is something the staff can do; insist they do it properly, especially any blood in the hair. You can do a great operation but the patient will not be impressed, nor should they be, if blood is left anywhere on them.

Summary:
Steps necessary to perform an operation correctly continued

Dressings
Waterproof dressings are best but blood can ooze through the central thin island gauze and distress, if not the patient, their spouse. If it is likely to bleed a thicker more opaque dressing, such as cutiplast, can be placed over the top as a disguise (with instructions not to remove the bottom waterproof).

Protecting the wound
Obviously, the potential for transmission from skin infections to open wounds is great. Delay any cryosurgery that may result in blister formation until all excisions are completed and healed. Cover any cuts and abrasions with a waterproof dressing and treat if infected and check regularly. Topical antibiotic is a suggested minimum with systemic antibiotics if inflammation and infection manifest.

Post-op check
When operating in a danger zone, check for intact motor function post-op. Local anaesthesia can cause temporary loss of function.

Recover the patient in theatre
Sit patients up slowly, let them settle and assess them. Help them up with support – especially the elderly. Watch for any loss of balance or vaso-vagal syncope (fainting). Help them out firmly but without rushing them.

Handouts
Ensure patients receive postoperative care handouts and an appointment for ROS.

Cleaning postoperatively
Clean the operating table and any spillage or debris immediately after the patient leaves. Most hospitals clean their theatres with 'soap and water'. Various 'antiviral' solutions are used to wipe down surfaces and the operating table, but most don't work for 10 minutes and are a waste of money if used as a wipe.

Re-excision
If re-excision proves necessary don't remove the original sutures as they are a marker of the original surgery. Do not worry if the original sutures have to be left in a long time and cause a reaction as this skin will be excised. Removing sutures may lead to confusion and head-scratching.

Sharps injuries
OT needlesticks and other sharps injury rates have increased 6.5%. In the operating room, just three devices accounted for most injuries: suture needles (43.4%), scalpel blades (17.1%) and disposable syringes (12.1%). Focusing on suture needles may present the greatest opportunity for improving operating room safety [85].

REFERENCES

[1] Gill JF, Yu SS, Neuhaus IM. Tobacco smoking and dermatologic surgery. J Am Acad Dermatol 2013;68:167–72.

[2] MacDonald NE, Hébert PC, Flegel K, et al. Working while sleep-deprived: not just a problem for residents. CMAJ 2011;183(15):1689.

[3] Klein AS, Forni PM. Barbers of civility. Arch Surg 2011;146(7):774–7.

[4] Bethune DW, Blowers R, Parker M, et al. Dispersal of *Staphylococcus aureus* by patients and surgical staff. Lancet 1965;1:480–3.

[5] Woodhead K, Taylor EW, Bannister G, et al. Behaviours and rituals in the operating theatre. A report from the Hospital Infection Society Working Party on Infection Control in Operating Theatres. J Hosp Infect 2002;51:241–55.

[6] Hayek LJ, Emerson JM. Preoperative whole body disinfection – a controlled clinical study. J Hosp Infect 1988;11(Suppl. B):15–19.

[7] Veiga DF, Damasceno CA, Veiga Filho J, et al. Influence of povidone–iodine preoperative showers on skin colonization in elective plastic surgery procedures. Plast Reconstr Surg 2008;121:115–18.

[8] McGinness JL, Goldstein G. The value of preoperative biopsy-site photography for identifying cutaneous lesions. Dermatol Surg 2010;36:194–7.

[9] Brach JP, Vergilis-Kalner I, Goldberg LH. Update to where was that biopsy taken? Dermatol Surg 2010;36(6):963–4.

[10] Thakkar SC, Mears SC. Visibility of surgical site marking: a prospective randomized trial of two skin preparation solutions. J Bone Joint Surg Am 2012;94:97–102.

[11] Erkkilä J, Punkanen M, Fachner J, et al. Individual music therapy for depression: randomised controlled trial. Br J Psychiatry 2011;199:132–9.

[12] Lung DC, Man JH-K, Tang TH-C, et al. Surgical hand-washing. Ann Coll Surg Hong Kong 2004;8(3):71.

[13] Dodds RD, Guy PJ, Peacock AM, et al. Surgical glove perforation. Br J Surg 1988;75(10):966–8.

[14] Beltrami EM, Williams IT, Shapiro CN, et al. Risk and management of blood-borne infections in health care workers. Clin Microbiol Rev 2000;13(3):385–407.

[15] Weiss ES, Makary MA, Wang T, et al. Prevalence of blood-borne pathogens in an urban, university-based general surgical practice. Ann Surg 2005;241(5): 803–7.

[16] Centers for Disease Control and Prevention. NIOSH Publication no. 2004–146. 2004. Worker Health Chartbook.

[17] Ministerial Advisory Committee on AIDS, Sexual Health and Hepatitis C Sub-committee. Hepatitis C Virus Projections Working Group: Estimates and projections of the hepatitis C virus epidemic in Australia 2006. Available: <http://www.health.gov.au/internet/main/publishing.nsf/content/A6B2E9BE0AE3A249CA2572020003E1D2/$File/hcvpwg.pdf>; 2006 [accessed 14 Nov 2012].

[18] Royal Australasian College of Surgeons. Advisory Committee on Infection Control in Surgery. Infection Control in Surgery Policy. Available: <http://catalogue.nla.gov.au/Record/2700098>; 1998 [accessed 14 Nov 2012].

[19] Department of Health and Ageing, Australian Government. Infection control guidelines for the prevention of transmission of infectious diseases in the health care setting. Commun Dis Intell 2004;28(2). Available: <http://www.health.gov.au/internet/main/publishing.nsf/Content/cda-pubs-cdi-2004-cdi2802-htm-cdi2802b.htm>; [accessed 14 Nov 2012].

[20] Australian College of Operating Room Nurses (ACORN). ACORN standards for perioperative nursing. Available: <http://www.acorn.org.au/about-acorn-standards/standards-index.html>; 2010 [accessed 14 Nov 2012].

[21] Berguer R, Heller PJ. Strategies for preventing sharps injuries in the operating room. Surg Clin N Am 2005;85:1299–305.

[22] Thomas S, Agarwal M, Mehta G. Intraoperative glove perforation – single versus double gloving in protection against skin contamination. Postgrad Med J 2001;77:458–60.

[23] Smoot EC. Practical precautions for avoiding sharp injuries and blood exposure. Plast Reconstr Surg 1998;101(2):528–34.

[24] Tunevall TJ. Postoperative wound infections and surgical face masks: a controlled study. World J Surg 1991;15:383–8.

[25] Bahli ZM. Does evidence based medicine support the effectiveness of surgical facemasks in preventing postoperative wound infections in elective surgery? J Ayub Med Coll Abbottabad 2009;21(2):166–70.

[26] Lipp A, Edwards P. Disposable surgical face masks for preventing surgical wound infection in clean surgery. Cochrane Database Syst Rev 2002;(1):CD002929.

[27] White MC, Lynch P. Blood contact and exposures among operating room personnel: a multicenter study. Am J Infect Control 1993;21:243–8.

[28] Wen JC, McCannell CA, Mochon AB, et al. Bacterial dispersal associated with speech in the setting of intravitreous injections. Arch Ophthalmol 2011;129(12):1551–4. doi: 10.1001/archophthalmol.2011.227.

[29] National Institute for Occupational Safety and Health. Control of smoke from laser/electric surgical procedures. Publication No. 96–128. Centers for Disease Control and Prevention; 1996. Available: <http://www.cdc.gov/niosh>; [accessed 6 January 2000].

[30] American Sleep Disorders Association. Practice parameters for the use of laser-assisted uvulopalatoplasty. Available: <http://www.guidelines.gov>; 1994 [accessed 10 October 1999].

[31] Baggish MS, Elbakry M. The effects of laser smoke on the lungs of rats. Am J Obstet Gynecol 1987;156:1260–5.

[32] Capizzi PJ, Clay RP, Battey MJ. Microbiologic activity in laser resurfacing plume and debris. Lasers Surg Med 1998;23:172–4.

[33] Eisen DB. Surgeon's garb and infection control: what's the evidence? J Am Acad Dermatol 2011;64:960.

[34] Darouiche RO, Wall MJ Jr, Itani KM, et al. Chlorhexidine–alcohol versus povidone–iodine for surgical-site antisepsis. N Engl J Med 2010;362(1):18–26.

[35] Bode LG, Kluytmans JA, Wertheim HF, et al. Preventing surgical-site infections in nasal carriers of Staphylococcus aureus. N Engl J Med 2010;362(1): 9–17.

[36] Hospital Infection Society. Behaviours and rituals in the operating theatre: A report from the Hospital Infection Society Working Party on Infection Control in Operating Theatres. J Hosp Infect 2001;51(4):241–55.

[37] Grey JE, Healy B, Harding K. Antibiotic prophylaxis for minor dermatological surgery in primary care. BMJ 2009;338:a2749.

[38] Eriksen NH, Espersen F, Rosdahl VT, et al. Carriage of Staphylococcus aureus among 104 healthy persons during a 19–month period. Epidemiol Infect 1995;115(1):51–60.

[39] Whyte W, Hambraeus A, Laurell G, et al. The relative importance of routes and sources of wound contamination during general surgery. I. Non-airborne. J Hosp Infect 1991;18(2):93–107.

[40] Byrne DJ, Phillips G, Napier A, et al. The effect of whole body disinfection on intraoperative wound contamination. J Hosp Infect 1991;18(2):145–8.

[41] Centers for Disease Control and Prevention. Guideline for prevention of surgical site infection. Am J Infect Control 1999;27:98–134.

[42] Coldiron B. Office surgery incidents: what seven years of Florida data show us. Am Soc Dermatol Surg Inc 2008;34:108.

[43] Lipsky BA, Tabak YP, Johannes RS, et al. Skin and soft tissue infections in hospitalised patients with diabetes: culture isolates and risk factors associated with mortality, length of stay and cost. Diabetologia 2010;53(5):914–23. doi: 10.1007/s00125-010-1672-5.

[44] Centers for Disease Control and Prevention. MRSA infections: People at risk of acquiring MRSA infections. Available: <http://www.cdc.gov/mrsa/riskfactors/index.html>; 2010 [accessed 13 May 2012].

[45] Tacconelli E, De Angelis G, Cataldo MA, et al. Does antibiotic exposure increase the risk of methicillin-resistant *Staphylococcus aureus* (MRSA) isolation? A systematic review and meta-analysis. J Antimicrob Chemother 2008;61(1):26–38. doi:10.1093/jac/dkm416.

[46] David MZ, Daum RS. Community-associated methicillin-resistant *Staphylococcus aureus*: epidemiology and clinical consequences of an emerging epidemic. Am Soc Microbiol 2010;23:616–87.

[47] Weiss EA, Oldham G, Lin M, et al. Water is a safe and effective alternative to sterile normal saline for wound irrigation prior to suturing: a prospective, double-blind, randomised, controlled clinical trial. BMJ Open 2013;3:ii. doi: 10.1136/bmjopen-2012-001504.

[48] Cruse PJ, Foord R. The epidemiology of wound infection. A 10-year prospective study of 62,939 wounds. Surg Clin North Am 1980;60(1):27–40.

[49] Cruse PJE. Classification of operations and audit of infection. In: Taylor EW, editor. Infection in surgical practice. Oxford: Oxford University Press; 1992. pp. 1–7.

[50] Leaper DJ, Gottrup F. Surgical wounds. In: Leaper DJ, Harding KG, editors. Wounds: biology and management. Oxford: Oxford University Press; 1998. pp. 23–40.

[51] Gottrup F. Wound closure techniques. J Wound Care 1999;8(8):397–400.

[52] Thomas S. Wound management and dressings. London: Pharmaceutical Press; 1990.

[53] Mangram AJ, Horan TC, Pearson ML, et al. Guideline for prevention of surgical site infection. Infect Control Hosp Epidemiol 1999;20:250–78.

[54] Nguyen D, MacLeod WB, Phung DC, et al. Incidence and predictors of surgical-site infections in Vietnam. Infect Control Hosp Epidemiol 2001;22:485–92.

[55] Furtoryan T, Grand D. Postoperative wound infection rates in dermatologic surgery. Dermatol Surg 1995;21:509–14.

[56] Dettenkofer M, Wilson C, Ebner W, et al. Surveillance of nosocomial infections in dermatology patients in a German university hospital. Br J Dermatol 2003;149:620–3.

[57] Amici J, Rogues AM, Lasheras A, et al. A prospective study of the incidence and complications associated with dermatological surgery. Br J Dermatol 2005;153:967–71.

[58] National Primary Care Research and Development Centre and Centre for Public Policy and Management, University of Manchester. Outpatient services and primary care. A scoping review of research into

strategies for improving outpatient effectiveness and efficiency. Manchester: NPCRDC; 2006. Available: <http://www.npcrdc.man.ac.uk/Publications/final_report.pdf>; [accessed Jan 2006].

[59] Lathlean S. Skin cancer in general practice in South Australia. A five-year study. Aust Fam Physician 1999;28(Suppl. 1):S28–31.

[60] Sylaidis P, Wood S, Murray DS. Postoperative infection following clean facial surgery. Ann Plast Surg 1997;39:342–6.

[61] Heal C, Buettner P, Browning S. Risk factors for wound infection after minor surgery in general practice. Med J Aust 2006;185(5):255–8.

[62] Dixon AJ, Dixon MP, Dixon JB. Prospective study of skin surgery in patients with and without known diabetes. Dermatol Surg 2009;35:1035–40.

[63] Messingham MJ, Arpey CJ. Update on the use of antibiotics in cutaneous surgery. Dermatol Surg 2005;31:1068–78.

[64] Cho CY, Lo JS. Dressing the part. Dermatol Clin 1998;16:25–47.

[65] Erel E, Platt AJ, Ramakrishnan V. Chloramphenicol use in plastic surgery. Br J Plast Surg 1999;52:326–7.

[66] Heal CF, Buettner PG, Cruickshank R, et al. Does single application of topical chloramphenicol to high risk sutured wounds reduce incidence of wound infection after minor surgery? Prospective randomised placebo controlled double blind trial. BMJ 2009;338:a2812.

[67] National Institute for Health and Clinical Excellence. Surgical site infection. Available: <http://www.nice.org.uk/nicemedia/pdf/CG74NICEGuideline.pdf>; 2008 [accessed 14 Nov 2012].

[68] Smack DP, Harrington AC, Dunn C, et al. Infection and allergy incidence in ambulatory surgery patients using white petrolatum vs bacitracin ointment. A randomized controlled trial. JAMA 1996;276:972–7.

[69] Draelos ZD, Rizer RL, Trookman NS. A comparison of postprocedural wound care treatments: do antibiotic-based ointments improve outcomes? J Am Acad Dermatol 2011;64:S23–9.

[70] Taylor SC, Averyhart AN, Heath CR. Postprocedural wound-healing efficacy following removal of dermatosis papulosa nigra lesions in an African American population: a comparison of a skin protectant ointment and a topical antibiotic. J Am Acad Dermatol 2011;64:S30–5.

[71] Trookman NS, Rizer RL, Weber T. Treatment of minor wounds from dermatologic procedures: a comparison of three topical wound care ointments using a laser wound model. J Am Acad Dermatol 2011;64:S8–15.

[72] Mills SJ, Holland DJ, Hardy AE. Operative field contamination by the sweating surgeon. Aust NZ J Surg 2000;70:837–9.

[73] Dixon AJ, Dixon MP, Askew DA, et al. Prospective study of wound infections in dermatologic surgery in the absence of prophylactic antibiotics. Dermatol Surg 2006;32:819–27.

[74] McHugh SM, Collins CJ, Corrigan MA, et al. The role of topical antibiotics used as prophylaxis in surgical site infection prevention. J Antimicrob Chemother 2011;66(4):693–701.

[75] Bencini PL, Galimberti M, Signorini M, et al. Antibiotic prophylaxis of wound infections in skin surgery. Arch Dermatol 1991;127(9):1357–60.

[76] Goldsmith CE, Moore JE, Murphy PG. Pneumococcal resistance in the UK. J Antimicrob Chemother 1997;40(Suppl. A):11–18.

[77] Patel JB, Gorwitz RJ, Jernigan JA. Mupirocin resistance. Clin Infect Dis 2009;49:935–41.

[78] Ohlsson K, Attewell RG, Pålsson B, et al. Repetitive industrial work and neck and upper limb disorders in females. Am J Ind Med 1995;27:731–47.

[79] Kilbom A, Horst D, Kemfert K, et al. Observation methods for reduction of load and strain on the human body: a review. Arbetarskyddsstyrelsen Publikation Service. 1986;171(84):92.

[80] Kilbom A, Persson J. Work technique and its consequences for musculoskeletal disorders. Ergonomics 1987;30:273–9.

[81] Schibye B, Skov T, Ekner D, et al. Musculoskeletal symptoms among sewing machine operators. Int J Ind Ergon 1988;3:1–12.

[82] National Institute for Occupational Safety and Health (NIOSH). Low-back musculoskeletal disorders: evidence for work-relatedness. Publication No. 97–141. Atlanta: CDC; 1987. Available: <http://www.cdc.gov/niosh/docs/97-141/pdfs/97-141f.pdf>; [accessed 14 Nov 2012].

[83] Park A, Lee G, Seagull FJ, et al. Patients benefit while surgeons suffer: an impending epidemic. J Amer Col Surg 2010;210(3):306–13. doi: 10.1016/j.jamcollsurg.2009.10.017.

[84] Pronovost P, Needham D, Berenholtz S, et al. An intervention to decrease catheter-related bloodstream infections in the ICU. N Engl J Med 2006;355:2725–32.

[85] Jagger J, Berguer R, Phillips EK, et al. Increase in sharps injuries in surgical settings versus nonsurgical settings after passage of national needlestick legislation. J Am Coll Surg 2010;210:496–502.

Flaps 8

Always measure twice and cut once.

Carpenters' axiom

Everybody has a plan, 'til they get hit.

Mike Tyson

Classification, principles and blood supply

Definitions:

- Flappe (1522, Dutch): anything that hangs broad and loose fastened only on one side.
- Flap (1807, surgical): a portion of skin or flesh, separated from the underlying part, but remaining attached at the base.

Flaps are essentially a technique for closing an excised defect by mobilising adjacent tissue from the donor to the recipient site with the donor site base still attached in situ. They are used to close wounds that cannot be closed because of size or poor cosmetic or functional results from a simple closure. They are especially useful on the face, across joints and distal to the wrist and knee.

CLASSIFICATION

All of the flaps described in this text are classified as being **local random flaps**:

- local – using adjacent skin
- random – surviving via its own blood supply (subdermal plexus)
- movement (ART) – advancement, rotation, transposition
- design – individual name/description.

Mostly they are just referred to by their individual names: A-T, O-S, bilobed, rhomboid etc.

> **NOTE**
>
> Local random flaps use adjacent skin that has its own attached, usually subdermal, blood supply.

Other flaps (not covered in this text):

- **axial flap** – supplied by a known artery or group
- tissue type
  - **composite** (e.g. myocutaneous)
  - **innervated** (e.g. flap with nerve)
- **distant** donor site – noncontiguous sites.

Terminology

Elements of a flap:

- Recipient site or **primary defect**: the excised lesion site
- **Secondary defect** or donor site: where the flap is excised or harvested
- **Base of the flap**: that skin remaining attached and not excised (except in an A-T)
- **Pedicle**: the base and tongue of the flap where the blood supply enters
- **Tip**: that part of the flap furthest from the base

There is no standard terminology for flaps. What is described here as an A-T flap, some surgeons legitimately call a double Burow's triangle flap, a T-plasty, a bilateral advancement flap or something else. In the end most flaps are referred to by their design only, as in A-T, O-S, rotation, bilobed, rhomboid. These five would account for well over 90% of flaps performed.

SCAR SHAPES

The surgeon should know what the end result scar will look like before it is inflicted on a patient. Figure 8.2 shows the resultant scars from most skin surgery techniques. They are self-explanatory. However, good technique and hiding the incisions in skin lines can further disguise these scars. Note that the nose heals remarkably well and even trilobed flaps become almost invisible. In most instances operations can be done discreetly but unsightly grafts on the nose where a flap is possible or a rhomboid angular branding on a woman's cheek or a huge 'H' across a man's forehead when an A-T could have been done is difficult to reconcile or justify.

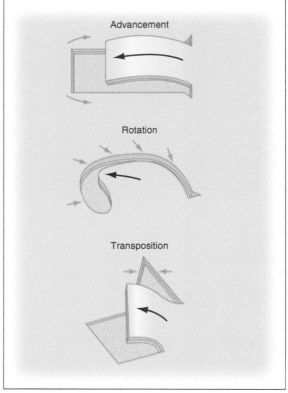

Figure 8.1 Types of flaps

PRINCIPLES

The aims or goals are:

- TOP:
  - **T**otal excision of the skin cancer – correct margins or slow Mohs (see box below)

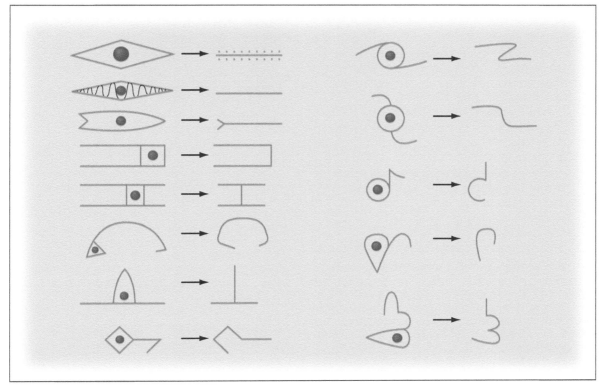

Figure 8.2 Incisions and resulting scar shapes

– **O**ptimal aesthetic outcome – cosmesis
– **P**reservation of function, maximising healing (good blood supply)

or

• Complete, discreet and beat:
  – Complete – **excise the whole cancer**
  – Discreet – use the most elegant and cosmetic flap design
  – Beat – ensure a good blood supply to make it 'beat' and be viable

Details of the procedure

1 First and foremost, excise the tumour completely with adequate margins. Plan the closure so as not to compromise this adequate excision.
2 Size and the depth of the wound: can the defect be closed or is there a good chance at least? BCCs, SCCs and non-infiltrating melanoma should be excised to include some fat. Invasive lesions should be taken down to the deep fascia.
3 Always have plans B and C if plan A cannot be done due to the size of the deficit.
4 If the defect obtained in excising the tumour cannot be closed, help is always at hand. The wound should be dressed and reconstruction reconsidered, delayed or the patient referred to another surgeon specialising in such repairs. Establish such a back-up with a colleague.
5 Sites:
    A Facial defects present particularly visible and potentially functionally detrimental reconstructions relative to wounds elsewhere.
    B Below the knee is a special problem with impaired healing.
    C The scalp when and where the skin is tight needs consideration.
6 Anatomy:
    A Dangerous areas are documented in Chapter 2, 'Essential anatomy for skin surgery'.
    B Unique anatomical structures and areas to avoid distortion:
        i defects approaching the eyelids, the nasal openings, the oral commissure and the external auditory meatus
        ii free margins such as the nostril, which need to be reconstructed to avoid distorting the anatomy unique to those areas.
7 Design: when designing flaps try and stay within the same cosmetic units to maximise tissue match

151

and minimise distortion. The ramus, preauricular and temporal areas have loose facial skin that makes flaps easier.

8   Consider the quality of the surrounding skin: young, tight and elastic or aged, dry and lax.

A   Wrinkled skin offers less obvious scarring and the opportunity to conceal scars.

B   Consider premalignant satellite lesions.

C   Pigmented or oily skin generally yields a less favourable scar.

9   Minimise tip or flap necrosis:

A   Ensure adequate length-to-base ratio to provide essential blood supply.

B   Use bipolar cautery.

C   Minimise handling and be gentle.

D   Minimise tension.

E   Use the smallest possible needle gauge/sutures.

Understanding where there is appropriate excess tissue to mobilise, the potential lines of tension, the blood supply and where the scar(s) can naturally be best hidden is essential in the planning and selection of what flap to use. Think of what closures are possible (frequently four present themselves – including side-by-side) and then choose the best.

Some flaps are contraindicated in certain areas, some result in very ugly scars, some ensure inbuilt safeguards as to blood supply and others depend on a ratio formula to minimise complications. This basic knowledge is explained in the sections below.

HINTS AND TIPS

- To help decide which flap, draw the surrounding subunits and assess loose tissue and movement.
- Close any donor site first. This reduces the tension on the actual flap and makes closure easier.

Guidelines

In Australia, the government guidelines for performing flaps are given in the Medicare Schedule of Fees and the PSR Report on the indications for flaps. Those from the *Medical Benefits Schedule*, Australian Government Department of Health and Ageing, 1 November 2007, Therapeutic Procedures Category 3, T8.97.1 p 237, are as follows:

FLAPS:
Needed to adapt scar position optimally with regard to
- skin creases or landmarks
- maintain contour of face or neck
- prevent distortion of adjacent structures or apertures

Only when required for adequate wound closure

And those from the *Report to the Professions 2005–06, Professional Services Review,* Commonwealth of Australia 2006, p 62, are:

FLAPS:
Flap procedures are typically indicated:
- where the defect is not closable primarily
- where there is a need to alter the tension vectors of closure
- to avoid crossing cosmetic boundaries
- to produce irregular scar lines which may settle better than a single line closure

The above recommendations are excellent guidelines. One referral doctor performs 65% of his operations by simple ellipse whereas an exclusive skin clinic doctor performs 11% of operations by flaps. It is also difficult to reconcile some of the amazing (flap) scars found on patients that have been executed by specialists and GPs alike. That said, a well-executed flap can be a wonderful advance with a fantastic result for a formerly difficult area where, invariably, an ugly graft used to be the usual procedure and result.

Fundamentals of flap survival

Flap survival depends on:

- Blood supply
- Perfusion pressure
- Tension
- Oedema
- Revascularisation/angiogenesis
- Inflammation
- Reperfusion injury
- Capillary obstruction
- Infection

Dzubow's principle states that: 'Any flap transposed or rotated around a pivot point will be tethered at the base of the pedicle' [1]. What this means practically is that, as the flap is rotated towards the defect, the distance from the pivot point effectively decreases. This can lead to a gap between the leading edge of the primary flap and the distal edge of the defect. To avoid this potential shortfall, make the primary flap longer.

Design flaps to avoid (minimise) tension on the pedicle, so as not to compromise the blood supply, with careful attention to the skin tension by using loose skin, undermining and mobilising the flap, and considering the elastic properties of the skin and the flap's pivot point.

Common mistakes

- Under-sizing
- Tension
- Incorrect length-to-width (pedicle) ratio
- Back cuts into flap pedicle
- Cutting into pedicle when repairing a dog-ear

BLOOD SUPPLY

Flap survival is based on blood supply [2–4]. It used to be thought that it was possible to double the length of a flap by doubling the width of its base. This proved to be incorrect [5], but the correct length-to-base ratio does ensure an adequate blood supply if the length is not too long. This ratio diminishes from 3:1 on the face, where there is good blood supply, progressively down the body to <1:1 below the knee.

Knowing at what level the various vessel plexi run and, hence, at what level to undermine to preserve and optimise this blood supply is essential. It was not until 1970 that it was demonstrated that flap survival is based, not on the length-to-base ratio, but rather on the blood supply that is incorporated into the flap [5]. An adequate length-to-base ratio is still needed, however, to provide this blood supply whose source was defined in 1973 as either the musculocutaneous or the direct cutaneous vessels. Many factors affect blood supply such as perfusion pressure and even outlet obstruction. In random flaps the blood supply is from the subdermal plexus, and every precaution and technique possible must be utilised to provide good perfusion both in and out of the tip to prevent necrosis. If necrosis occurs, it is usually at the tip.

Flap and graft necrosis

The incidence of flap and graft necrosis ranges from 1.9% to 10.4%.

Cutaneous vascular patterns

The cutaneous tissues and their vessels form flat layers of horizontal, interconnected vascular plexi running in three main and two minor levels supplying the fascia, subcutaneous tissue and skin (Figure 8.3). These plexi include the following:

1. The **fascial plexus** is the deepest at the deep muscle fascia and is fed by musculo- and septocutaneous vessels. These have no direct involvement for random flaps but are the main deep arteries of supply.

2. The **subcutaneous plexus** lies in the superfacial fascia or SMAS. The subcutaneous vessels exit at the superficial fascia and divide the subcutaneous fat into superficial and deep layers. It is formed by both musculocutaneous and septocutaneous arteries and, again, has little direct involvement for random flaps.

3. The **subdermal (or upper fat layer) plexus** is the main blood supply to the skin. It runs like a flat mat of interconnecting vessels in a plane at the junction of the reticular dermis and the subcutaneous fat or upper fat layer or, more practically, the superficial to mid-subcutaneous fat. The subdermal vessels account for the dermal bleeding seen at the leading edge of flaps. *This rich blood supply/plexus is the most important and, in practical terms, means that a layer of fat, which contains this nourishing plexus, has to be attached to*

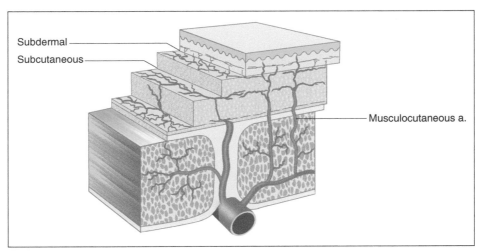

Figure 8.3 Cutaneous vascular plexus

The cutaneous vascular plexus forms a stacked series of interconnected vascular tissue planes that derive their blood supply from septocutaneous and musculocutaneous arteries. The fascial, subcutaneous and subdermal (cutaneous) layers are shown.

Adapted from Daniel RK, Kerrigan CI. Principles and physiology of skin flap surgery. In: McCarthy J, ed. Plastic Surgery, Vol 1. Philadelphia: WB Saunders, 1990; Fig 9.2.

Labels in figure: Subdermal, Subcutaneous, Musculocutaneous a.

153

the dermis and hence epidermis of any raised flap so as to provide and continue its essential blood supply and nutrients. Undermining too superficially, as in the dermis, runs the considerable risk of cutting off this blood supply with subsequent necrosis of the flap. The **subdermal plexus** consists of both arterioles and capillaries with enough perfusion pressure to nourish a random flap and the wad of fat containing it is all important, in fact critical, to the survival of the flap.

4 The **dermal plexus** provides thermoregulation. The intradermal plexus itself is not sufficient to support tissue viability (i.e. do not undermine in the dermis).

5 **Subepidermal plexus capillary bed** supplies nutrients to the skin. The subepidermal vessels are located at the papillary ridge.

Microcirculation of arteriovenous anastomoses or shunts between the arterial and venous systems within flaps allows communication between the arterial and venous systems.

Perfusion pressure/blood flow in flaps

Perfusion is the process of delivery of blood to a capillary bed. Whereas the length-to-base ratio of a flap is important to ensure an adequate number of vessels, sufficient perfusion pressure is also required. Until recently, it was thought that, for longer flaps, bases needed to be wider to provide more feeder vessels. However, rather than the number of blood vessels, survival is directly dependent on the perfusion pressure. Furthermore, all the vessels in any one flap have the same perfusion pressure, which is not altered by including more vessels. Adequate perfusion pressure is needed to maintain patency of the capillaries [3–7]. The perfusion pressure decreases with distance and, hence, flap length is critical. If the flap tip is not perfused and does not get nutrients, necrosis follows [4, 8]. The distal or tip perfusion pressure drops immediately the flap is raised [7, 9].

Perfusion pressures of random flaps vary with body location [4, 5, 10–15]. The blood flow through the facial skin is ten times higher than needed for basic metabolic needs [16–19]. This generosity diminishes towards the lower limbs, which is the reason why the length-to-base ratio of flaps has to alter from 3:1 on the face [20–22] to 2:1 on the trunk and thighs [14, 20, 21, 23, 24] and even less below the knee. In random pattern flaps, venous outflow is also impaired in the subdermal plexus, which can be more injurious to flap survival than a poor arterial supply.

Sufficient blood flow through the base of the flap is essential during the first 48 hours. There is a graded response with flow improving within 14–16 hours to the flap closest to the base, then within 24–48 hours to the

first 1 cm of flap skin and to 3 cm within 96 hours (4 days), with a gradient to day 14 [7]. Microvascular flow peaks at greater than preoperative levels between days 14 and 21 with opening of collaterals [7]. The trauma causes the release of catecholamines, noradrenaline and other humoral factors such as prostaglandins, which may help [18, 25, 26]. Adhesion molecules recruit neutrophils to the flap to clear metabolic debris and, finally, endothelial progenitor cells allow the ingrowth of new vascular channels to supply the flap [27].

Undermining

It is necessary to undermine flaps so as to mobilise them to be repositioned. In doing so it is essential the subdermal plexus of blood vessels is not compromised. The skin, especially on the head and neck, varies and knowledge of this aids successful surgery. Undermining 2–4 cm [28] or 50–100% [29] of the defect diameter is recommended to decrease wound tension and minimise compromising blood supply.

Flap tension

Wound tension is arguably one of the most critical determinants of poor flap results. Pre-planning and extensive undermining are the best ways to provide a wound with minimal tension. No tension is unavoidable but minimal 'controlled' tension, lack of twisting and distortion are essential. Closure tension results in wound edge necrosis and dehiscence; however, it seldom results in necrosis of the entire flap [30–32].

Tension vectors (TV)

These are the resultant sum of all tension forces. Every closure, from an ellipse to a flap to a graft to a second intention healing contraction, has a resultant TV (Figure 8.4). Understanding the TV allows better planning to reduce excess tension with its inherent complications.

The practical importance is to undermine where there is tension and so reduce it. Pull the flap and feel or even see where it is tethered and tensioned and undermine there.

Summary: Retaining flap blood supply

- Flaps need a good blood supply to survive.
- A poor or compromised blood supply is the greatest cause of flap necrosis and failure.
- Poor undermining, excess wound tension and an incorrect length-to-base ratio are the greatest causes of failure.
- Knowing at what level and in what tissue plane the feeding blood vessels run is essential. Random flaps are supplied by the subdermal (upper fat) plexus, which is in the mid- to superficial subcutaneous fat. Undermining must preserve this plexus for the flap to survive by including a layer of fat in which the blood vessels run.
- Undermining 50–100% of the defect width [29] or to 2–4 cm [28] beyond the wound edge has been recommended to decrease the wound tension, but this is a guide only.
- Do not undermine superficially. Undermine in the mid-fat layer. Always leave a wad of fat attached to the skin flap.
- It is imperative there is a wide enough base to provide sufficient blood vessels to the tip of the flap.
- The recommended length-to-base ratio to provide a good blood supply and sufficient perfusion pressure decreases from the face (3:1) to the body (1:1) to below the knee (<1:1). A ratio of 3:1 starts to compromise and risk the blood supply.
- Do not risk it! Always provide a good base.

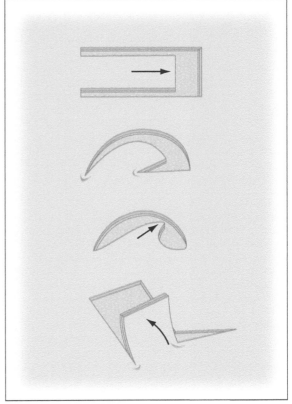

Figure 8.4 The arrows show the resultant tension vectors (TV)

For rhomboid flaps (bottom drawing) the TV is the furthest margin away from the horizontal. When the flap is raised to move across to the recipient site, this now becomes obvious and further undermining can lessen this tension and facilitate flap movement. Knowing the TV and the final scar also allows best placement of incisions.

Other factors affecting flap survival

Oedema

Oedema can increase the pressure on the capillaries, reducing the blood flow [33]. Rat studies showed that oedema alone will not cause flap necrosis [34], but it is a compounding and additive complication.

Revascularisation/angiogenesis

Within 2 days a fibrin layer forms between the flap and the recipient base [35], and angiogenesis, revascularisation and neovascularisation begin by day 3 or 4 [27, 36–40]. Endothelial cells move out, followed by capillary sprouts that form loops and then new blood vessels. Although it occurs earlier in animal models [36, 41, 42], revascularisation in humans allowing division from the pedicle has been demonstrated by day 7 [36, 43, 44].

Inflammation

Surgery causes tissue injury, ischaemia and an inflammatory cascade with the release of histamine, prostaglandins, kinins and serotonin with increased capillary permeability and oedema. Thromboxane A_2, a potent vasoconstrictor, is released [45, 46] as are free radicals that cause direct tissue injury [35, 47]. However, the hypoxaemia and cascade products also induce pre-capillary sphincter relaxation with consequent increased blood flow [18, 26, 48].

Reperfusion injury

As the flap reperfuses this seems to cause the release of free radicals from neutrophils and further cellular injury with lactic acid build-up.

Capillary obstruction

This 'no-flow' phenomenon develops when flaps are kept in an avascular state that exceeds their critical ischaemia time. Erythrocytes sludge, leukocytes adhere, oedema causes pressure and the microcirculation is obstructed permanently.

Infection

Infection causes partial or total flap necrosis and, although most infective agents are from the patients themselves, it is devastating to both the patient and the surgeon to have a great job slough because of infection. Infection releases toxic free radicals and increases oedema [49]. There is local tissue destruction and vascular compromise. Collagen production and deposition decrease [50]. Thrombosis of vessels can occur [51]. The end result is lack of adhesion, breakdown and sloughing.

Smoking

Cigarette smoking has a deleterious effect on the survival of reconstructive flaps and grafts. Smoking results in vasoconstriction, increased blood viscosity, hypoxia and increased platelet aggregation, which promotes microvascular thrombosis. Patients who smoke more than 1 pack of cigarettes per day have 3 times the risk of necrosis of flaps and full-thickness grafts when compared with persons who have never smoked, low level smokers (<1 pack/day) and ex-smokers. When necrosis does occur, the median area involved tends to be greater in smokers (approximately 3-fold) than in patients who never smoked. Many of the adverse effects of cigarette smoking on the microvasculature are reversible; benefits in flap and graft survival may be realised by stopping (or decreasing) smoking for at least 2 days before surgery and for 1 week after surgery. Treatment with parenteral pentoxifylline and topical nitroglycerin has been shown to improve skin flap survival in animal models [52–54].

Elsewhere it has been noted that smoking does not affect healing. Any practitioner who has seen the coronary artery spasm induced by smoking or who has seen smokers with peripheral vascular disease must, however, feel that smoking would certainly compromise the microvascular blood flow in a flap or graft. Perhaps for normal straight line wounds/simple ellipses smoking is not that important.

Conclusions

Most of these problems can be avoided by correct undermining, careful selection of the correct flap and its design to minimise tension, handling the tissues gently and attention to a sterile technique. Asking the patient to cease smoking 2 weeks prior helps.

 NOTE

Certain flaps by their very design ensure a good length-to-base ratio or an adequate blood supply. The rhomboid flap ensures a ratio of 1 : 1 or less.

The A-T and O-Z flaps also provide generous adequate bases, whereas island flaps are fraught with potential problems.

TISSUE BANK: HARVEST AREAS

Flaps depend on the Robin Hood principle: 'rob from the rich to give to the poor' (i.e. take from loose skin to fill the defect). It is essential to find some mobile, loose skin that can be transferred to the excision site without tension (Figure 8.5). Do this during planning, with a plan B if plan A fails.

The lower leg and the scalp are notoriously donor tissue poor with tight skin and little to spare.

Plan B may well entail leaving some of the defect open to heal by secondary intention, which is often forgotten but usually gives excellent results. Warn the patient that there may not be enough skin to fully close the hole but that it will heal over a matter of weeks.

MONITORING OF SKIN FLAPS AND FOLLOW-UP

After successful flap design and implementation, monitor the flap for viability, as early recognition of ischaemia is important in preventing subsequent flap necrosis and failure. Clinical observation is the best method to assess a flap. An extremely pale flap may signify arterial insufficiency, whereas a blue flap may be secondary to a failure of venous outflow. Two additional tests often used to assess viability are capillary refill and warmth. Assessment of bleeding from the flap after stabbing it with a small needle is believed to be one of the most reliable methods of clinical assessment. Surface temperature monitoring is another dependable technique. Sophisticated hospital techniques include pH monitoring and trans-cutaneous PO_2, doppler and laser doppler, fluorescein dye and illumination with a Wood lamp.

Optimal appearance begins at 3–6 months. Scars can continue to improve. Alternatively, some scars thin and stretch and can look worse.

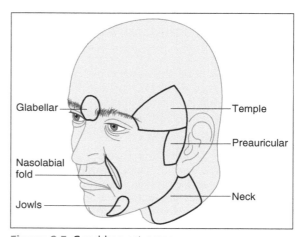

Figure 8.5 Good harvest areas
Adapted from Chatrath V. Transposition flaps. eMedicine. Picture 2, Reservoirs of extra skin. Available at: emedicine. medscape.com (accessed 1 Feb 2007).

Advancement flaps

An advancement flap moves skin directly forwards with no lateral movement. The lesion is excised, then two incisions are made usually parallel on either side of the defect to form a corridor or pedicle of tissue. These incisions and undermining of this pedicle release the flap from all tension except where it remains tethered to the base, distal to the defect.

It is initially a difficult concept, which amounts to pushing or advancing a shorter pedicle into a corridor that is longer due to the excision of the lesion and questions arise. What happens to the skin at the side? Doesn't it bunch and crinkle up?

Advancement depends on the elasticity and laxity of both pedicle and surrounding tissue, the latter undermined if and as necessary. The pedicle itself is undermined, leaving a layer of fat to ensure the subdermal plexus of blood supply. The leading free edge is advanced and secured to the far end of the defect, and the edges are sutured to equate out the uneven lengths of the pedicle and the sides. With lax tissue this 'takes up' and no bunching actually occurs. Earlier techniques created Burow's triangles at the base end to shorten the sides of the defect to the length of the pedicle, but these have been found in practice not to be needed as the pedicle stretches and the sides take up. However, Burow's triangles may still be added for larger flaps. Tension is focused on the relatively narrow pedicle and there has to be a decent width of base to ensure a good blood supply. The following maximum length-to-base ratios are recommended:

- forehead/scalp = 3 : 1
- face = 2 : 1
- neck = 1.5 : 1
- hips = 1 : 1
- below knee = <1 : 1.

Adequate tissue laxity and mobility are required to move an advancement flap in the desired direction. This is best assessed by the finger pinch test (i.e. trying to approximate the planned wound edges pinched between the thumb and the finger). Advancement flaps are not good where there is too much tension. They are used mainly on the forehead and then, to allow more mobility and less tension, as double advancement flaps, from either side of the defect, with the end result looking like a horizontal 'H'. The raised flap is moved in a linear progression to fill the defect. The skin is moved in the direction of closure parallel to the incision(s). These flaps are arguably the simplest design, but they have limited coverage potential and limited utility.

A variation is the V-Y island flap, which is a combination of an advancement flap and an island flap. In this case, the pedicle is *not* undermined as the base is cut (forming the island) and the only blood supply then comes up from perforators to the subdermal plexus of the island. The island is then advanced. Island flaps per se are not used much any more except as this V-Y variation and then mostly for mid-helical ear excisions and mucosal lip lesions.

SINGLE ADVANCEMENT FLAP

Mastering this basic flap is fundamental to progressing to the more complex flaps.

These flaps are mostly used on the forehead as they do not lead to eyebrow elevation but, from the author's point of view, an A-T flap can do the same job with fewer scars. They require a wide length-to-base ratio.

Technique

1   Mark the tumour and draw a square around it at the appropriate margins (Figure 8.6).
2   Extend long arms from the appropriate sides. On the forehead it is often possible, and preferable, to place and thus hide these in the corrugator grooves.
3   Advancement flaps derive blood supply from subdermal vessels and a thin layer of fat is mandatory. The thickness of the flap should match the depth of the excision. Make longer flaps thicker, especially at their base, so as to include larger subcutaneous vessels that can nourish the distal tip of the flap. Ensure the length-to-width ratio does not exceed 3 : 1 to avoid tip necrosis. Twin or bi-pedical flaps survive better than a single pedicle.
4   Undermine widely the flap skin as well as the surrounding skin, ensuring a good wad of fat is left attached to the skin of the now raised flap.
5   'Advance' the raised flap into the tumour defect. The wider the surrounding skin undermining, the less corrugating and puckering as the flap is advanced, but Burow's triangles may still be needed to untether and help the flap advance.

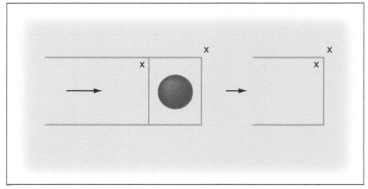

Figure 8.6 Single advancement flap (arrow on the left indicates direction of tissue movement)

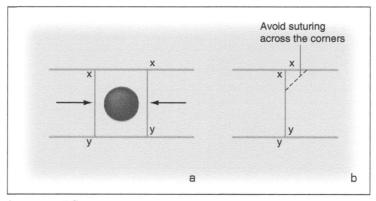

Figure 8.7 Double advancement flap
a Mark-up and flap movement. **b** 'x' moves to 'x' (and 'y' to 'y'). The flaps are then sutured together, but avoid suturing across the corners as in undermining.

6 Accommodate puckering and corrugating by suturing the sides by the rule of halves, thereby equally distributing the tension and allowing the side and flap skin to stretch and accommodate.

DOUBLE ADVANCEMENT FLAP OR H-PLASTY

For this type of flap, the lesion and the arms of the 'H' are marked and incised and the flaps are advanced, necessitating considerable undermining (Figure 8.7).

A major problem is that four Burow's triangles may need to be excised to eliminate dog-ears (Figure 8.8). These can often be avoided by suturing the sides by the law of halves and skin stretch, but this is not always possible or predictable.

Note the flap corners have not been sutured. If this leaves a gap or a 'gate', a Gilles or corner stitch can be used without cutting off the blood supply. The corner or Gilles suture goes from the surface of the side to exit in the dermis, enter the dermis of flap 1 then across in the dermis of the other leading edge of flap 2, across to enter the dermis of the side then up to the surface next to the original entry point.

A curvilinear lateral flap incision obviates these dog-ears but also reduces the tissue movement granted by the Burow's triangles (Figure 8.9). Excessive stretching, tension and resultant thinning of the flap are to be avoided.

Figures 8.10 and 8.11 show rather obvious double advancement flap scars.

The double advancement flap is mostly used on the forehead as it moves the skin across the forehead and thus does not incur brow lift.

Technique

1 Mark the lesion and margins with a square or rectangle.
2 Make the long horizontal incisions to their extremities, preferably in obvious skin creases. Long

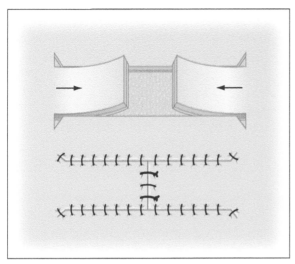

Figure 8.8 Double advancement flap with four Burow's triangles (arrows indicate the direction of tissue movement)

In practice Burow's triangles are now not used much.

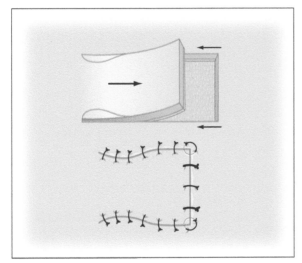

Figure 8.9 Curvilinear lateral flap incision to avoid standing cone formation (arrows indicate the direction of tissue movement)

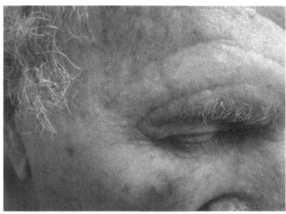

Figure 8.10 H-plasty scar

The procedure was performed so many years prior the patient couldn't remember what for or when, but he still bitterly resented the rather obvious scar. It is difficult to conceive why an A-T flap could not have been done with better cosmetic results.

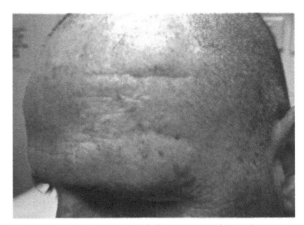

Figure 8.11 The central dehiscence and scarring was even more obvious in vivo

An A-T would do as well, if not better, as there are only two scar lines and not, as here, three. The vertical incision, however, would have to be generous but no more so than these horizontal ones.

incisions need not be straight but can curve and follow skin furrows and creases.

3 Excise the lesion (with a locator suture before being detached) by making the two vertical incisions.
4 Minimal haemostasis to bed.
5 Undermine the flaps between the horizontal incisions, working towards and meeting in the centre.
6 Suture placement is important.

BUROW'S TRIANGLE FLAPS

Burow's triangle

Burow's triangles are used to shorten the skin on one side of an excision to aid in closure or cosmesis and in rotation flaps (Figure 8.12). Extensive undermining is needed and a length-to-width ratio of 4:1.

A Burow's flap is a good choice when one arm can be hidden, such as preauricular lesions where the Burow's triangle is excised under the lobe. It has also been used

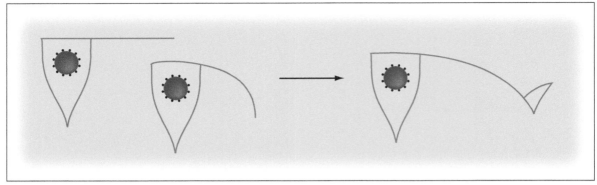

Figure 8.12 A Burow's triangle flap can be straight (advancement) or curved (when it may well be termed a rotation flap)

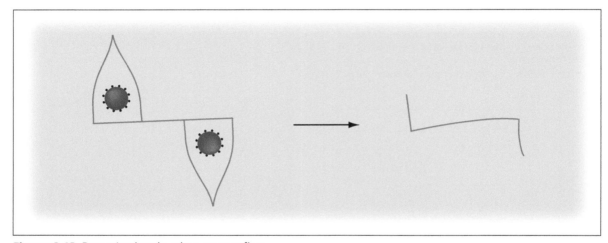

Figure 8.13 Burow's triangle advancement flap

for lesions on the nasal lateral supratip (but only for small lesions), on the infraorbital area as it does not cause tension on the lower lid and, finally, on the temple and forehead with the Burow's triangle hidden in the hair line.

Technique
1 Excise the lesion as a triangle.
2 Place an equal Burow's triangle at the other end of the incision line on the opposite side, the length of which is determined by tissue movement and cosmesis. They may well be next to each other.
   Large dog-ears/standing cones can result.

Burow's triangle advancement flap (AA or O-Z flap)

Here the confusion of terms and mixed movement may result in classification as either a double A-T flap using a common base or rotational flaps. The type illustrated in Figure 8.13 has been described as two rotation flaps

away from each other, contralateral, with each providing a Burow's triangle for the other.

Another way to think of these is as alternating, contralateral A-T flaps. This technique allows at least three lesions to be so excised (Figure 8.14).

This type is of most use where the 'T' or the horizontal arm can be drawn to provide a common base between a number of lesions.

A-T FLAP (BILATERAL T-PLASTY)

Cadaver studies indicated that the ideal A-T flap (Figure 8.15) is designed to be twice the height of the original defect, with base extensions one defect diameter in each direction, and undermined to three times the diameter of the defect [55].

The A-T flap is arguably the most versatile and useful of all flaps. As well as being applicable over most of the body, it also has the distinct advantages of excellent perfusion, few complications and good cosmesis.

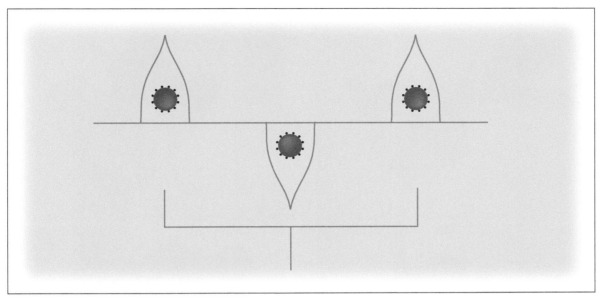

Figure 8.14 Excision of three lesions via alternating, contralateral A-T flaps

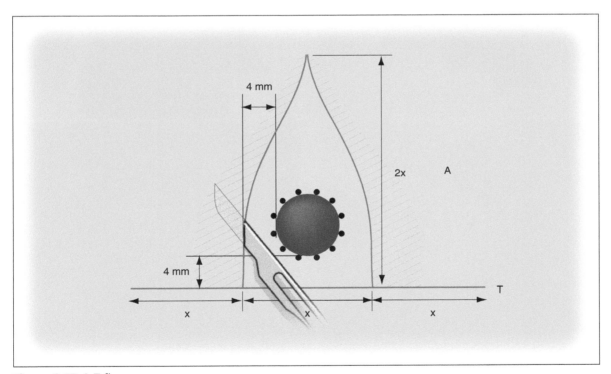

Figure 8.15 A-T flap

It is shaped more like a pear than an 'A'. It can be elongated at both ends to facilitate greater movement with less tension and can be curved onto the 'T' base to varying degrees. The cadaver-recommended undermining would seem excessive based on in vivo experience.

Its greatest use is on the forehead where the horizontal T ensures there is no eyebrow lift.

The procedure is illustrated in Figures 8.16, 8.17 and 8.18. The Reader is also referred to Figures 6.14 to 6.17 inclusive, for greater detail.

161

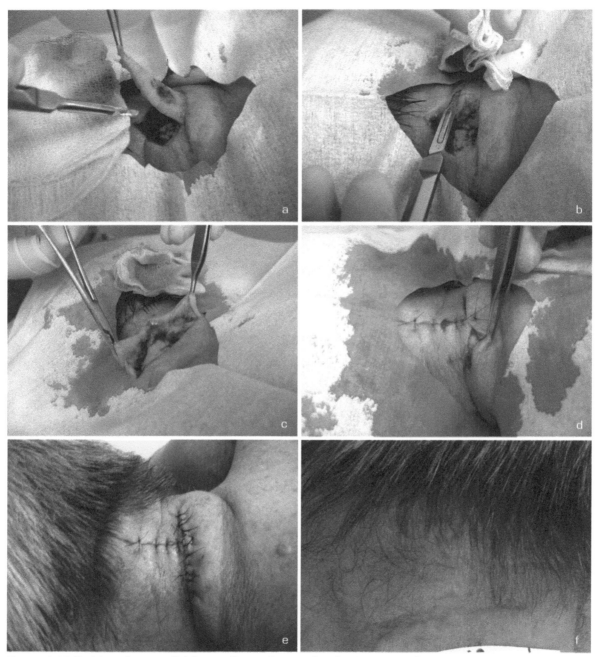

Figure 8.16 Excision of a superficial spreading melanoma (SSM) using an A-T flap

a Mark out the lesion and margins, in this case an SSM not invading through the basement membrane, thus necessitating 5-mm margins. Try and find a skin crease for the base incision and draw it. This is the horizontal arm of the 'T'. Then draw the 'A' to end on it (but curve it like the hull of a ship or a pear). The T can be as long as you like but a good rule is to make each arm the same width as the base of the excision and no shorter. Excise the lesion. **b** Undermine the side flaps and mobilise. Here, sharp scalpel undermining is done in the mid-fat plane. This is a significant defect to have to close. **c** Pull the flaps together. If there is a problem, undermine further and extend the vertical incision. Undermine under visual control, freeing the adhesions or where the skin is tacked down. The length of this vertical incision and the undermining should be such as to minimise wound tension. **d** Suture the vertical wound first. Where the vertical incision meets the base, a corner stitch is usually employed but with good apposition may not be necessary. **e** The finished operation with the base hidden in a horizontal neck crease. Although a vertical simple ellipse may have been attempted, the central defect would have been difficult to close with the distinct possibility of dehiscence. Allowing the hair to grow longer will hide the scar – impossible with a long ellipse. **f** Removal of sutures. The inflammation will subside and the scars fade.

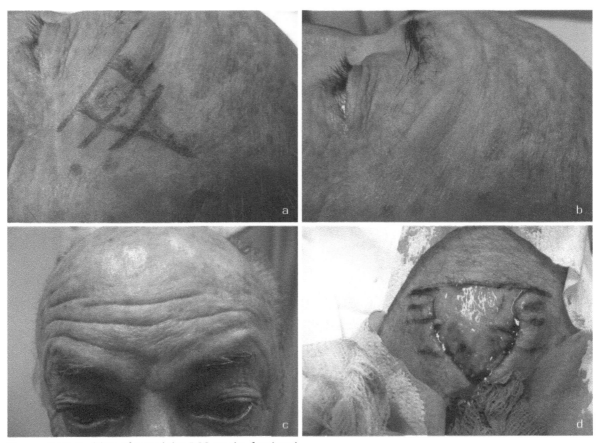

Figure 8.17 Excision of a nodular BCC on the forehead

a A-T map with marker lines for incisions in skin creases. **b** 6 weeks later. For the best cosmesis subcuticular sutures can be performed, but with 6/0 inert sutures, sharp needles and minimal tissue handling excellent results can be obtained with just interrupted sutures. **c** No deformities, no complications, excellent cosmesis. Certainly better than the double advancement flap. **d** Match-up lines are of great help when the wound spreads apart. Why not use every trick and aid to get the best result and minimise problems?

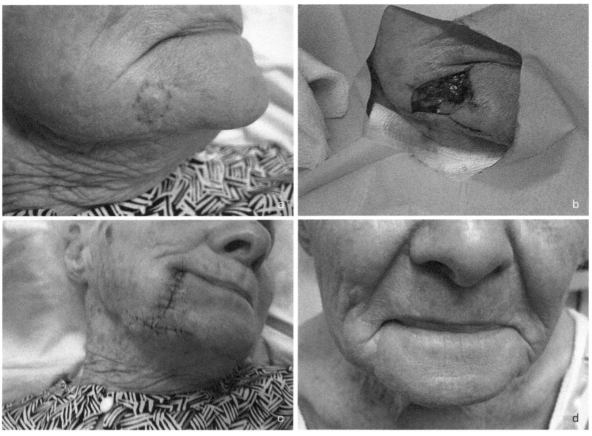

Figure 8.18 Excision of a micronodular/invasive BCC

a This micronodular/invasive BCC necessitated 6-mm margins. **b** The versatility of the A-T flap is that it allows such wide margins. **c** A rather extensive operation for an elderly lady but done under local anaesthetic without the inherent dangers of a general anaesthetic with no worries as to tip necrosis or an ugly scar. **d** 4 months later it is difficult to see which side was involved.

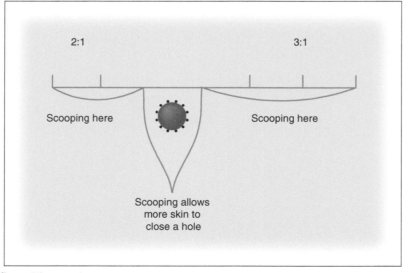

Figure 8.19 A-T flap with scooping

L-Plasty, hatchet or 7 flap

The 7 flap is really an A-T flap done on one side (Figure 8.20). Although the hatchet flap is classed here as an advancement flap it may equally well be regarded and classified as just an extension/modification of the rotation flap but with a mirror cut at the opposite end plus undermining allowing greater tissue movement. Do not make the reverse cut too acute or this developed Burow's triangle will be too hard to close.

High preauricular lesions lend themselves to the hatchet flap, especially when the horizontal incision can be hidden in the hairline (Figure 8.21).

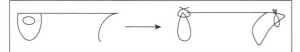

Figure 8.20 Hatchet or 7 flap

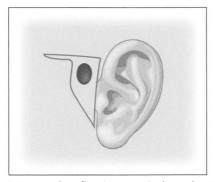

Figure 8.21 Hatchet flap is extensively undermined and the preauricular sutures and scar seldom seen

Mercedes flap

This is a handy flap when there is a circular defect (that can be quite large) where closure will create dog-ears or unwanted TV (Figure 8.22). It is also used to reduce the bald spot in male crown baldness. It is, of course, named after the car logo seen when three A-T flaps are created from the defect circumference.

A purse string suture connecting the base ends provides an elegant closure.

M FLAP

Best described as an attenuated ellipse or where an ellipse has to be shortened and compromised by a vital structure such as an eye, the lip or an ear lobe. The (vital) end of the ellipse is cut back towards the centre of the ellipse, thus allowing a wedge of the vital structure to intrude. This end of the ellipse then forms an 'M' (Figure 8.23).

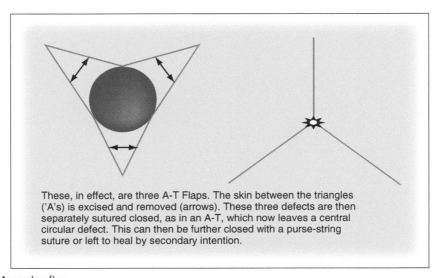

These, in effect, are three A-T Flaps. The skin between the triangles ('A's) is excised and removed (arrows). These three defects are then separately sutured closed, as in an A-T, which now leaves a central circular defect. This can then be further closed with a purse-string suture or left to heal by secondary intention.

Figure 8.22 Mercedes flap
Adapted from Salasche S, Orengo IF, Siegle RJ, Dermatologic Surgery Tips and Techniques. Philadelphia: Mosby, 2007.

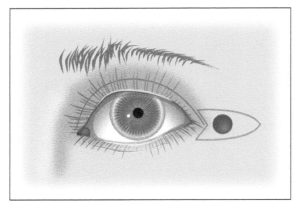

Figure 8.23 M flap

It has also been used for cancers of the central upper lip where the 'V' of the M prevents the columella from intruding and the arms of the M go somewhere towards recreating the philtral ridges.

V-Y ISLAND FLAP

Island flaps transposition an island of skin that is raised on its blood supply. The skin island is moved into the defect, and the donor site is closed primarily. This can involve tunnelling the flap under adjacent skin on its vascular pedicle, when it is called an interpolation flap.

Island flaps

Island flaps per se are not described here as they are not used much because of multiple problems. The V-Y island flap, however, has uses on the ear and the lateral upper lip. In selected other areas, such as the lateral malar prominences or inferior nasal sidewall above the superior alar groove, it is more easily camouflaged as it is smaller than a standard advancement flap.

Island flaps have no base and obtain blood from the fat or perforators in and under the island. Hence they are more precarious and vulnerable. Island and advancement flaps depend on there being lax surrounding tissue that can be undermined to allow the flap or island to be moved forwards. Island pedicle flaps are not only pulled but pushed into place.

Technique

1 Excise the tumour.
2 Cut one or two triangles using the tumour excision as the triangle base.
3 Undermine the skin *outside* the 'V' island (not under the island). Undermining *the surrounding skin* (and not the island itself which needs its blood supply) allows the island to then be moved with its underlying fat still attached to the deeper structures.

In the classic island flap, two such islands can then be butted to meet.

V-Y plasty

In a V-Y plasty, the skin flap is not elevated; it remains attached to the underlying subcutaneous tissues from which it derives its essential blood supply. This flap lends itself to disguising the scar in natural crease lines.

Technique

* A: Cut the lesion out as a square or rectangle (**A** in Figure 8.24), which forms the base of the triangular or V-shaped flap (**B** in Figure 8.24).
* B:
  1 Using its margin as the leading edge, cut a 'triangle' (see Figure 8.25). Make this billow out at the sides to enlarge the flap so as to provide as much blood supply as possible. On the ear this usually extends to the ear-mastoid junction; on the upper lip it extends at least to an equilateral

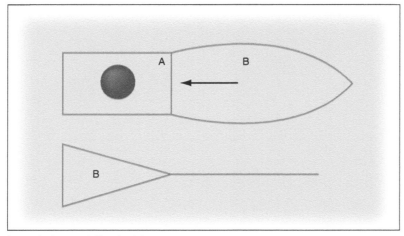

Figure 8.24 V-Y plasty: lesion and flap incisions

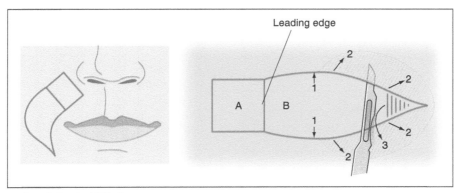

Figure 8.25 Undermining in V-Y plasty

triangle and goes below the lower part of the lip. On the upper lip do not cross the philtrum.

2 Elevate the skin surrounding (outside) the flap, *not* the flap itself as this is where it gets all its blood supply. Undermine the outsides as widely as possible. This undermining allows the lateral edge skin to move back (rather than the island moving forwards).

Do not undermine the triangle/island except the tail to untether it (hatched area in Figure 8.25). *Do not undermine the leading edge.*

3 Try to end with an island on a mobile fat pad. The connection and preservation of this fat pad maintains the all-important blood supply.

4 Advance the V-shaped flap into the wound. If the island is not moving, undermine outside *not* inside.

5 Close the donor site primarily, yielding a Y-shaped closure.

Alternative ways to elevate a V-Y flap include central undermining and lateral pedicles or partially undermining the central attachment while ensuring a good pedicle is left to supply flap blood.

correcting the whistle deformity of the lip, but can be applicable to many defects elsewhere on the skin.

Technique
1 Although the standard advice is not to undermine the leading edge, on the helix this is undermined, leaving a wad of fat to fold over the helical rim. If possible, make this the same dimensions as the excised defect. But ensure a good island remains as this is now the only blood supply.

2 On the mid-helix advance the island from postauricular to over and under the internal helix.

3 Suture this advanced, now internal helical edge and secure in place. The 'trick' is to use a horizontal mattress suture from the posterior corner of the tumour excision but go 2 mm down the island, to exit and again come up 2 mm on the ear. This provides a helical 'roll' by pulling the island up.

The ear will now look quite distorted. Do not panic. Cartilage and tissue have great memory and the ear will look great at ROS. Initially, there may be some tightness and pull on the ear but this soon stretches.

> ⚠️ **WARNING** ⚠️
>
> The island pedicle/V-Y flap is not undermined. Only the surrounding tissue is undermined.

> ⚠️ **WARNING** ⚠️
>
> Do not cross sutures at the two free edge corners. This is a common mistake by even the experienced (e.g. a suture from the superior helix to secure the flap crosses or is crossed by the suture at 90°, securing the flap anteriorly). This cuts off the blood supply to the corner(s) and tip necrosis is inevitable.
>
> Using only a horizontal mattress suture avoids this possibility as well as providing a better cosmetic result.

V-Y flap for helical repair
The V-Y flap is not used much any more but is good for helical repairs from post auricular over the helix. It is also well suited to elongating the nasal columella and

Rotation or pivotal flaps

Rotation flaps are semicircular flaps that 'rotate' tissue around a pivot point to form the flap into an adjacent triangular defect from which the lesion has been excised. As it pivots the flap draws skin at right angles to the incision. Extensive undermining is required to reduce skin tension. Most rotation flaps constitute a quarter of a circle with the defect an isosceles triangle at one end.

After the flap is rotated into the defect, the donor site is closed primarily, yielding an arcuate scar. Rotation flaps require a great degree of planning, and little gain is realised relative to the size of the flap. In some cases, the donor site cannot be primarily closed and may require a skin graft. However, depending on the location of the defect to be repaired, rotation flaps may be preferable to transposition or advancement flaps.

TENSION

Considerable tension may be present in rotation flaps, which needs to be anticipated, recognised and dealt with by identifying the pivot point and tension lines and then undermining extensively as excessive tension may result in ischaemia and subsequent necrosis of the flap. Although the line of maximal tension is theoretically directly opposite the pivot point, practically the tension is seen by folds at the base around the pivot area and when pulling the flap so as to close. Keep undermining in these areas until the flap closes without tension.

SITES

- Lateral face
- Large medial cheek lesions [56]
- Scalp
- Temple
- Nose (selected cases)

Rotation flaps have, to a large extent, been replaced by better designs. Perhaps their greatest use is now for large lesions on the medial cheek but they also remain the fallback procedure for difficult wounds.

PROS

- No blood supply problem (good length-to-base ratio) – the wide base provides an excellent blood supply.

- Blood supply is more from dermal vessels than subdermal. Haematomas are a more common complication and meticulous haemostasis is necessary and pressure dressings used.
- A narrow base (<3 cm) results in a higher risk of flap necrosis.
- Heal well.
- Can be incised along RSTL and cosmetic borders.

CONS

- Extensive undermining needed.
- Large scar for size of lesion.
- Tissue wasteful.

PLAN

Ensure the ratio of the length of the flap to the defect is greater than 4 : 1.

PIVOT POINT

Both rotation and transposition flaps have a fixed point at one side of their base around which the flap pivots. For rotation flaps it is at the furthest point from the defect. For transposition flaps it is at the opposite side of the base from the direction the flap moves. Tightness at the pivot point compromises the blood supply and flap necrosis. This is best avoided by ensuring that the length of the flap from the pivot point to the tip of the flap is the same as from the pivot point to the furthest side of the defect by measuring both while drawing the operation design.

UNDERMINING

The larger the flap, the greater the undermining needed. Extensive undermining is the 'secret' key to easier rotation flap surgery.

S-PLASTY

Refer to Chapter 5, 'The basics'.

CLASSIC OR CONVENTIONAL ROTATION FLAP

A problem with rotation flaps is that the excised flap falls short of the far margins as it is rotated (i.e. there will be a defect created along the superior margin). Dzubow recommended, therefore, that the actual height of the flap be greater than the defect height [1]. To minimise the tension short-fall, the arc of the flap can be made oversized and offset to extend more than the defect [1, 57]. This effectively minimises tip tension.

Technique

1 Mark the lesion with appropriate margins as an isosceles triangle using available cosmetic or wrinkle lines, usually at the lateral edge of this triangle (see Figure 8.26). The triangle may be visualised as part of a half semicircle and its size as well as the laxity of the donor skin dictates the size of the semicircle, which can always be enlarged if need be.
2 As a working rule, the base of the flap is three to four times the side of the triangle. Draw an arc with a high tangent to curve onto the base.
3 Excise the lesion/triangle.
4 Incise the arc from the distal tip of the isosceles triangle to define the flap.
5 Back cut but limit as this cuts off the flap blood supply.
6 Undermine extensively in the fat layer, ensuring the flap has fat attached that contains its blood supply, and raise the flap [29].
7 Rotate the flap towards the triangular defect.
8 Place the first suture at the point of maximum rotation.
9 Place the second suture at the bottom of the defect.
10 Trim.

There is always some tension in bringing the tip of the flap to the distal extent of the excision. Undermining should help this but, if the flap tip doesn't reach the defect distal point, there is then a rim of defect between the flap and the circular excision line. If there is a shortfall and the surrounding skin is lax the defect may well be able to be closed. If, however, it is immobile, the tip must be pulled to the distal point creating tension that may not be acceptable.

As distinct from the area of maximal tension, the area of maximum restraint is at the pivot point and undermining here optimises flap mobility. Sometimes, a small back cut can be made from the apex of the triangle along the base to increase mobility (especially useful on the scalp) [58] but cutting across the incision line beyond 90° incurs backwards tension.

Medial cheek

This rotation flap is good for large lesions >1 cm or 2-cm deficit holes of the medial cheek (Figure 8.27). A 7 flap can be used for lesions <1 cm.

The downside is that this is a very large flap proportional to the size of the lesion. The resulting scar is large and permanent.

Technique

1 Excise the lesion.
2 Incise a standing cone running parallel to or in the nasolabial fold. This, in effect, makes an isosceles triangle defect.
3 Make the superior margin of the excision continuous with the medial edge of this cone and

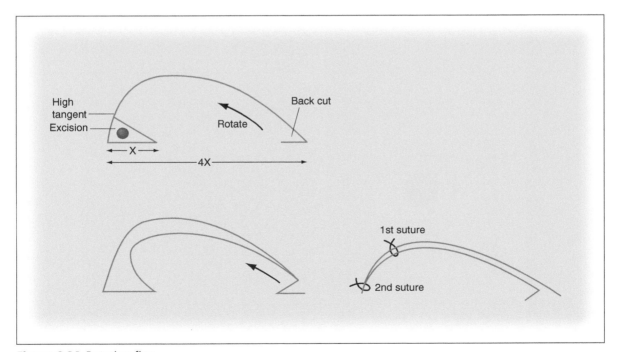

Figure 8.26 Rotation flap

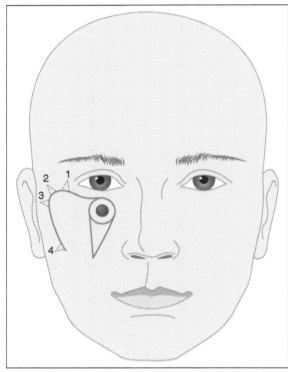

Figure 8.27 Rotation flap on the medial cheek

sweep under the eye, following the contour of the orbit, then down the lateral cheek.

4 Burow's triangle(s) can be positioned anywhere along this lateral incision to facilitate greater rotation/lengthening, but probably the best place is beside the eye to hide in the crow's feet.

5 Caution is needed where the incision crosses the zygomatic arch as the neurovascular bundle is very superficial here.

O-S OR O-Z FLAP

These are two opposing rotation flaps (Figure 8.28). They have an intrinsic coil or Z-plasty effect in that the resultant scar is S- or Z-shaped, which allows the central limb to stretch in every direction but mainly along the long axis. This design therefore prevents long-term contraction problems (see Figure 8.29). Thus, if placed over a joint, the incision limbs should run down the limb (e.g. on the shoulder, one limb of the 'S' or 'Z' would run down the arm while the other would run towards the spine).

Sites
- Scalp
- Pectoral
- Over joints
- Trunk
- Lower leg

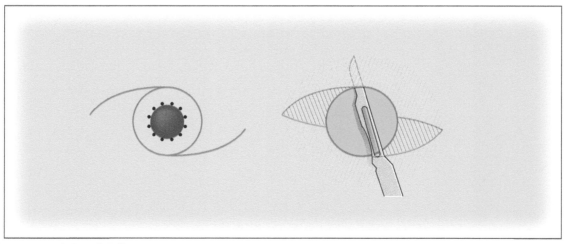

Figure 8.28 O-S or O-Z flap

Red = incision/excision lines; grey = undermining of flaps; blue = undermining everywhere else as necessary to get mobilisation.

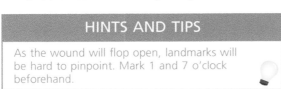

Figure 8.29 A finished O-Z (-S) flap

If the scar then contracts, the central arm acts like a coil allowing the scar to extend, preventing or compensating for long-term contraction. Scars can contract up to 30% of their length over time.

Technique

1 Mark the margins as a circle around the lesion.
2 Draw two tangential arms, roughly half the length of the circumference of the circle, in an arc to meet the circle at 12 o'clock and 6 o'clock (i.e. opposite each other).
3 Excise the lesion with a locator at 12 o'clock.
4 Incise the arcs to form two flaps, which are in effect two rotation flaps.
5 Undermine the flaps first but then everywhere else if necessary. Extensive undermining is usual and necessary.
6 Move the tips of the flaps from 12 and 6 o'clock to 1 and 7 o'clock and secure (suture).

HINTS AND TIPS

As the wound will flop open, landmarks will be hard to pinpoint. Mark 1 and 7 o'clock beforehand.

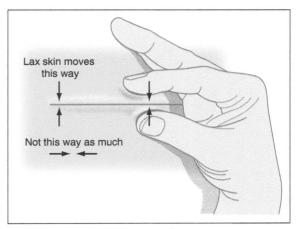

Figure 8.30 Pinch test

Where to place incisions

Use the pinch test (Figure 8.30): squeeze in every direction between thumb and index finger (some use three fingers) to find where skin is loosest and moves more. Align the incision(s) with the creases or wrinkles made by pinching this loose(r) skin.

The long axis goes from the end of one incision limb to the other. It should run down the arm or leg to provide a hinge over the joint, allowing it to flex and extend.

Closure

1 Suture at 1 o'clock (Figure 8.31).
2 Suture at 7 o'clock.
3 Suture centre.
4 Fill in the middle.
5 Then work out to the ends.
   Often, dog-ears result.

O-Z or O-S?

There is no difference between the O-S and the O-Z flaps, just personal preference with clinicians dividing 50/50. The O-S is formed when the flap incisions are more vertical than tangential (Figure 8.32). The O-S flap is favoured on the limbs and trunk. The technique is exactly the same.

See Figures 8.33, 8.34–8.36 for further examples.

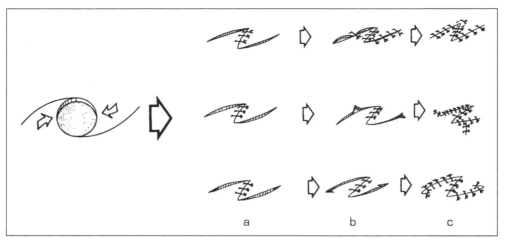

Figure 8.31 Closure of a circular defect

a Unequal edges are closed with the halving technique. **b** O-Z flap with Burow's triangles used to close uneven edges.
c O-Z flap with Z-plasties to close unequal sides.

Source: Roenigk R, Roenigk H (eds). Dermatologic Surgery, 2nd edn. New York: Marcel Dekker Inc, 1989; Fig 33.

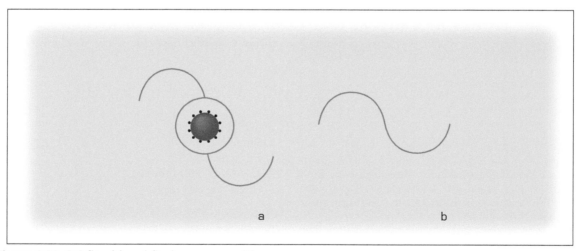

Figure 8.32 O-S flap (**a**) and final appearance (**b**)

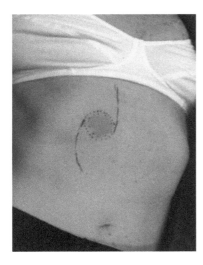

Figure 8.33 A quite large superficial BCC treated in the UK with imiquimod, which had such severe systemic side effects the patient requested surgery

She returned to the UK the day after surgery but wrote to say she was now feeling healthy and the wound had healed well. It is hard to imagine any flap other than a rhomboid but the circular shape of the lesion made an O-Z more tissue-sparing.

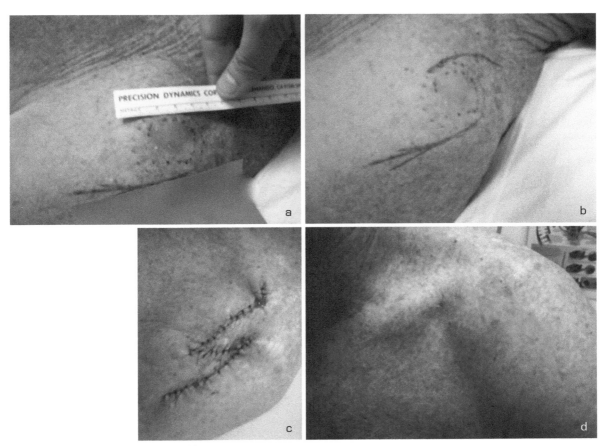

Figure 8.34 O-Z flap on the shoulder

a A 25-mm (+) superficial and nodular BCC left shoulder. **b** Flap arms orientated to go along the limb. **c** Dog-ear/standing cone formation medial and posterior tip. This 'Z' scar is in effect a coil that can stretch and open by elongating the centre limb. It is also ideal over the knee where it allows flexion and extension whereas a straight scar may form an impeding fibrous band. **d** One month later. The skin stretches. No dog-ears and an in-built spring allowing full use of the arm with no impeding scar contraction.

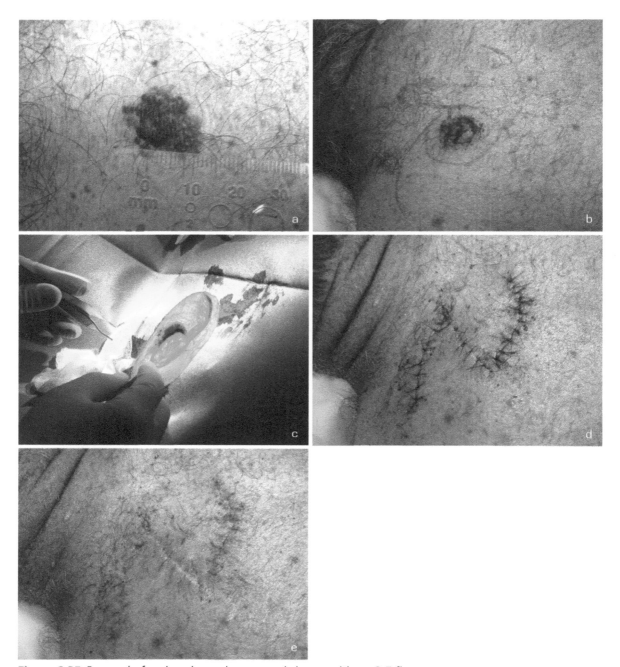

Figure 8.35 Removal of an invasive melanoma and closure with an O-Z flap

a An invasive melanoma >20 x 15 mm on a male back. An O-Z flap is arguably the flap of choice here. With 10-mm margins this equates to a 40-mm defect. **b** The 10-mm margins are drawn, then two tangential lines, approximately half the circumference of this margin circle, are drawn. Pinching the skin to find the most mobile skin was equal but the tangents were relocated so that the superior tangent ran toward the patient's arm, thus providing an extension 'spring' made by the central arm of the resultant 'Z'. These curved tangential arms result in a 'Z' whereas, if they enter at right angles or vertically, an 'S' results. This latter the author prefers on lower limbs as the incisions do not cut across the blood supply as much as a 'Z' does. **c** The melanoma with 10-mm margins is excised down to the deep fascia. Extensive undermining is now done in every direction until the points of the flaps can be moved without undue tension to their final position. The point of the upper right flap in the photo is at 6 o'clock on the drawn plan and is now taken across to 7 o'clock and sutured. The 12 o'clock point of the flap is immediately above the surgeon's index finger and is sutured to 1 o'clock on the excised margin/plan. These flaps sometimes distort or fall apart such that locating 1 o'clock and 7 o'clock is difficult and it is a good idea to mark these beforehand. **d** The final sutured 'Z'. Mohs pathology found it to be completely clear at all margins. **e** The final scar at ROS. Not the prettiest of scars but it in no way interfered with his mountain-biking with the central arm of the Z allowing full movement of his very active left arm (with the top of the 'Z' pointing towards his left arm). The scar subsequently settled extremely well with no spread but this can never be guaranteed. What can be 'guaranteed' or at least the very best job done, is to ensure Mohs pathology.

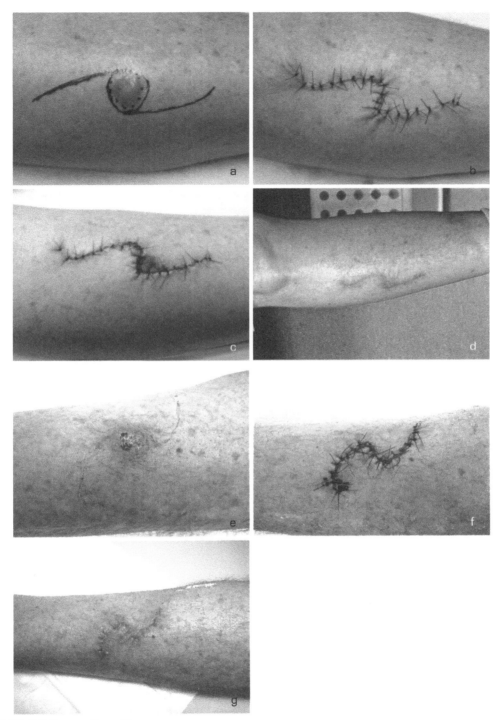

Figure 8.36 O-Z flap on the calf

a A 20-mm nodular BCC anterior calf. **b** O-Z flap. Note excessive tension at tips of centre. **c** Threatened tip necrosis – no surprises here. **d** Three months later no necrosis – thank goodness. But lessons to be learned: do an O-S, not an O-Z, so as to angle the centre down so blood vessels are not cut across as much as with this horizontal middle O-Z. Undermine, undermine, undermine. No tension at tips. **e**, **f** Here a similar site and sized SCC as in **a**–**d**, but an O-S done angling the limbs more vertically with good healing and no complications at 3 weeks (**g**).

theme. They involve meticulous planning/design. They can become quick and easy with experience.

PIVOT POINT

Transposition flaps have a fixed point at one side of their base around which the flap pivots. It is at the opposite side of the base from the direction the flap moves. Tightness at the pivot point compromises the blood supply and flap necrosis ensues. This is best avoided by ensuring that the length of the flap from the pivot point to the tip of the flap is the same as from the pivot point to the furthest side of the defect by measuring both while drawing the operation design. There is a case for also making the primary flap longer.

RHOMBOID FLAP

The rhomboid flap is an excellent flap to begin with as it follows a strict geometric plan and, if meticulously mapped out (Figure 8.37), ensures everything falls into place. Rhomboid-shaped skin flaps are transposed into like-shaped defects, leaving an angulated donor site that can then be closed primarily. The strict design removes any guesswork or conceptual problem and the final appearance can be predetermined. Its length-to-base ratio of 1:1 also ensures good blood supply. It is used for large defects on the trunk and shoulders but not below the knee where a length-to-base ratio <1:1 is needed. There is minimal tissue wastage. The rhomboid flap scar is incredibly ugly; although well-respected authorities may recommend it for the face, select more discreet flaps if possible. The side of the nose, however, heals well.

Transposition flaps

Transposition flaps move laterally in relation to a pivot point to be positioned into an adjacent defect. This involves moving a random skin and subcutaneous tissue flap as an adjoining raised flap into the excised primary deficit. The flap has to be raised and then taken across areas, isthmuses or intrusions of normal tissue (usually remaining from the primary incision site). In other words, the flap is transpositioned as distinct from rotation flaps, which rotate across an excised area. Although they arguably began with the angulated rhomboid flap, they have evolved into a family of flaps with increasing curves and more extended lobes, allowing for greater harvesting and coverage. This redirects the direction and tension of wound closure. As a group, they are regarded as the most complex of all flaps even though the rhomboid may be one of the simplest. They are versatile solutions to many coverage problems. Rhomboid flaps, Z-plasties and W-plasties are variations on this basic

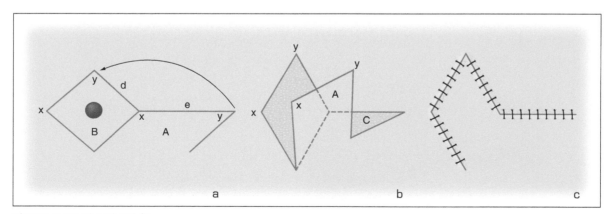

Figure 8.37 Rhomboid flap

a B = the lesion, which is excised with appropriate margins as a rhomboid with all sides equal. This is the recipient site. A = an exact duplicate, which is cut as flap A. This is the donor site. A is then transposed into B: 'y' to 'y', 'x' to 'x'. The 'tail' ('y') is always secured first. This rotational movement has a pivot point and considerable undermining is needed to mobilise the flap. **b** Here flap A is transported across to fill the now excised defect B. In doing so, it narrows the defect C that it leaves. With extensive undermining all can be sutured closed. **c** The resultant sutured scar.

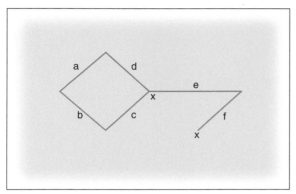

Figure 8.38 Geometric requirements of the rhomboid flap

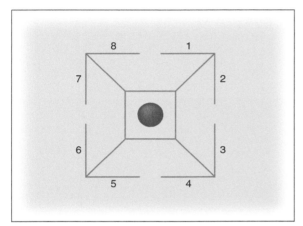

Figure 8.39 Eight possible rhomboid flaps can close a rhomboid defect

There are four geometric requirements (see Figure 8.38):

1 Six lines – all the same length
2 'a', 'c' and 'f' all parallel
3 'b' parallel to 'd'
4 'e' perpendicular to the rhombus abcd.

Eight flaps are possible from any primary excision (rhomboid) site by taking the secondary site incision in any straight (perpendicular) direction from the four rhomboid corners and defining the secondary tail site by a second incision to be parallel with the rhomboid sides, which can go two ways (Figure 8.39). This makes the rhomboid flap extremely versatile and allows for 'last minute' adjustment.

Rather than the customary angles of 60° and 120° in the rhomboid flap, variations using 30° and 150° angles are possible. This allows coverage of rhomboid defects with unequal sides. Because this approach involves more meticulous planning, first converting the defect into a rhombus of 60° and 120° angles is sometimes simpler.

Sites

Although the ugly scar may prompt the practitioner to seek another option, the following give the rationales for choosing a rhombic flap in certain locations [59].

- Dorsum of the nose and the nasal sidewall: free margins of the lower eyelid and nasal ala are particularly susceptible to distortion. Tension vectors should be directed away from the free margins.
- Medial and lateral canthi: owing to their close proximity to the highly mobile free margins of the eyelids, care is needed to redirect tension vectors to ensure that distortion of these structures does not occur on closure of the defect. Patients with lid margin laxity are particularly prone to distortion, which can lead to functional impairment of the eyelid. In addition, because some contraction occurs along the long axis of any wound, design closures to minimise lines going across the concave contours of the inner canthus to avoid webbing. The acute angles of the crow's feet of the lateral canthi offer excellent camouflage for the acute angles generated by transposition flaps in this location.
- Temple: occasionally, transposition flaps may be used to take advantage of the reservoir of excess skin over the cheeks, temple and preauricular areas when closing larger defects. They can also be designed to

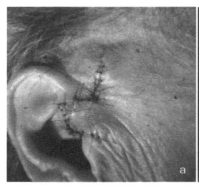 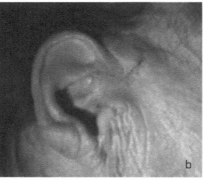 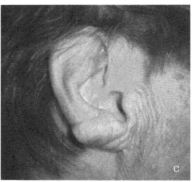

Figure 8.40 Rhomboid flaps are not usually recommended for ears but here was a cancer on the crux of the helix with a generous harvest area reservoir of mobile skin pre-auricular

a This demonstrates the need to have a number of design options and, in this case, the rhomboid worked well. A banner flap may have been an alternative except for the extent of the cancer. **b** The nodular BCC on the crux was excised leaving an exposed curved ridge rather than a flat surface. The rhomboid flap donated such a generous amount of tissue that this was able to be draped over the ridge of the crux and down the far internal side. ROS 7 days. **c** Some months later.

keep the closure of defects in the medial temple from entering the periorbital cosmetic unit.

- Cheeks: best designed laterally with the redundant tissue inferior to the primary defect. Positioning the scar laterally makes the scar less visible to the patient in a mirror and to onward-looking observers, whereas an inferiorly based flap provides good dependent lymphatic drainage to minimise the risk of flap engorgement and pincushioning.
- Perioral: a good option for repairing certain perioral cutaneous defects. The adjacent skin folds and wrinkles in various orientations provide ample camouflage for the geometric scars of transposition flaps. The proximity of the medial cheek can provide a good reservoir of lax skin. Take care to properly orient the flap to ensure that the closure does not result in tension, which may distort the lateral lip.
- Chin: like the perioral area, repairs of defects of the lateral chin can take advantage of the laxity of the medial cheek and submandibular area and the many natural lines in this area to hide the resulting scar. Take care to minimise lines across the convex contour where the chin and neck meet.
- Dorsal hand: although, in certain positions, there appears to be significant laxity of the dorsal hand, when a fist is made and the wrist is flexed downwards, this laxity all but disappears. If a vertically oriented closure is not possible and the defect is on the radial aspect of the dorsal hand, a transposition flap may be used to tap into the laxity in the region between the thumb and the first finger. This area often offers the only reservoir of tissue on the dorsal hand.

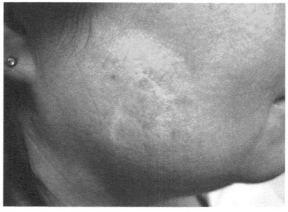

Figure 8.41 It is difficult to reconcile why a rhomboid flap was performed for such a small area in such a prominent position

The patient stated that it was done 11 years prior by a plastic surgeon for a BCC. With this amount of loose skin, a simple ellipse may have been possible or certainly an A-T flap, both of which would have resulted in less obvious scars.

LOBED FLAPS

These are a natural progression from the rhomboid flap, in which the straight lines of the rhomboid are replaced by more elegant curves. They start with just a single lobe which, like the rhomboid, replaces the excised deficit from a single secondary 'tail', now a 'lobe' site. To get more harvest area this single lobe can be augmented by creating a second and even a third lobe. Further, these lobes can vary in diameter, site of origin, take-off point and excision cone length. The primary excision site is usually close to a circle, as dictated by the lesion and the necessary margins. Then, to establish the full primary excision to facilitate a flap, this circle is extended to a point making a standing cone or dog-ear. The concept of stitching the tail first applies for all of these flaps.

Single lobe flap

There are themes and variations of this transposition flap in which the lobe can be either side and vary in diameter, take-off point, cone and lobe length (Figure 8.42).

Sites:

- Face
- Cheek next to the nose
- Upper nose
- Trunk
- Limbs

Banner flap

Banner flaps are, in effect, single lobe flaps. They are designed as a pendant of skin tangential to the edge of a round defect. They are triangular (banner) or finger-shaped flaps that borrow from adjacent lax skin to fill a defect to produce a long, linear scar. To achieve the best cosmesis this scar is best placed at the junction of two cosmetic units.

Sites:

- Ala: nasolabial fold – the classic nasolabial transposition flap
- Superior helix – the flap is taken behind the superior aspect of the ear
- Medial anterior ear (concha, tragus, crus of helix) – the flap is taken in the preauricular area

Technique

1 Two triangles or banners are created (Figure 8.43). One is to excise the lesion, which dictates its greatest

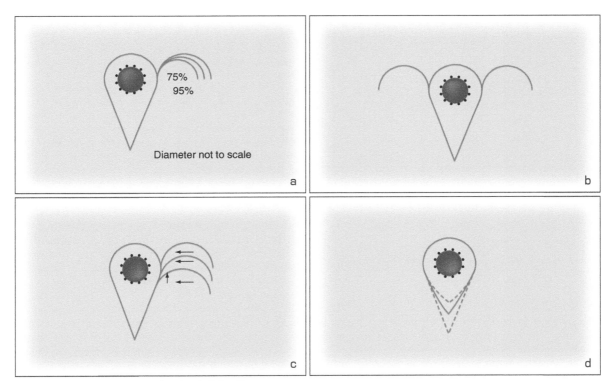

Figure 8.42 Variations on the single lobe flap

a Diameter reduction variable: the lobe can vary from a 'total' replacement 100% lobe to some 70%, depending on the mobility of the harvest area. **b** The lobe can be placed either side of the standing cone as the site and lesion dictate. This may seem obvious but to some it is not. Place the donor lobe where there is the most laxity to harvest and for cosmesis. **c** The take-off point need not be an exact shadow/mirror image but can be as far down as the harvest area laxity allows. This lobe may then have to be pulled up and over more. **d** The standing cone length can be extended or shortened so as not to cross a cosmetic border or so as to fall better into a cosmetic border and hide the incision.

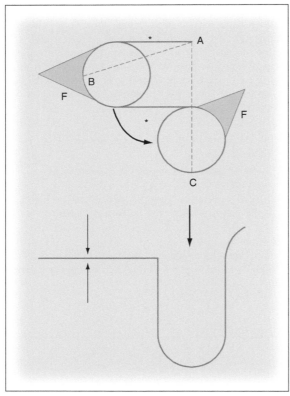

Figure 8.43 Banner flap
Adapted from Grekin RC. Flap surgery. In: Lask GP, Moy RD (eds), Principles and Techniques of Cutaneous Surgery. New York: McGraw-Hill, 1996; p 322.

width and base; the donor banner is a mirror image of this defect.

2 Elevate the flap.
3 Close the donor site.
4 Trim the flap edges to better fit the defect.
5 Close the recipient site.

For further details, refer to Chapter 9, 'Ear, nose, lip, scalp and digits'.

Bilobed flap

Bilobed flaps are covered in greater detail in Chapter 9, 'Ear, nose, lip, scalp and digits', as they are most commonly used in the closure of nasal defects.

The basic concept is for three touching circles (Figure 8.44). The traditional description is for diminishing diameters from the first, where the lesion is to be excised, forming a lower case 'm' plan. The first circle marks the margin around the lesion, and then a cone or dog-ear is extended so it looks like an ice cream in a cone. This standing cone or dog-ear (so called because of its shape) is actually excised to *prevent* a standing cone or

dog-ear when finally sutured up. This was a deliberate modification and improvement.

The lesion and the cone are excised as the recipient site.

Most advice is for the second (donor site) circle to be smaller than the first (recipient site). Although these are called transposition flaps, there is considerable rotation. Early attempts at these flaps resulted in a dog-ear and pin-cushioning, and this second donor flap often fell short of the recipient site far margin. In all such flaps the tail, which in this case is the apex of the donor flap, is always sutured first and it is there the shortfall occurs. This places greater and undesirable tension on the flap. As discussed in Chapter 9, there may be an argument for enlarging, not shortening, this second lobe.

The final lobe, if peaked like a bishop's hat and slightly elongated, also may become easier to approximate and suture (Figure 8.45).

Trilobed flap
More lobes can be added to provide greater mobility and coverage if there is enough lax tissue.

PINWHEEL OR MULTIPLE RHOMBOID FLAP
Multiple O-Z flaps are the simplest way to do a pinwheel flap, but they can also be formed by multiple transposition rhomboid flaps (Figure 8.46).

When a larger wound needs to be closed, the circular defect can be converted into a hexagon and closed with three rhomboid flaps (Figure 8.47). This procedure is even more complicated to plan, and it leaves a stellate scar. The scar is difficult to merge into natural crease lines and is consequently noticeable as a geometric scar. Use this technique with caution.

Z-PLASTY
The Z-plasty is a double transportation flap (but with rotation and advancement elements) of two equal triangles – the 'V's of the 'Z'. It is not used in skin cancer surgery but for lengthening scars, especially those that cross relaxed skin tension lines.

The incision consists of a 'Z' with a central slanted limb and two horizontal limbs, all of which are the same length. The length of the central limb dictates the gain in length. The classic Z-plasty has 60° angles (Figure 8.48), resulting in a gain in length of 70% relative to the central limb, but the angles may range from 30° to 90° (Figure 8.49). Although theoretically these may promise gains in length of 25% and 120%, respectively, the actual gains are smaller because of skin restriction factors. The final position of the central limb is plotted first and made perpendicular to the original central limb incision, and it should be oriented parallel to the skin lines. This central line of the Z-shaped incision is thus made along

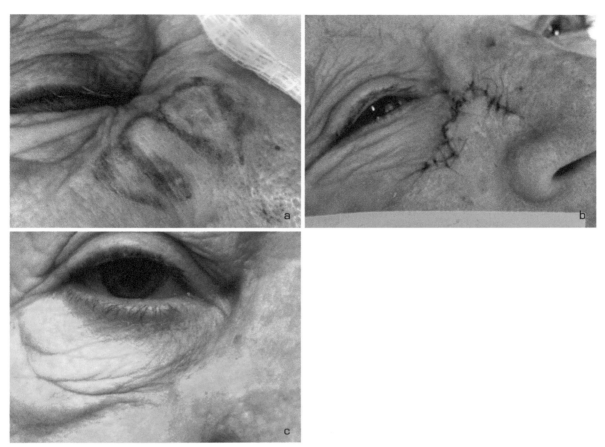

Figure 8.44 Bilobed flap
a Three circles with cones. **b** Sutured bilobed flap. **c** 7 weeks post-op.

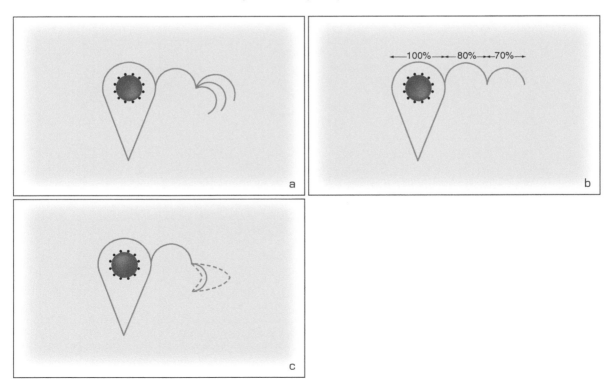

Figure 8.45 Bilobed added variants
a Angle between transpositions. **b** Reduction in diameter. **c** Peaked final lobe.

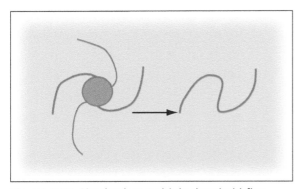

Figure 8.46 Pinwheel or multiple rhomboid flap

In an O-Z flap (thick red lines), rotation flaps are incised on opposite sides of the primary defect. In this way each rotation flap can harvest loose tissue from different sides of the defect. Additional rotation flaps may be added in a pinwheel-like fashion (thin red lines) around the primary defect.

Adapted from Buchen D. Skin Flaps in Facial Surgery. New York: McGraw-Hill, 2007; Fig 3.4.

the line of greatest tension or contraction, and triangular flaps are raised on opposite sides of the two ends and then transposed. The length and angle of each flap must be precisely the same to avoid mismatched flaps that may be difficult to close. The changed axis of the final scar often provides a more aesthetic result in facial scar revision. However, as the Z-plasty relies on healthy adjacent skin, it is a poor choice for the correction of burn contractures. As a prerequisite, the skin has to be loose at right angles to the scar.

The W-plasty is similar to a Z-plasty in its ability to break up a linear scar, but in this case multiple smaller triangular flaps are interposed among one another. The base of each triangle is aligned with the vertex of the one opposite it. However, unlike the Z-plasty, the W-plasty does not confer any gain in length to the contracted scar line. The W-plasty increases rather than decreases lateral tension, and skin is sacrificed in its construction. Therefore, only undertake this procedure in areas of scar with excess adjacent skin. As the ends of the scar are approached, make the triangles smaller in size and the limbs of the triangles shorter as well.

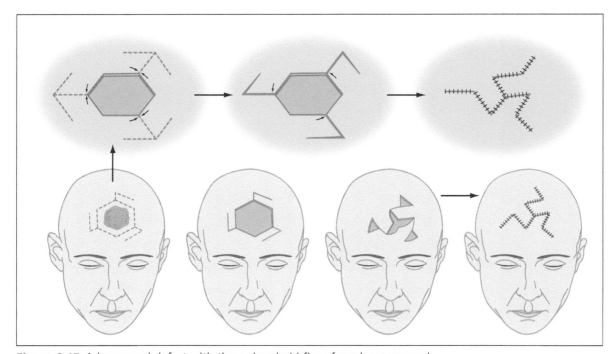

Figure 8.47 A hexagonal defect with three rhomboid flaps for a larger wound

Adapted from Roenigk R, Roenigk H (eds). Dermatologic Surgery, 2nd edn. New York: Marcel Dekker Inc, 1989; Fig 47.

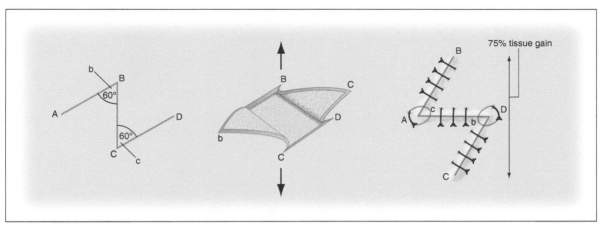

Figure 8.48 60° Z-plasty

a The central scar is the common diagonal. **b** Incisions result in two triangular flaps that are lifted and transposed. **c** 60° Z-plasty results in a 75% gain in tissue length.

Adapted from Robinson JK, Hanke WC, Sengelmann R et al (eds). Surgery of the Skin. Philadelphia: Mosby, 2005; Fig 20.6.

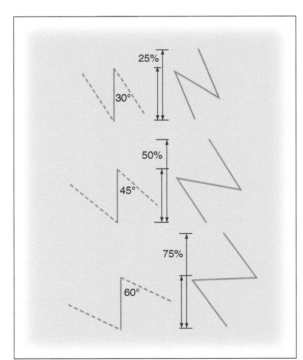

Figure 8.49 Different angles used in Z-plasty to adjust the final length of the scar

Adapted from Kotler HS. Scar revision surgery treatment and management. eMedicine. Available at: emedicine.medscape. com (accessed 4 Feb 2014).

REFERENCES

[1] Dzubow LM. The dynamics of flap movement: effect of pivotal restraint on flap rotation and transposition. J Dermatol Surg Oncol 1987;13:1348–53.

[2] Patterson TJ. The survival of skin flaps in the pig. Br J Plast Surg 1968;21:113–17.

[3] Patterson TJ. Study of the blood-supply of skin flaps by close-up thermography. Br J Surg 1969; 56:381.

[4] Stell PM. The pig as an experimental model for skin flap behaviour: a reappraisal of previous studies. Br J Plast Surg 1977;30:1–8.

[5] Milton SH. Pedicled skin flaps: the fallacy of the length:width ratio. Br J Surg 1970;57:502–8.

[6] Cutting C. Critical closing and perfusion pressures in flap survival. Ann Plast Surg 1982;9:524.

[7] Marks NJ. Quantitative analysis of skin flap blood flow in the rat using laser Doppler velocimetry. J R Soc Med 1985;78:308–14.

[8] Cutting C, Ballantyne D, Shaw W, et al. Critical closing pressure, local perfusion pressure, and the failing skin flap. Ann Plast Surg 1982;8:504–9.

[9] Pearl RM. A unifying theory of the delay phenomenon – recovery from the hyperadrenergic state. Ann Plast Surg 1981;7:102–12.

[10] Kernahan DA, Zingg W, Kay CW. The effect of hyperbaric oxygen on the survival of experimental skin flaps. Plast Reconstr Surg 1965;36:19–25.

[11] Baran NK, Horton CE. Growth of skin grafts, flaps, and scars in young minipigs. Plast Reconstr Surg 1972;50:487–96.

[12] Daniel RK, Williams HB. The free transfer of skin flaps by microvascular anastomosis. An experimental study and a reappraisal. Plast Reconstr Surg 1973;52:16–31.

[13] Donovan WE. Experimental models in skin flap research. In: Grabb WC, Myers MB, editors. Skin flaps. Boston: Little Brown; 1975. pp. 11–20.

[14] Daniel RK. The anatomy and hemodynamics of the cutaneous circulation and their influence on skin flap design. In: Grabb WC, Myers MB, editors. Skin flaps. Boston: Little Brown; 1975. pp. 111–31.

[15] Neligan P, Pang CY, Nakatsuka T, et al. Pharmacologic action of isoxsuprine in cutaneous and myocutaneous flaps. Plast Reconstr Surg 1985;75:363–74.

[16] Guyton AC. Textbook of medical physiology. 6th edn. Philadelphia: WB Saunders; 1981. pp. 344–56.

[17] Pearl RM, Johnson D. The vascular supply to the skin: an anatomical and physiological reappraisal – Part I. Ann Plast Surg 1983;11:99–105.

[18] Meyers B. Understanding flap necrosis. Plast Reconstr Surg 1986;78:813–14.

[19] Midy D. A contribution to the study of the facial artery, its branches and anastomoses: application to the anatomic vascular basis of facial flaps. Surg Radiol Anat 1986;8:99–107.

[20] Mathes SJ, Naha F. The reconstructive triangle: a paradigm for surgical decision making. In: Reconstructive surgery: principles, anatomy and technique. New York: Churchill Livingston; 1997. pp. 9–36, 37–160.

[21] Fazio MJ, Zitelli JA. Flaps. In: Ratz JL, et al., editors. Textbook of dermatologic surgery. Philadelphia: Lippincott-Raven; 1998. pp. 225–7.

[22] Heniford BW, Bailin PL, Marsico RE. Field guide to local flaps. Dermatol Clin 1998;16:65–74.

[23] Hartwell SW Jr. Local flaps of the leg and foot. In: Grabb WC, Myers MB, editors. Skin flaps. Boston: Little Brown; 1975. pp. 497–506.

[24] Stranc MF, Sanders R. Abdominal wall skin flaps. In: Grabb WC, Myers MB, editors. Skin flaps. Boston: Little Brown; 1975. pp. 419–26.

[25] Sasaki GH, Pang CY. Experimental evidence for involvement of prostaglandins in viability and acute skin flaps: effects on viability and mode of action. Plast Reconstr Surg 1981;67:335–40.

[26] Kerrigan CL, Zelt RG, Daniel RK. Secondary critical ischemia time of experimental skin flaps. Plast Reconstr Surg 1984;74:522–6.

[27] Park S, Tepper OM, Galiano RD, et al. Selective recruitment of endothelial progenitor cells to ischemic tissues with increased neovascularization. Plast Reconstr Surg 2004;113:284–93.

[28] Leach J. Proper handling of soft tissue in the acute phase. Facial Plast Surg 2001;17:227–38.

[29] Boyer JD, Zitelli JA, Brodland DG. Undermining in cutaneous surgery. Dermatol Surg 2001;27: 75–8.

[30] Myers MB. Wound tension and vascularity in the etiology and prevention of skin sloughs. Surgery 1964;56:945–9.

[31] Myers MB, Combs B, Cohen G. Wound tension and wound sloughs – a negative correlation. Am J Surg 1965;109:711–14.

[32] Larrabee WF. Design of local skin flaps. Otolaryngol Clin North Am 1990;23:899–923.

[33] Mellow CG, Knight KR, Angel MF, et al. The biochemical basis of secondary ischemia. J Surg Res 1992;52:226–32.

[34] Demirseren ME, Yenidunya MO, Yenidunya S. Island rat groin flaps with twisted pedicles. Plast Reconstr Surg 2004;114:1190–4.

[35] Goding GS Jr, Horn DB. Skin flap physiology. In: Baker SR, Swanson NA, editors. Local flaps in facial reconstruction. St Louis, MO: Mosby; 1995. pp. 15–30.

[36] Tsur H, Daniller A, Strauch B. Neovascularization of skin flaps: route and timing. Plast Reconstr Surg 1980;66:85–93.

[37] Jonsson K, Hunt TK, Brennan SS, et al. Tissue oxygen measurements in delayed skin flaps: a reconsideration of the mechanisms of the delay phenomenon. Plast Reconstr Surg 1988;82:328–36.

[38] Pickett BP, Burgess LP, Livermore GH, et al. Wound healing. Arch Otolaryngol Head Neck Surg 1996;122:565–8.

[39] Liu PY, Wang XT, Badiavas E, et al. Enhancement of ischemic flap survival by prefabrication with transfer of exogenous PDGF gene. J Reconstr Microsurg 2005;21:273–9.

[40] Simman R, Craft C, McKinney B. Improved survival of ischemic random skin flaps through the use of bone marrow nonhematopoietic stem cells and angiogenic growth factors. Ann Plast Surg 2005;54:546–52.

[41] Serafin D, Shearin C, Georgiade NG. The vascularization of free flaps: a clinical and experimental correlation. Plast Reconstr Surg 1977;60:233–41.

[42] Gatti JE, LaRossa D, Brousseau DA, et al. Assessment of neovascularization and timing of flap division. Plast Reconstr Surg 1984;73:396–402.

[43] Klingenstrom P, Nylen B. Timing of transfer of tubed pedicles and cross flaps. Plast Reconstr Surg 1966;37:1–12.

[44] Cummings C, Trachy R. Measurement of alternative blood flow in the porcine panniculus carnosus myocutaneous flap. Arch Otolaryngol 1985;111: 598–600.

[45] Kay S, Green C. The effect of a novel thromboxane synthetase inhibitor dazmegrel (UK38485) on random pattern skin flaps in the rat. Br J Plast Surg 1986;39:361–3.

[46] Kerrigan CL, Stotland MA. Ischemia reperfusion injury: a review. Microsurgery 1993;4:165–75.

[47] Angel MF, Narayanan K, Swartz WM, et al. The etiologic role of free radicals in hematoma-induced flap necrosis. Plast Reconstr Surg 1986;77:795–803.

[48] Kerrigan CL, Daniel RK. Skin flap research: a candid view. Ann Plast Surg 1984;13:383–7.

[49] Salasche SJ. Acute surgical complications: cause, prevention, and treatment. J Am Acad Dermatol 1986;15:1163–85.

[50] Salasche SJ, Grabski WJ. Complications of flaps. J Dermatol Surg Oncol 1991;17:132–40.

[51] Myers MB. Investigation of skin flap necrosis. In: Grabb WC, Myers MB, editors. Skin flaps. Boston: Little, Brown; 1975. pp. 3–10.

[52] Lawrence WT, Murphy RC, Robson MC, et al. The detrimental effect of cigarette smoking on flap survival: an experimental study in the rat. Br J Plast Surg 1984;37(2):216–19.

[53] Aker JS, Mancoll J, Lewis B, et al. The effect of pentoxifylline on random-pattern skin-flap necrosis induced by nicotine treatment in the rat. Plast Reconstr Surg 1997;100(1):66–71.

[54] Karacaoğlan N, Akbaş H. Effect of parenteral pentoxifylline and topical nitroglycerin on skin flap survival. Otolaryngol Head Neck Surg 1999;120(2):272–4.

[55] Stevens CR, Tan L, Kassir R, et al. Biomechanics of A-to-T flap design. Laryngoscope 1999;109(1):113–17.

[56] McGregor IA. Local skin flaps in facial reconstruction. Otolaryngol Clin NA 1982;15:77–98.

[57] Ahuja RB. Geometric considerations in the design of rotation flaps in the scalp and forehead region. Plast Reconstruct Surg 1988;8:900–6.

[58] Kroll SS, Margolis R. Scalp flap rotation with primary donor site closure. Ann Plast Surg 1993;30:452–5.

[59] Rohrer TE, Bhatia A. Transposition flaps in cutaneous surgery. Derm Surg 2005;31(8 Pt 2):1014–23.

Ear, nose, lip, scalp and digits

Ear

This, with more tender logic of the kind,
He pour'd into her small and shell-like ear.

Thomas Hood, Bianca's Dream *(1827)*

The type and the technique for ear excisions and repairs are determined by the size and location of the lesion and the subsequent defect. The aim is to first completely excise the lesion with adequate margins and to then restore the shape, size and alignment of the ear so that it is not noticed. Recognition that the ears are important for supporting spectacles is important; a difference in size is seldom noticed but deformities are obvious. The surgical procedures covered here are for primary, one-stage operations.

SURGICAL LOCATIONS

1 **Helix**: is the rigid, semicircular, posterosuperior rolled border of the ear formed by the auricular cartilage but does not extend into the lobe (see Figure 9.1). Maintaining the shape and contour of the helix is most important in any repair (refer to Figure 9.2 for site distribution of SCCs). Meticulous alignment and apposition must be achieved. Wedge resections, flaps or full-thickness skin grafts (FTSG) are the usual operations with simple linear ellipses often possible for small lesions. Wedge resections are probably the most performed operation.

2 **Anterior surface**: consists of the areas inside the helical rim, viz: the triangular fossa, scaphoid fossa, antihelix and concha. Here skin grafts are useful but secondary intention most often gives excellent results – see the section on 'Secondary intention – healing of bare cartilage' below.

3 **Posterior surface**: includes of the postauricular sulcus. Skin cancers in this region can go undetected and thus the backs of the ears must always be examined. Excisions can usually be closed with simple ellipses or flaps and occasionally grafts.

4 **Preauricular surface**: includes the tragus, helical root, preauricular sulcus and the bare skin free of hair to the sideburns. This skin is loose and lax and provides a good reservoir and harvest area for flaps and also allows for long generous ellipses. Removal of the tragus or helical root is not noticed.

5 **Lobe/lobule**: is often a site for epidermoid cysts but, increasingly, the site of tears from earrings. Repair can be by primary closure or a wedge resection wherein 50% can be excised without it being noticeable. Wound edge eversion is important. Keloid formation may be a common complication from earrings.

OPERATIONS/TECHNIQUES

HINTS AND TIPS

Hydrodissection

To discern if a cancer of the ear has infiltrated the cartilage, hydrodissection with local anaesthetic can often provide the answer. Lignocaine with adrenaline is injected under the cancer (to where it can be best judged, just above the cartilage/perichondrium) and the area pumped up. If the cancer hasn't infiltrated the perichondrium, it should become evident that the cancer lifts off. It can then be excised or dissected and sutured or secondary intention healing may be possible if so desired and applicable.

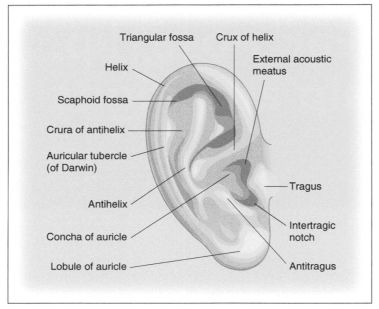

Figure 9.1 Anatomy of the ear
Adapted from Hansen JT. Netter's Clinical Anatomy, 2nd edn. Philadelphia: Saunders, 2009; p 93.

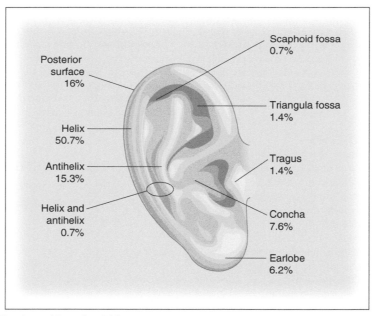

Figure 9.2 Site distribution of invasive SCC
Adapted from Silapunt S, Peterson SR, Goldberg LH. Squamous cell carcinoma of the auricle and Mohs micrographic surgery. Dermatol Surg 2005; 31(11):1423–27.

Surgical site preparation

Preoperative cleansing of the patient's skin with chlorhexidine–alcohol is superior to cleansing with povidone–iodine for preventing surgical-site infection after clean-contaminated surgery [1].

> **NOTE**
>
> Chlorhexidine is damaging to the tympanic membranes (and conjunctiva) and, if used, care must be taken to ensure none trickles down the external auditory meatus (EAM). A recommended practice for all ear surgery to prevent blood or other liquid running into this natural channel is to insert a pledget of cotton wool firmly into the EAM. It may even be secured with paper tape to prevent its inadvertent dislodgement.

Simple ellipse

Small lesions on the helix can be excised by longitudinal ellipses. Although this may thin the helix this is seldom noticeable. Many lesions on the posterior surface and most on the anterior surface can be excised and repaired this way (see Figures 9.3, 9.4 and 9.5).

Wedge resection

This is mostly used on the lateral helix (Figure 9.6). A wedge resection is less optimal on the superior helix than on the lateral helix due to the smaller dimension of the superior helical rim [2].

A good wedge resection of the helix is seldom noticed. Although one ear becomes smaller this is not perceived, especially with lesions <1.5 cm. Larger ears allow for wider wedges. Multiple Burow's triangles allow for extensive resection/wedges but the ear is then considerably smaller, but again, seldom noticed.

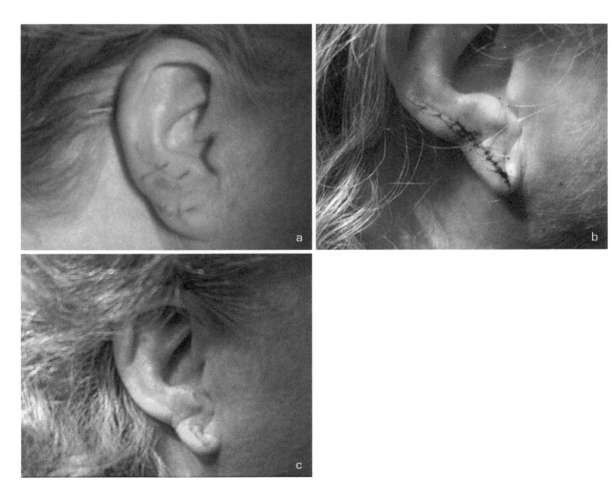

Figure 9.3 Excision of an SCC on the lobe

a Always do the simplest excision possible. Don't forget the simple ellipse. **b** A long ellipse allowed 4-mm margins. **c** Removal of sutures at 7 days. The scar subsequently became virtually invisible.

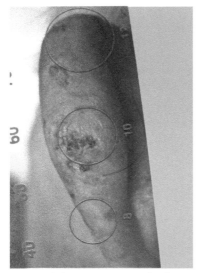
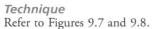

Figure 9.4 A nodular BCC >10 mm in diameter
Quite large lesions can be excised from the helical rim with a simple ellipse. Local anaesthetic is pumped under the BCC. If it rises off, free of the cartilage, this indicates that it hasn't invaded the cartilage and that a simple ellipse rather than a wedge resection can be attempted. Nevertheless, Mohs pathology should be requested to ensure clearance.

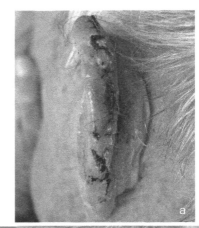
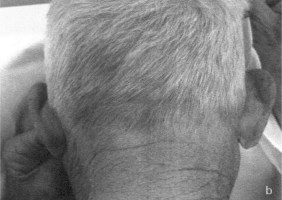

Figure 9.5 Excision of the nodular BCC in Figure 9.4
a A long ellipse allows the wound edges to be drawn together. **b** The result is a complete excision and good cosmesis with no discernible differences between his ears (9 months later).

Technique

Refer to Figures 9.7 and 9.8.

1 Mark appropriate margins. The ear wedge always makes the ear smaller; therefore, the size of the defect is the limiting factor. 1.5 cm has been the traditional recommended maximum for an excision but, with experience, wider wedges can be taken.

2 Draw a wedge towards the external auditory meatus or an isosceles triangle as defined by the helical base. Its length is determined by the size of the lesion and ensuring the wedge apical angle is approximately 30°.

3 Infiltrate with 1% lignocaine (with adrenaline 1:200,000) (2%/1:80,000 provides no advantage), generously including either side of the wedge and, if necessary, either side of the ear (anterior and posterior). Wait! 15 minutes provides maximum vasoconstriction. Test for sensation – prick the area to be excised and sutured.

4 Be bold and cut the wedge out with either a scalpel or best quality sharp scissors. The cartilage obviously provides greater resistance than skin but the excision must have clean and defined edges.

5 Punch a 4-mm hole right through the ear at the apex of the triangle. This prevents a flap-door

deformity where the ear can click back and forth like a door on spring hinges.

6 The wedge is repaired by carefully re-approximating each layer. Assess in toto, then:

A Suture the cartilage first. Pull the wedge together to assess where the first cartilage suture should go. Use absorbable sutures, usually 4/0, to align and suture together the cartilage. Although it is not important as they resorb, if possible place the knots posteriorly. Use more sutures than you would normally, *at least six*, as this cartilage will want to pull apart and use medium- to long-term absorbable sutures (Monosyn/Maxon).

B Place a couple of strategic tacking sutures at the front – usually 6/0 nylon interrupted – to align the helix.

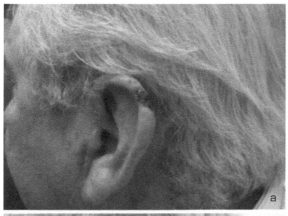

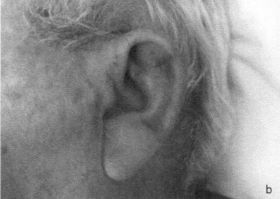

Figure 9.6 A relatively large basilo-squamous carcinoma of the helix

a This necessitated at least 4-mm margins and prophylactic inclusion of cartilage. Therefore, a wedge resection was ideal with Mohs pathology requested. **b** Seven days later at ROS an initially hesitant but now very grateful patient with no one noticing any differences between his ears. Excision complete as confirmed by Mohs pathology.

C Meticulously align the rim of the helical defect to match and marry to the other side to prevent notching or noticeable misalignment. A vertical mattress suture at the helical rim/curve to accentuate eversion and avoid any dimpling/notching is traditionally recommended. However, if pulled too tight or with too much eversion a join lump can result, and a meticulously performed interrupted 6/0 nylon suture with just the correct eversion and pulled firmly, but not tightly, can give the best result.

D Suture the posterior wound edges with 6/0 interrupted sutures.

E Use minimal (6/0) sutures to tack the front.

The dressing is also important. Although antibiotic ointment is not recommended if sterility is guaranteed,

the ear is prone to *Pseudomonas* infections, which can be rapid and serious. Consider a chloramphenicol ointment cover and even oral antibiotics for diabetics and the unkempt (invariably single males living alone). Place a non-stick wrap (Cutelin, Melolin) over the helix to drape over the wedge anterior and posterior. Add some sterile gauze padding and finally some Fixomull adhesive tape to bind it all down. Multiple strips provide greater security. A useful ear dressing is described with images in the 'Dressings' section of Chapter 12, 'Postoperative care'.

Sutures can be removed at 7 days but there is no rush and leaving them for up to 10 days provides additional security. Apply security strips after ROS as, if the patient is a disturbed sleeper, turning the head on the pillow can cause shear forces and potentially open the wound. Ear operations are remarkably pain free (as indeed are most skin cancer operations), but the patient should be cautioned to sleep on the good ear side before and after ROS, as much as possible.

> **Essentials**
>
> - Make a 4-mm punch hole right through at the apex of the wedge that will function as a pivot point so that the cartilage won't buckle or form a 'spring-flap'.
> - Some advocate a wedge apical angle of <30° to avoid distortion, but an apical punch obviates this.
> - Put as many sutures as possible at the back of the ear so that, if it points, it can't be seen.
> - Most importantly, always securely suture the cartilage together with medium- to long-term absorbable sutures; otherwise the wedge will part and separate.

> **HINTS AND TIPS**
>
> Cartilage takes a long time to heal together – longer than most absorbable sutures – and, with a wedge resection, there are constant separation forces, so use at least six sutures and the longer acting absorbable (e.g. polyglyconate/polytrimethylene carbonate [Maxon] or poliglecaprone 25 [Monocryl, Monosyn]) and not the shorter duration ones such as polyglycolide or polyglycolic acid (PGA; Dexon, Safil, Assucryl).

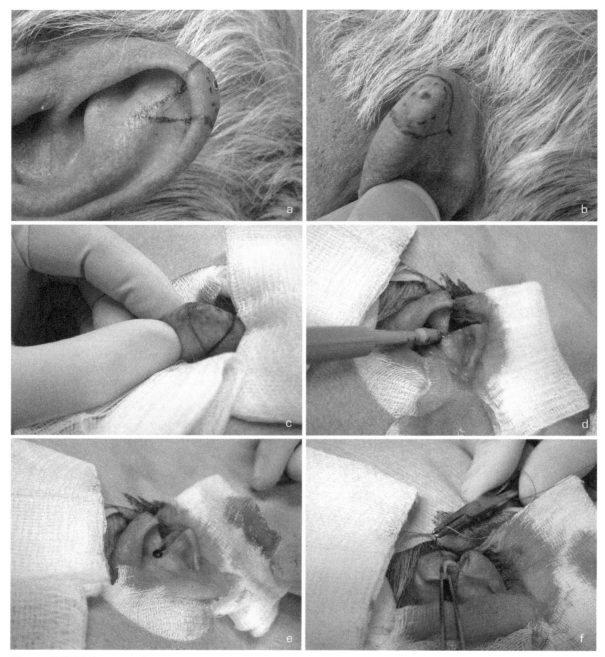

Figure 9.7 Wedge resection

a Dot out the lesion and 4-mm margins from the visual edge (seen on the superior surface of the helix in **b**). Draw a wedge from this lateral margin to form a 30° angle. This denotes the extent of the wedge. **b** Mark the posterior surface. This is arguably the easiest to cut as it is a plane surface. Cut through to the external surface. **c** Cut along the wedge. Here a scalpel was used. Some prefer scissors. Ultra-sharp scissors make it easier. **d** At the apex of the wedge bore out the cartilage with a 4-mm biopsy punch. **e** The result should look like this. This prevents the cartilage flexing and flapping like a spring 'flap door' or 'spring-back' complication. **f** Pull the wedge together so as to align where the cartilage sutures should go. Then sew up the cartilage from the posterior surface. Here 4/0 absorbable has been used.

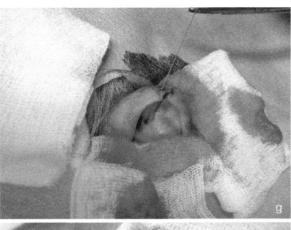
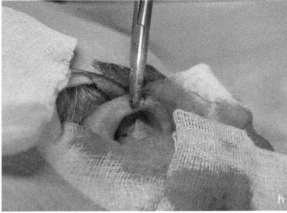
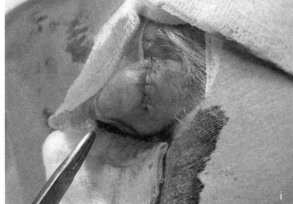
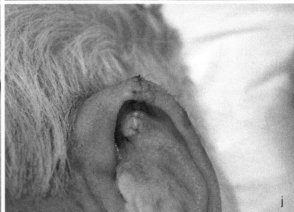

Figure 9.7 continued

g The knots of these absorbable cartilage sutures are at the back of the ear. Tying the knot pulls the wedge together. Don't stint. Ensure a minimum of four cartilage sutures that pull the cartilage surfaces together to abut and join. Use medium-to-long duration absorbable sutures. **h** One or two tacking sutures may be used to align the helix so as to allow a suture to be meticulously placed on the inferior surface margin of the helix. Most recommend a vertical mattress suture as this is where the first wide bite can be seen; this will then return to evert the edges. However, this can cause 'too much' eversion with a joint lump. A careful interrupted suture that everts the edge can provide an excellent result. Neither should be pulled too tight. **i** Once the helix is meticulously matched the posterior of the wound is sutured, here with 6/0 blue nylon. The use of blue nylon in hairy areas makes it easier to see. **j** The external surface is then sewn using the minimum number of sutures.

Flaps

Helical rim repairs

Direct closure or simple advancement flaps have the disadvantage of placing great tension on the wound margins, either edge-to-edge or leading edge, which thins the flap, flattens the rim and may uncurl the natural roll of the helix.

Reconstruction of the upper one-third of the ear may be achieved using several strategies such as full-thickness skin grafts, wedge resection, helical advancement flaps and one-stage preauricular or postauricular transposition flaps such as a banner flap taken behind the superior aspect of the ear. Multi-stage tubed flaps are also used.

When defects are smaller than 1.5 cm, wedge conversion of the defect followed by primary closure is aptly suited with no distortion of the anatomy. When the defect is 1.5–2.5 cm, the best choice is a helical advancement flap.

Advancement flaps

Standard advancement flap

The helical advancement flap (Figure 9.9) is used as a standard repair for defects of the lateral portion of the helical rim but not the superior helix. The lesion is excised and the flap is constructed by incising from the superior margin of the excision along the helical crease down to the earlobe. Undermining along the helical rim and widely over the posterior ear is needed. A Burow's

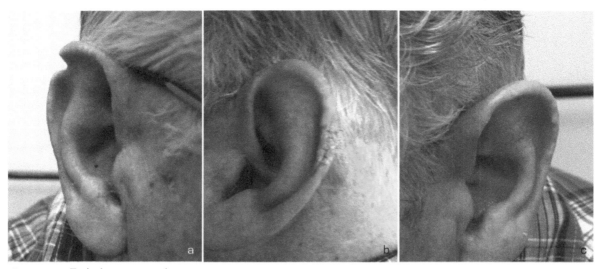

Figure 9.8 Technique comparison

a This patient had had a lesion previously excised from his right ear. Obviously, the cartilage was not sutured, or not sutured adequately, resulting in this preventable unsightly deformity. He was never told what the lesion was or given a pathology report. When he presented with a lesion on his left ear it was biopsied and reported as an SCC. **b** SCC L mid-helix (2 to 4 o'clock). The defect here would be significantly larger than the residual defect on his R ear, yet this cancer was completely excised without a residual deformity. **c** Post-op L ear. The SCC was excised with the cartilage sutured and with meticulous matching of the helical rim with most sutures on the posterior surface and Mohs pathology to ensure complete clearance. The differences between **a** and **c** demonstrate how a good result can be achieved. This time his results were given to him, thus helping any other doctor he might attend and reassuring him as to clearance margins.

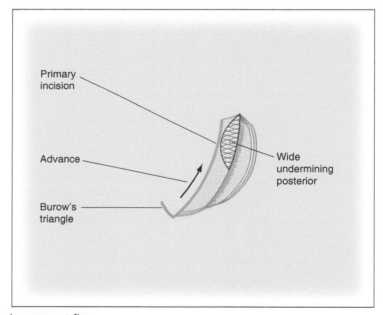

Figure 9.9 Helical advancement flap

triangle from the earlobe is often necessary. This flap can also be devised as a chondrocutaneous flap, including the cartilage of the inferior helix to replace missing cartilage along the helical rim [3]. Generally, defects up to 2 cm along the lateral helical rim can be repaired in this fashion. Larger defects of the lateral helical rim have also been repaired using bilateral helical chondrocutaneous advancement flaps in which the traditional earlobe-based helical advancement flap is performed in conjunction with a superior helical chondrocutaneous advancement flap [3, 4]. Surgical defects of the auricular helix generally require reconstruction to maintain the contiguous border of the helical rim.

A-T flap

Lesions towards the posterior of the helix can be repaired by an A-T flap where the T base runs longitudinally along the helix and the apex of the A is towards the postauricular sulcus. This is a good flap when there is not enough skin for a bilobed flap.

V-Y island flap

This flap can provide very good helical repairs. The lesion is excised as a rectangle on the helix and the V-Y is taken right down to the posterior sulcus. Some recommend

horizontal mattress sutures where the flap is rolled over the helical edge as this reinstates the natural roll.

Transposition flaps

Banner flap

- Superior helix: for defects greater than 2.5 cm, the banner flap can be taken pre- or postauricular.
- Anterior helix: refer to Figure 9.10.
  Note: as with most flaps there is considerable rotation needed around a pivot point, even though this is classed as a transposition flap. The anterior superior pivot point should be extensively undermined to facilitate this rotational element.
- Posterior helix: the anterior edge of the flap is cut along the retroauricular sulcus. The flap is designed to have a length-to-width ratio of $1:4$ (exceeding the length of the defect). A Burow's triangle is added to the flap near the lobe to allow easy closure of the secondary defect by tapering its tip. As the postauricular skin is thin, undermining should be done with care. After trimming the flap to fit the defect, the first suture is placed at the (anterior) tip

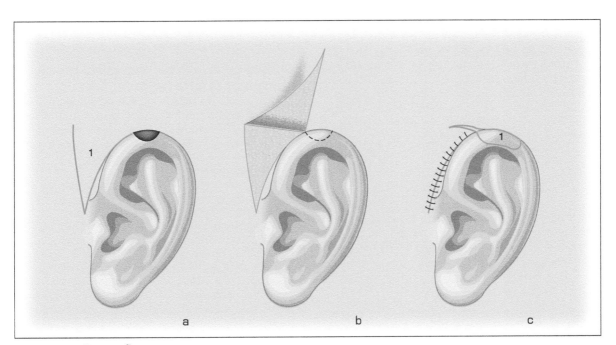

Figure 9.10 Banner flap

a Measure the helical defect (black). A 'V' or banner to duplicate this defect is drawn from the leading inferior margin of the helical defect down the preauricular sulcus, returning to form the base of the V. This base of the banner is as wide as the helix roll (or perhaps somewhat wider as it can be trimmed). That is, there are two triangles or banners created: one is to excise the lesion, which dictates its greatest width and base, and the other is the donor banner, *which is a mirror image of this defect*. **b** The flap is elevated. **c** The donor site closed. The flap edges are trimmed to better fit the defect, and the recipient site is closed.

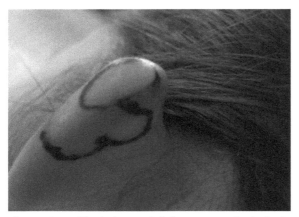

Figure 9.11 The lesion and defect are on the helical rim; the primary lobe is drawn slightly larger and the two lobes are undermined and moved into the defect

of the flap and secured to the remaining helix with a vertical mattress suture to allow good eversion and avoid notching of the rim. The rest of the flap is then sewn into place with routine simple interrupted sutures.

Bilobed flap
2-cm defects can be repaired with a bilobed flap. The donor site is the posterior surface, which can be extensively and easily undermined (Figure 9.11).

The technique for the bilobed flap is best and fully explained in the section on the nose below. The same technique is applied to the ear. Preferably, the helical cartilage is intact but it need not be. In the latter case, elongating and enlarging the donor lobe may be considered so as to provide enough donor flap to form a helical roll.

Grafts
Ensure intact perichondrium for grafts – not bare cartilage – or punch holes through the cartilage until it 'gives', which signals the junction between it and its perichondrium. Remove the plugs of cartilage and the perichondrium from the other side will grow through to nourish the graft.

Keys
1 Good blood supply to base
2 Haemostasis
3 Stab graft
4 Button suture
5 Pressure dressing

> **WARNING**
>
> Ears are prone to *Pseudomonas* infections and diabetics are especially prone with the distinct problem of a severe mastoiditis. The clinical clue to this is severe pain not commensurate with the appearance of the relatively mild inflammation of the external auditory meatus or tympanic membrane. This is a medical emergency. Consider covering all diabetic ear operations with ciprofloxacin, especially if cartilage is exposed, but treat immediately for 2 weeks.

Secondary intention – healing over bare cartilage
Healing of grafts or by secondary intention will not occur over bare cartilage (or bone), i.e. where the perichondrium/periostium has been removed. This can be fixed in the ear by punching through the (usually inner) ear cartilage to the perichondrium on the opposite (external) side (Figure 9.13). Granulation tissue then migrates through these holes to re-colonise the denuded (inner) cartilage.

The threat of *Pseudomonas* infections must always be kept in mind for the ear. The key is usually pain disproportionate to the clinical signs. In the case of surgery such signs are confused in any event. Chloramphenicol ointment is usually ineffective against *Pseudomonas* and systemic ciprofloxacin is needed.

Chondrodermatitis nodularis helices chronicus (CNH/CNC)
CNH presents as a solitary painful nodule up to 10 mm on the external ear. Although it is encountered mostly in middle-aged, sun exposed males' right (sleeping side) ears, it is considered a problem due to pressure and a derogatory cycle ensues where sleeping on the raised nodule exacerbates it.

Numerous treatments have been tried, including ear pads, cryosurgery, intralesional steroids, antibiotics, wedge resection, curettage and electrocautery, CO_2 laser ablation and excision. Excision of the nodule, although giving good results, frequently has recurrence at the edges. The current recommendation is to excise the nodule as well as the cartilage below and on both sides, smoothing such that no pressure point(s) remain. A scalpel has traditionally been used to do this, but a sharp curette also achieves an excellent result provided caution is exercised to prevent the curette incising rather than planing. The aim is to plane the cartilage to one smooth surface with no rises, falls, bumps or nodules, making it co-planar with, and indecipherable from, the continuing helical cartilage.

Technique
The aim is to excise the nodule and then the underlying cartilage.

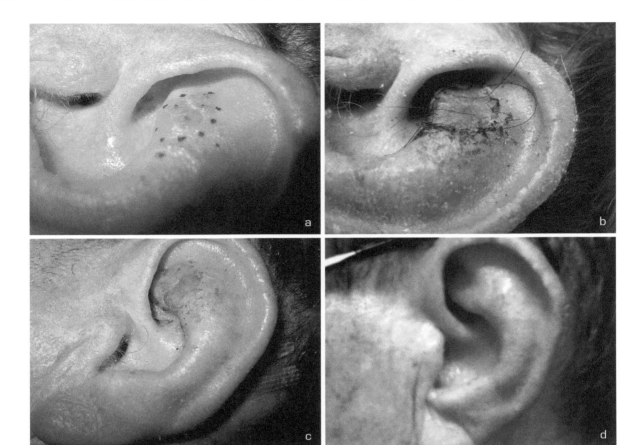

Figure 9.12 Skin graft to the ear

a The 'inside' of the ear is one site where a graft has to be done. The lesion, here on the crux of the anti-helix, is mapped and excised and a template made of the deficit. Haemostasis is secured. The template is transferred to the postauricular area and an exact copy made and excised to fill the deficit. **b** The graft is sutured in place, usually by alternating opposite sutures, entering through the graft first. These are left long so that they can tie across to each other, tethering the dressing in place. A central 'button suture' is stitched right through the ear to tether the centre of the graft down. Its depression can be seen in **c**. Lance or stab the graft to allow any fluid to escape so that it does not lift off the graft. A non-stick dressing the size of the graft with a pressure plug bolster gauze on top is then tied down. **c** Removal of sutures at 7 days. **d** 3 months post-op.

1 Infiltrate with 1%:200,000 adrenaline lignocaine.
2 Make a narrow ellipse around the nodule with a 15 blade scalpel.
3 Undermine both sides in the perichondrial plane to expose the cartilage.
4 Excise the nodule to a depth of 2–3 mm using curved (side up) scissors, a scalpel or a sharp 4-mm curette.
5 Smooth the cartilage surface to be co-planar (Figure 9.14). This may mean extending so that there is no obvious dip.
6 Close with 6/0 interrupted nylon sutures.
7 ROS 7 days with security strips.

Cure rates of 90.4% for helical lesions and 62.5% for anti-helical lesions have been recorded [5]. A 39% recurrence rate has been recorded with just nodule excision with a small bit of underlying cartilage [6].

Summary: Ear lesions

Most ear lesions can be excised by a simple ellipse.
Always insist on Mohs pathology to ensure margins and that there is no cartilage involvement.
A wedge resection can usually fix everything.
Use a banner flap for the anterior helix.
Use a graft or secondary intention inside the ear.

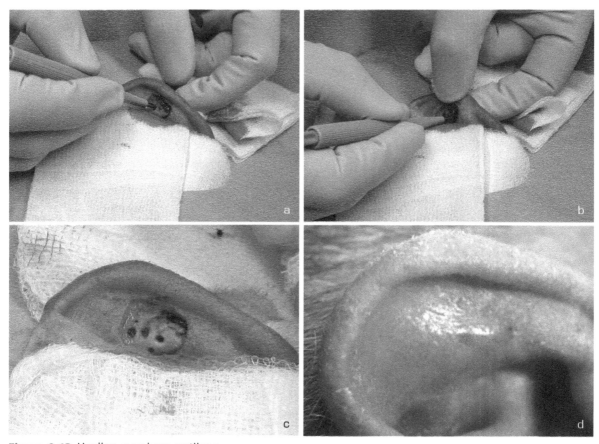

Figure 9.13 Healing over bare cartilage

a A 2-mm punch is pushed through the bare cartilage of the inner ear until it is felt to 'give'. The tube of cartilage is removed. **b** Holding the helix with the thumb and supporting the external ear surface with the index finger allows greater feel and control. Do not punch too hard – ensure the perichondrium is intact and not injured on the far side. **c** A number of holes are punched out to provide generous access for the viable external side perichondrium. An alginate dressing such as Kaltostat is cut to size and placed on the wound bed to promote coagulation. A non-stick dressing is placed over this pressure gauze. This is soaked off with normal saline in 1–3 days and the wound cleaned. Chloramphenicol ointment is then applied plus a non-stick dressing and changed regularly to prevent it drying out until healed. Healing can then be by secondary intention or a delayed graft applied. **d** 4 weeks later.

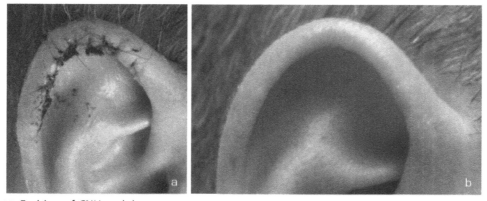

Figure 9.14 Excision of CNH nodule

a A simple ellipse is made around the nodule(s) and the cartilage is then planed flat. A scalpel, punch biopsy or sharp curette can be used. The aim is to smooth the cartilage flat so that there are no rises to create pressure points which are thought to be the aetiology. **b** Although many treatments are documented this simple ellipse and cartilage smoothing has consistently given good results such as this, even in patients who have suffered recurrences from other modes of treatment.

Nose

Although most people nominate other parts of their anatomy as the focus of their attention, it is my experience that more anguish is to be found in all patients with noses deformed by operations and grafts. It is, after all, our most prominent feature and the surgeon is obliged to perform the best cosmesis possible.

ESSENTIAL ANATOMY

The nasal subunits should be known and appreciated so as to provide the basis for planning excisions and flaps (see Figure 9.15). In general, if more than 50% of a subunit has to be excised then all of the subunit should be removed so as to best provide optimal camouflage with reconstruction. The greatest potential problem is the free margin of the ala/nares where contraction can cause deformity or extensive deep excision can cause ala collapse and airway obstruction (Figure 9.16).

NERVES AND ARTERIES

The sensory nerves and how to anaesthetise the nose with blocks are covered in Chapter 3, 'Local anaesthesia'. The author routinely blocks the infratrochlear, external nasal and maxillary nerves (Figure 9.17).

It is also my experience that the ala branch of the facial or lateral nasal artery winds around in the ala groove and forewarned is forearmed as it seems the most common vessel encountered. Have some absorbable tie-off sutures always ready for nasal surgery.

FLAPS VS GRAFTS

Many nose lesions can be excised by a simple ellipse but surgery on the nose has improved with the development of newer flaps. In the past, grafts were commonly used but they were invariably ugly and disfiguring and caused the patient ongoing embarrassment. Grafts, in the main, have now been superseded and should be avoided unless there is a very good reason. As a Mayo Clinic study concluded: 'For defects on the nose where flap and graft repair may both be technically possible, a flap may be more likely to result in superior cosmetic outcome' [7].

POSSIBLE OPERATIONS

The following are the most performed operations with the bilobed flap being most performed on the lower nose.

1 Simple ellipse
2 Wedge resection
3 Nasal banner flap
4 A-T flap
5 Cheek advancement flap
6 Note flap
7 Melo (naso)-labial flap
8 Bilobed transposition flap
9 Axial nasolabial flap
10 Dorsal nasal flap
11 Rhomboid flap
12 Graft
13 Secondary intention

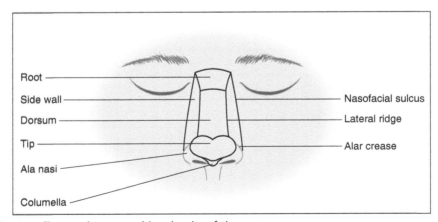

Figure 9.15 Contour lines and topographic subunits of the nose
Adapted from Roenigk R, Roenigk H (eds). Dermatologic Surgery, 2nd edn. New York: Marcel Dekker Inc, 1989; Fig 7.

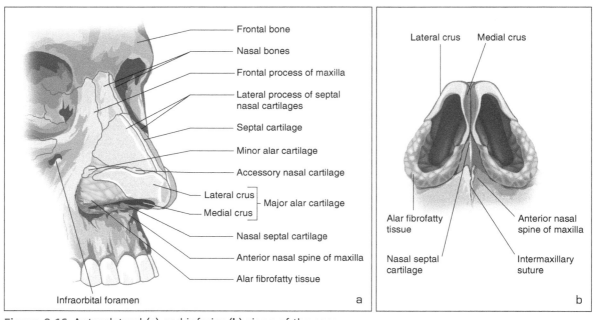

Figure 9.16 Anterolateral (**a**) and inferior (**b**) views of the nose
Adapted from Netter FH. Atlas of Human Anatomy, 5th edn. Philadelphia: Saunders, 2010.

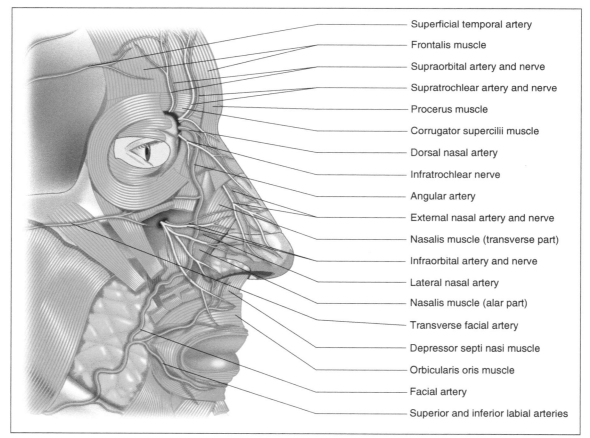

Figure 9.17 Nerves and arteries relevant to nasal surgery
Adapted from Hansen JT. Netter's Clinical Anatomy, 2nd edn. Philadelphia: Saunders, 2009.

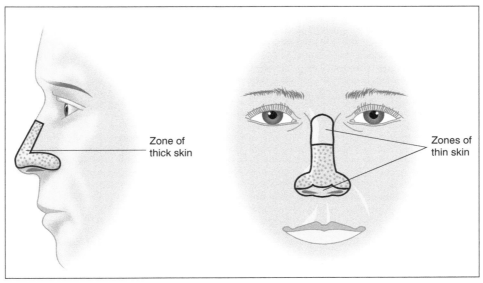

Figure 9.18 Upper and lower zones of skin on the nose

Undermining

In the main, undermining on the nose is done just above the perichondrium, which results in less bleeding than the more superficial intramuscular plane. This also incorporates the richly blood supplied muscle in the mobilised flap and ensures viability. The supra-perichondrial plane also affords the most tissue movement while minimising scar formation [8]. Some small nasal flaps may be undermined above the nasal musculature.

Nostril antibiotic ointment

A protein located on the bacterial surface of *Staphylococcus aureus* called clumping factor B (ClfB) has high affinity for the skin protein loricrin with the result that *S. aureus* persistently colonises about 20% of the nasal cavity of humans [9].

Decolonising of nasal carriers of *S. aureus*, by treatment with mupirocin nasal ointment and chlorhexidine soap, reduces the risk of *S. aureus* infection [10]. Given the increasing resistance of *S. aureus* to mupirocin (Bactroban®), the author now instils the nares/nostrils with chloramphenicol ointment preoperatively.

TWO SURGICAL AREAS

For excisions the nose divides into upper/top and lower areas (Figure 9.18).

1 Upper nose: the top has loose excess skin that can be moved for flaps.

2 Lower nose: the lower part is unique and needs special attention and techniques.

Upper nose

The glabella provides an area of loose skin that can be donated to most areas of the nose by a variety of flaps: simple transposition flap, rhomboid flap, nasal banner flap and A-T flap.

Simple transposition flap
Refer to Figure 9.19.

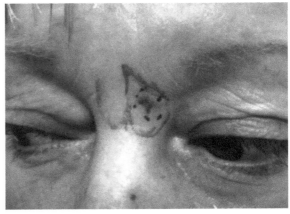

Figure 9.19 A simple transposition flap

Rhomboid flap

Rhomboid flaps on the nose or inner canthus are more like the simple transposition flap but drawing the plan makes the flap a rhomboid shape.

Although this is a modified rhomboid flap, any flap can be modified to suit the circumstance and situation. A transposition lobe, a banner or even an A-T flap would work equally well here.

Nasal banner flap

Refer to Figure 9.20.

A-T flap

With the emphasis on bilobed flaps an A-T may not be thought of as an option but works very well (Figure 9.21).

Lower nose

Repair of the nasal tip and lower third of the nose is particularly difficult. The lower nose is unique with thick pilosebaceous tissue conferring an inelastic texture not found elsewhere and with no RSTL, that can be either difficult or useful (or both) to disguise reconstruction scars. The main problem is preventing alar deformity from contraction or even alar collapse and airway closure. Just the slightest narrowing of the nostril can make breathing difficult. The lateral alar is composed of unique, firm connective tissue that lacks cartilage. It is its own inherent strength that maintains the patency of the nostril and the nasal valve.

Nasal skin gets looser the more superior and this fact must be utilised.

Options include:

- simple ellipse
- asymmetrical ellipse
- wedge
- single-lobe transposition flaps
  – note
  – nasolabial banner
  – advancement
- bilobed flap
- trilobed flap
- dorsal nasal flap
- forehead flap.

Asymmetrical ellipse

This technique is possible where the lesion is to one side of the nasal tip. One incision is made straight to align with the centre of the columella. The incisions on the other side are two tangents from the proximal end of the incision to the mid-point of the lesion and then to the distal end of the incision (Figure 9.22).

Note flap

This is the simplest of the lobe flaps and looks like a musical note. It is a good flap for closing an alar defect with a piece of cheek skin. The apex of the V cheek skin is trimmed to fit the defect (Figure 9.23). There is very little difference between this and the banner flap.

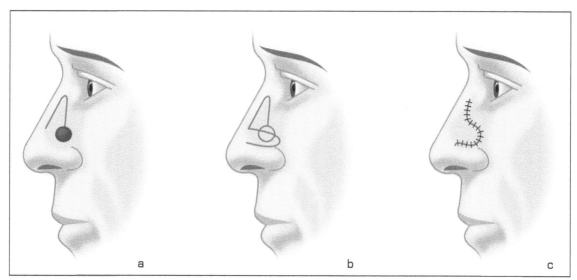

Figure 9.20 Nasal banner flap
a The lesion is excised. A triangle is marked such that the base is wide enough to provide a flap that will cover the defect. **b** The superior donor defect is widely undermined and closed. The elevated flap is then rotated to cover the defect. There will be tension at the pivot point and this can be undermined, but be careful not to undermine the base and compromise the flap blood supply. Trim the excess skin and fit the flap into the defect. **c** The resultant scar is often difficult to see.

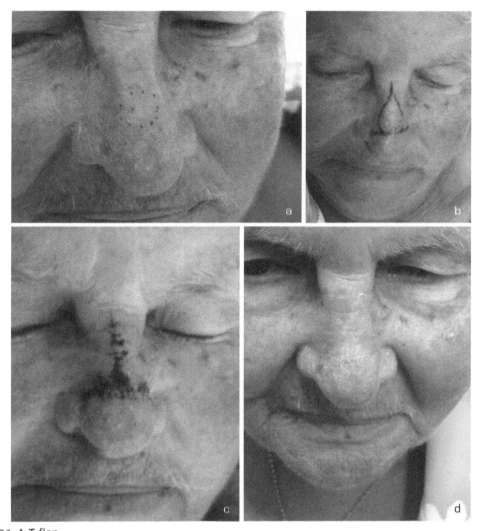

Figure 9.21 A-T flap

a A nodular BCC. **b** With 4 mm margins this leaves a relatively big deficit to try and close. The horizontal arm is sited in the natural sulcus between the mid nose and the tip. By raising and mobilising the lateral edges of the nose flaps with extensive undermining they come together. **c** 7 days later at ROS. Excision complete. **d** 14 days post-op an acceptable cosmetic result. Certainly better than a graft.

Melo (naso)-labial banner flap

This flap is excellent for alar defects as it preserves the lateral part of the alar groove (Figure 9.24). The secondary defect scar hides in the cosmetic boundary between the cheek and the nose. It also provides a very good blood supply.

See also the section 'Banner flap' under 'Single lobe flap' in Chapter 8, 'Flaps'.

Advancement flap

Refer to Figure 9.25.

Bilobed flap

The bilobed flap consists of two cone-shaped flaps that share a pedicle. It recruits the loose skin of the proximal nose to transpose and rotate into defects of the nasal tip and ala. The first (donor site) flap is moved into the excised defect and the second flap is moved into the donor site (see Figure 9.26). There is considerable rotation in moving these lobes, and knowing this and understanding the pivot point and restraint is critical and helpful as to undermining and achieving tissue mobility. As this is the most performed operation on the distal nose it is covered here in detail.

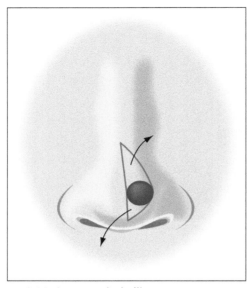

Figure 9.22 Asymmetrical ellipse

The use of a bilobed flap is indicated for lesions less than 1.5 cm in diameter when the tissue adjacent to a cutaneous defect is insufficiently mobile to close the defect without causing tissue distortion.

The **key** is wide undermining as far as possible towards the glabella and inner canthus so as to equally distribute tension over both lobes with the apical lobe pointed vertically so that, when sutured, it does not pull the lower lobes up (leading to ala deformities). It is a one-stage procedure that can be performed with local anaesthesia and provides predictable functional as well as good aesthetic results. The colour match is excellent and the flap reliable with few complications.

Although particularly used for defects on the distal nose, this technique can be used elsewhere (chin, lateral cheek, hand, posterior ear) [11]. The bilobed flap can be used instead of most other repairs and flaps for the nasal ala, distal nose and nasal tip where skin is less mobile, supplying matching skin and a better cosmetic result than grafts where colour matching is the main problem.

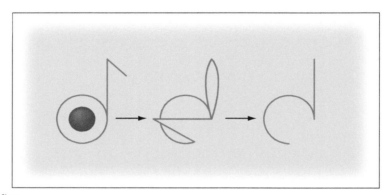

Figure 9.23 Note flap

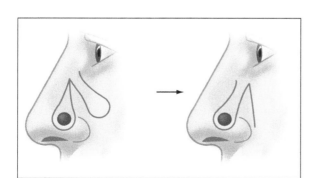

Figure 9.24 Melo (naso)-labial banner flap

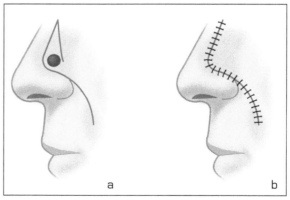

Figure 9.25 Advancement flap

a An elegant flap for lesions above the ala is to draw a cone towards the glabella/inner canthus with the lower incision following the ala and nasolabial groove. **b** There is some suggestion that this may depress the ala and some surgeons curve the ala incision as per the thinner lines.

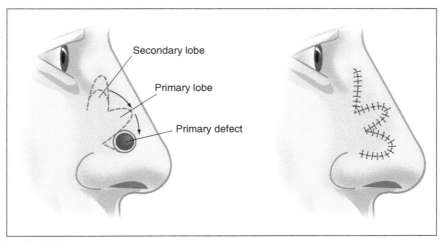

Figure 9.26 A bilobed flap
Adapted from a drawing by David Low, MD.

The base of the flap is placed laterally on the side wall of the nose for nasal tip defects, whereas the base is medial or central on the dorsum of the nose for repairing ala defects. The modified bilobed flap (designed by Moy) is an excellent choice for reconstruction defects of the lower nose because of the good skin match and low incidence of complications [12].

Larger defects can pose a problem because of the limited amount of lax donor skin from the upper nose. If 4-mm margins are taken, as they should be unless slow Mohs is done, this means, in effect, that only lesions <7 mm are suitable. With experience, however, by increasing the number of lobes and extensive undermining, larger lesions can be excised and repaired this way (see the section 'Trilobed flap' below).

The bilobed flap cannot place incisions in RSTL or between cosmetic units; the nasal tip doesn't have such units or lines. The fact that the flap uses adjoining like skin, however, can (and should) lead to excellent cosmetic results.

Where the skin thickens to become pilosebaceous is not a definite line. With a bilobed flap this thick sebaceous skin can 'bulldoze' or push down the ipsilateral (inferior) ala margin. This can be minimised by pointing the tertiary defect towards the medial canthus (see Figure 9.27). The skin on the upper dorsum and sides of the nose is thin and loose and provides an excellent reservoir for flap donation.

It is usually best suited for defects less than 1 cm, although it may be useful up to 1.5 cm if located on the middle or lower third of the nose in patients who have mobile proximal loose skin for the secondary lobe. Defects larger than 1.5 cm and on the distal nasal tip or ala, or arising on patients with rigid sebaceous nasal skin, present problems especially ala rim distortion. For the latter the trilobed flap is recommended

The nasal alae are supplied by the maxillary nerve and can usually be anaesthetised with a maxillary nerve block.

Bilobed flap on the nose

ADVANTAGES
- One stage
- Supply of sufficient tissue to sebaceous distal nose defects
- Predictable viability
- Good aesthetics
- Good colour match
- Good function
- Few complications

POTENTIAL PROBLEMS
- Not advised for defects >1.5 cm
- Distortion of tip symmetry (especially if the defect is <10 mm from the alar margin)
- Trapdoor defect (depression)/pin-cushioning (elevation)
- Bulldozing (depression of the ipsilateral alar rim)
- Scars difficult to camouflage in RSTL

Technique
Some advocate meticulous planning with measuring and arcs, but in practice these are somewhat pedantic, complicating and unnecessary measures. Some also advocate excising the lesion and the Burow's triangle/cone as separate procedures. Again, this is unnecessary and this whole

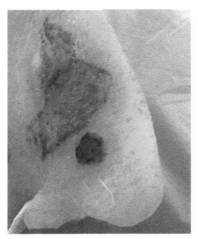

Figure 9.27 Bilobed flap sequence: 1) area outlined in red is excised; 2) green moves to red; 3) blue moves to green; 4) a third vertical lobe (if necessary) moves to blue

Black spot = cancer to be excised; red tear drop = excision margins (apex points medially and slightly up if possible); area from cancer to apex = Burow's triangle; red area after excision = primary defect; green = primary lobe; green area after excision = secondary defect; blue = secondary lobe; blue area after excision = tertiary defect.

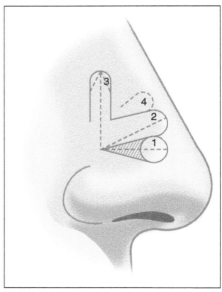

Figure 9.28 Alternative plans for a bilobed flap

1 = Excision defect; Burow's triangle cross-hatched = cone excised to prevent dog-ears (1–1.5 times the width of excision); 2 = donor flap, 90–100% the width of the excised defect but 10–20% longer than 1; 3 = second flap, 80–85% the width of 1 but 45–55% longer; apical dashes = arrow/extended ellipse/mitre hat – an often used plan; 4 otherwise, the third lobe runs off the second lobe to form a lower case 'm'.

section can be excised as one (i.e. lesion and cone, as demarcated in red in Figure 9.27). Furthermore, the Burow's triangle orientates the excision.

Initially, the length of the cone may need to be measured but, in practice, it is pretty obvious what the desired length is (as long as possible without exceeding the cosmetic nose unit). Placement should either use the ala groove as the lower margin or, if further caudal, angle the lower arm of the Burow's triangle slightly up to help reduce the pull on the free ala margin. Similarly, the donor flap can be drawn slightly larger without recourse to measures or arcs. The basic concept of three ice-cream cones prescribing a lower case 'm' at the free margin to be excised is the picture to keep in mind when planning and drawing, but then angle the top lobe as far towards the glabella or vertically as possible.

In essence:

1 Draw the edge of the lesion and the margins to be excised (Figure 9.28). Draw a cone horizontal or, preferably, one angled slightly upwards (cranial) that is 1.5 times longer than the excision.

2 Draw a second arc as a tangent from just above the centre of the excision circle and slightly larger and longer and more medial. This will be the primary donor flap that moves across into the excision defect.

3 Draw a third arc some 80% smaller than the second lobe. This should be pointed as vertically as possible.

It will be the second donor lobe. By making it considerably longer (50%) there will be enough skin to fill the defect but may have to be trimmed. Designing this as an ellipse or a pointed inverted 'V' makes it easier to close.

4 Excise the lesion with its cone. This invariably bleeds profusely on the distal nose from both the edges (the subdermal plexus) and the base. Bipolar cautery is most helpful but pressure, pressure and more pressure for 10 minutes without lifting to look works wonders.

5 Excise the other two lobes, lift and undermine.

6 Undermine and undermine – down to the nasal cheek border and as high as possible proximally.

7 Move the primary donor lobe into the excise defect. If there is a shortfall or tension, go back and undermine where it is pulling at the base until it meets and fits.

8 Although some advocate trimming and closing the proximal lobe first, it is my practice to secure this donor lobe first. My rationale is that this is the all-important cosmetic area, which the patient wants done best and will judge the surgery by, whereas the proximal lobe can be trimmed and altered 'as and when' (i.e. tidied up last).

Suture placement

- 1st suture: close the tertiary (ellipse) side to side – a mattress suture ensures eversion but is not necessary.
- 2nd suture: align the donor flap in the defect.
- 3rd suture: align the secondary lobe in the donor site.

Resume bilobed flap

Refer to Figure 9.29.

- Base the pedicle laterally (outside) in most cases.
- Plan as an arc.
- Point the primary defect horizontally or superiorly to avoid 'bulldozing'.

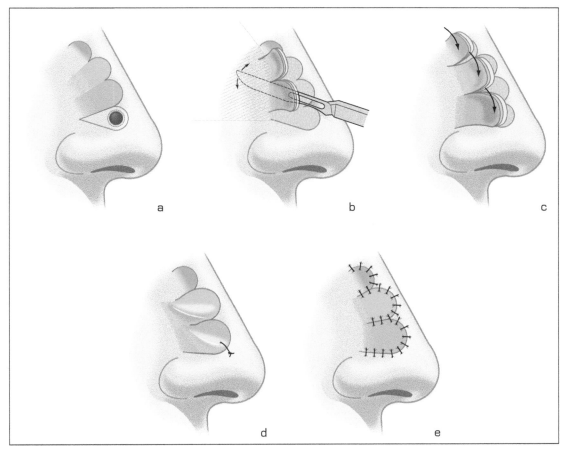

Figure 9.29 Resume bilobed flap

a The bi- or trilobed flap is mapped out. The lobes have been coloured for demonstration. The margins of the cancer (black spot) are dotted or inked in a solid line in red and adequate margins for excision are drawn (here as a red tear drop). The tear-drop excision consists of the actual excision of the cancer plus a cone or tail medially. This prevents dog-ear formation. If possible, the apex and lower margin should point slightly caudal to minimise ala pull. The green primary donor flap is made slightly larger than the red excision site. The proximal smaller lobe(s) progressively point towards the glabella or medial canthus. Here (coloured orange), the actual excision was made more vertical. **b** With only the lesion and (green) primary donor flap excised there is significant shortfall, rotation and tension. To free and mobilise, all of the donor lobes (green, blue, orange) are extensively undermined down to the nasal-cheek border and as far up into the inner canthus as one's experience allows. **c** These are then rotated into the excised defects. The sebaceous thick fatty layer of the primary donor lobe (green) may have to be thinned to prevent tip distortion (pin-cushioning). It is essential, however, that some blood-supplying fat is left attached to the skin. **d** Some surgeons advocate closing the proximal (orange) lobe first but the author has found a tethering first suture at the point of maximum tension for the primary donor lobe provides the essential information as to: 1) if it fits; 2) if it fills the defect or if there is a shortfall (and more undermining is needed); or 3) if there is too much tension with ala pull and elevation. **e** The lobes are now sutured. It is silly to be didactic. Each lobe may need an initial tethering suture to site and position it, which then allows the rest of the sutures to be placed as dictated by the lobe's architecture and needs.

- Make Burow's triangle long. Place above the ala groove or use as inferior margin.
- Minimise angle of transposition between flaps.
- Donor site lobe 100%, then 90%, then 80%.
- Make donor lobe longer and the secondary (apical) lobe a 50% longer ellipse.
- Point incision to between the inner canthus and the bridge of the nose or make it vertical.
- Thin flap – leave some/just enough fat but thin to prevent pin-cushioning.
- Trim and shape this apical ellipse to fit the primary defect.
- Align the lobes to prevent potential distortion.
- Undermine as far as possible, especially superiorly but also inferiorly and at the pivot area.
- Undermine just above the perichondrium.
- Suture in the above order.
- Consider nasal instillation of antibiotic ointment.

> **NOTE**
>
> With a punch biopsy only some 1–2% of the lesion is examined. With an excision some 30–40% is examined with the normal 'bread-loafing' pathology technique. This means some 70% is missed. It is the author's practice to always request Mohs pathology, which examines all margins, both lateral and deep, for any cancer on the face. The margins for lentigo maligna are notoriously difficult to find macroscopically; SCCs of the lip and ear have a very high metastatic rate and recurrences are more difficult to treat.

Improvements

Understanding the evolution of these design improvements and their application ensures a better result.

Esser first described the bilobed flap to repair nasal tip defects in 1918 [13]. This original design had two flaps of identical size at right angles to each other, which resulted in pin-cushioning (elevation) or trapdoor deformity (depression) and dog-ears. Zimany (1953) [14] is generally credited with popularising the use of the bilobed flap and showed the second cone could be smaller [14]. Zitelli (1989) [15] and Moy et al. (1994) [12] improved Esser's design and cosmetic results by making the lobes not identical in size but still of the same length and, importantly, making the angles between the lobes much reduced to even approximate a straight line with extensive undermining to reduce tension and pin-cushioning effect. Zitelli recommended wide undermining and dermabrasion 6 weeks after surgery if needed. Increasing the number of lobes reduces the angle even further, so that it is almost a straight line, and directing

this to a point between the bridge of the nose and inner canthus.

The cone extending from the actual round excision is a Burow's triangle. This was a deliberate modification to prevent a dog-ear deformity. Based on the location of the lesion it is based medially or laterally and extends 1–1.5 times the defect diameter. Lateral based cones are best directed towards the medial canthus and sited just above the ala groove. The ala groove is a fibrous band and involving or including it leads to bulldozing; however, it may provide a margin anchor that can be utilised. That is, the Burow's triangle/standing cone should not have this ala grooved sited in its middle but it may provide an already established margin for this triangle.

The Burow's triangle should be made as long as possible without encroaching on the cheek, which facilitates better movement of the flap.

Angle of lobe rotation

This can be individually adjusted to suit the patient. For a smaller area of transportation, movement is easier and there is less resulting tension. Design using small angles of <60° (50°) between the flaps to confine all scars within a small area.

Flap blood supply

The nose has a luxurious blood supply so flap necrosis should not occur. The reason it might is when the donor flap is trimmed of fat to prevent pin-cushioning but too much fat is taken and the essential subdermal plexus is cut off.

Hence, undermine leaving fat (i.e. raise the flap just deep to the subdermal plexus, leaving a small amount of subdermal fat on the undersurface of the flap).

> **HINTS AND TIPS**
>
> Thin the flap but always leave some fat.

Haemostasis

Stretch the bleeding area, then apply a gauze or cotton tip. Place the bipolar on either side of the bleeding point and/or apply pressure for 10–15 minutes without looking. Know the relevant anatomy. The lateral nasal branch of the facial artery seems to wind around the base of the lateral ala and, if working in this area, have some tie-off sutures and artery clamps ready.

Postoperative details

Scar dermabrasion can be used after surgery at 6 weeks to improve the cosmetic result.

Follow-up

Remove permanent cutaneous sutures 5–7 days after surgery.

Complications and prevention

1 Shortfall prevention and pivotal restraint

Dzubow's principle: any flap transposed or rotated around a pivot point will be tethered at the base of the pedicle [16]. What this means practically is that, as the flap is rotated towards the defect, the distance from the pivot point effectively decreases and it will fall short. This can lead to a gap between the leading edge of the primary flap and the distal edge of the defect. To close this gap requires a combination of further stretching, mobilisation and undermining, all of which have the potential to distort and can lead to retraction of the ala. A suggested modification to avoid this is to lengthen the primary lobe [17]. Note, however, that a large(r) flap can lead to trapdooring. The ultimate flap is one that just fits the defect with enough pull on the sutured edges to minimise trapdooring but does not cause a shortfall, undue tension or ala elevation. A slightly bigger flap can always be trimmed whereas, if it is too small, the aforementioned complications are encountered.

The primary donor flap should never be smaller than the excision site. One way to ensure this is to draw an arc pivoted on the apex of the primary cone. If the primary flap is then extended to the margins of this arc of rotation, it actually becomes longer than the primary defect. When it is rotated into the primary defect, the pivot point tethers it so that, unless it is designed on this arc, it will fall short. Making it slightly larger has much to recommend it.

2 Compromised blood supply

Thinning, if necessary to prevent pin-cushioning, should be done carefully leaving some fat and subdermal plexus so as not to compromise the blood supply.

Long length-to-width ratios increase the likelihood of tip necrosis because of inadequate perfusion, but this is unlikely on the nose as it is so well supplied with blood.

3 Trapdoor prevention

It is thought that scar contraction pushes the flap up. Wide undermining of all skin surrounding the flaps, including the area well beyond the base of the flap/pivot point and surrounds, creates a uniform area of contraction that doesn't push the flap up. Undermine widely beyond the base of the flap. This cannot be overemphasised in the pursuit of excellent flap performance. Wide undermining creates a uniform 'plate-like scar' and, therefore, does not push the flap tissue up [18]. De-fat the flap but take care to leave some fat for the subdermal plexus blood supply.

Slightly undersize the flap to prevent bunching but not enough to cause tension. Excess tension can increase the risk of flap necrosis at the edges. Secure contact between the flap base and the recipient site. As with grafts, this can best be obtained with an absorbable or buttonhole suture. Make sure this runs along the same axis as the flap/blood vessels and does not cut off any blood supply. Minimise transport/movement. Everting sutures may also help. Inferiorly based flaps facilitate better lymphatic drainage. Use straight lines and geometric angles and avoid curvilinear lines wherever possible to minimise circumferential contraction around the flap. Orient or position the flap to allow good lymphatic drainage and prevent lymphoedema. Pin-cushioning, rather than divot defects (trapdooring), is more common on the distal flap.

4 Dog-ears

These occur when flap lobes are transposed. A Burow's triangle included in the flap design at the base of the defect eliminates this complication.

Two other methods can be used to repair dog-ear defects. Excess tissue can be excised from the flap base, or it may be excised from the skin adjacent to the flap (Figure 9.30). Some believe that the cosmetic result is superior when tissue is excised adjacent to the flap because it breaks up the long, inferior scar line.

5 Ala pull

Ala pull or elevation can be minimised when the final lobe, as well as being longer (to be trimmed), also points vertically or towards the inner canthus so that, when sutured, the closed incision is perpendicular to the ala-free margin thus minimising pull (Figure 9.31). This lobe is usually cut as a pointed ellipse longer than the secondary defect that it moves to fill (i.e. it is longer and more

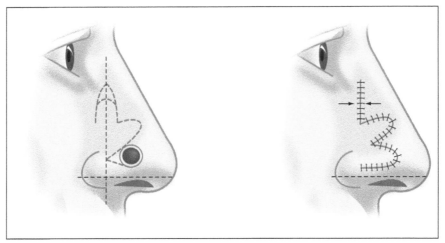

Figure 9.30 Three possible orientations for the excision of the dog-ear redundancy that will result from flap motion

By selecting a more superiorly oriented excision, the surgeon will minimise the likelihood of alar distortion. The arrows indicate flap motion.
(Adapted from a drawing by David Low, MD)

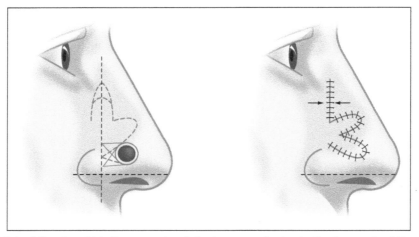

Figure 9.31 A bilobed flap in which the secondary lobe is perpendicular to the long axis of the ala margin

When the tertiary defect is closed on the nasal sidewall, the primary vectors of tension (arrows) are thus perpendicular to the alar margin, where they are unlikely to vertically distort this margin.
(Adapted from a drawing by David Low, MD)

pointed than the defect and as such has to be shaped and trimmed to fit).

Ala pull is also minimised if the axis of the cone (Burow's triangle) points horizontally or even upwards; then it does not create as much pull on the inferior margin, which in turn can pull and elevate the ala rim.

Good cosmesis
Good to excellent cosmetic results are obtainable (Figure 9.32).

Trilobed flap
The bilobed flap has limitations for larger lesions (>1.5 cm), with sebaceous skin and for the distal tip or ala. The trilobed flap addresses these problems and can facilitate a better result by increasing the range of the bilobed flap.

In the trilobed flap the secondary and tertiary lobes are made smaller. The angle of rotation should only be 45–50°, which reduces the pivotal torque. The third lobe proximal skin provides more mobility of the lobes to fill

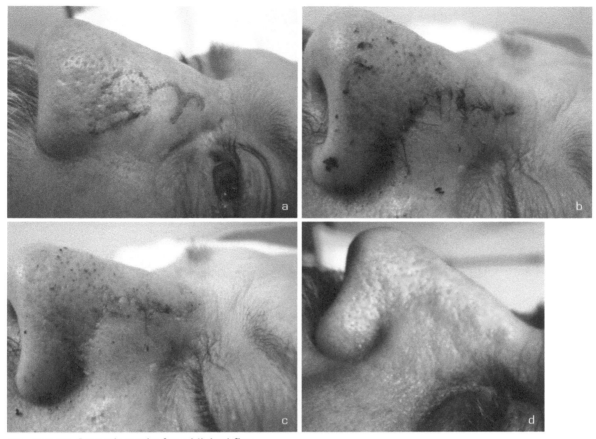

Figure 9.32 Cosmetic results for a bilobed flap
a Nodular BCC L distal nose. **b** 6 days post-op. **c** 6 days ROS. **d** 14 days post-op.

the distal defect (Figure 9.33). This reduces the tension and potential pin-cushioning and allows the tertiary lobe to be closed directly (side by side). This tertiary lobe (incision) should be at right angles to the horizontal or may point towards the medial canthus, which reduces the potential for ala rim elevation (Figure 9.34).

The secondary and tertiary lobes (and hence their defects) are usually best at 85% to 90% and 75% to 80%, respectively, of the diameter of the primary lobe. A smaller secondary and tertiary lobe size allows better tension on these lobes, which helps reduce pin-cushioning and also allows direct closure of the tertiary defect.

On the distal nose the bilobed flap can lead to ipsilateral ala depression with contralateral ala elevation but the trilobed flap can rectify these problems.

Wide undermining is essential to facilitate mobility of the lobes [19].

The trilobed flap allows the 45–50° per lobe rotation to be maintained, reducing bulldozing while keeping a favorable Burow's triangle orientation and horizontal tertiary lobe tension vector.

Dorsal and nasal sidewall nasal flaps – DNF (Reiger) and NAR

The dorsal and nasal sidewall flaps are not described here as they are not recommended for clinic or rooms procedures. Most proponents recommend sedation of the patient if local anaesthesia is used as the extensive elevation and undermining warrants this. The flap incision cuts through the ipsilateral branches of the angular artery; hence, the flap must be supplied by the contralateral branches of the angular artery, which run in the muscle layer. The preservation and incorporation of the contralateral angular artery also makes this a more risky procedure for one's rooms.

GRAFTS

Grafts are sometimes unavoidable. The aim is to achieve the best cosmetic result as to colour and texture match. The very best match, especially for the lower nose pilosebaceous skin, is from the concha of the ear. This is, in fact, the only other area of pilosebaceous skin. The donor

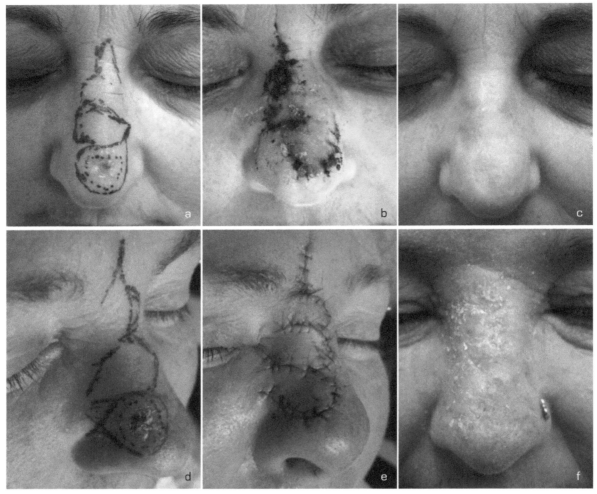

Figure 9.33 Trilobed flaps for primary defects on the nasal tip

a The preliminary plan for a trilobed flap for a significant lesion of the nasal tip. The third lobe was actually extended up the glabella crease. **b** At ROS. Note how the glabella crease has been used and how it is not then seen postoperatively. **c** 4 weeks later. She was advised to come back for dermabrasion (often recommended at 6 weeks), which would have improved the lower right edge somewhat but she went away for a year and, nevertheless, was delighted with the result and avoiding a graft. **d** Another large but lateral tip BCC. **e** Extensive tri-lobed flap elevation, large donor lobe and undermining. **f** 6 months later. No ala lift. Satisfactory cosmetic result – better than a graft. Trilobed flaps facilitate greater mobility and, as here, avoid ala lift, which would have occurred with a bilobed flap.

site is then left to heal by secondary intention. The use of chloramphenicol ointment is recommended as the ear is prone to infections, especially in diabetics, with *Pseudomonas* needing to be identified and treated early. Again, the key is pain not commensurate with appearance and the treatment is ciprofloxacin – urgently.

Other areas are used but, as seen in Chapter 11, 'Grafts', they invariably end in a poor cosmetic result. Post- and preauricular skin is mostly used.

It is essential that no hair is inadvertently harvested in the graft.

One advantage of grafts is that they allow for slow Mohs: the site is left open, then freshened up when clearance is reported, and the graft can then be taken and sutured in place.

Nasal grafts are usually able to be secured by button sutures through the nose to maximise take.

Refer to Chapter 11, 'Grafts', for further details.

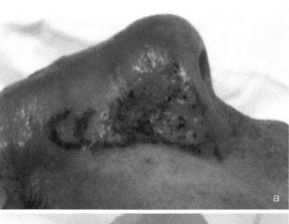
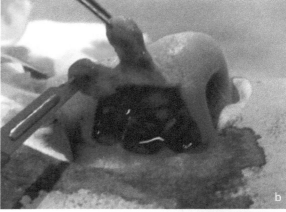
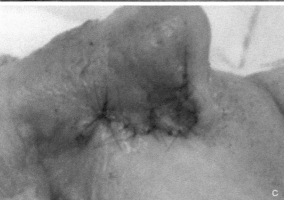
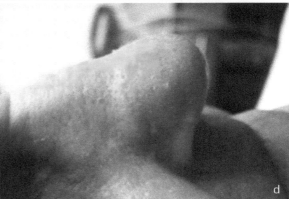

Figure 9.34 Trilobed flap for a primary defect close to the alar edge
a Although the base was originally drawn laterally, with time to plan this was altered to medial. **b** It would be hard to get much closer to the ala edge but, even with the need to resect involved cartilage (Mohs), this proved possible. **c** Clearance was complete and there was no airways incontinence or ala distortion. **d** A satisfactory result and certainly better than an ugly graft. Finally, while the incisions between the lobes can be quite long, as here, the good blood supply of the nose and the wide base, as in **b**, allows this.

SECONDARY INTENTION HEALING

The conventional wisdom is that secondary intention healing works well on concave but not convex surfaces. On the nose the concern is that scar contraction will lead to retraction of the ala tip. Nevertheless, secondary intention healing may be considered for small, non-perforating defects on the distal, sebaceous third of the nose. The ala groove obviously lends itself to such a technique and, in any event, is a difficult area to repair to maintain the groove. The placement of purse-string absorbable subcutaneous sutures to elongate the defect to a narrower ellipse has been found to be arguably better than secondary intention alone. This also recreates the groove and allows monitoring of the ala tip when they are placed [20].

In addition, however, secondary intention healing may similarly cautiously be tried on selected patients on the convex surface of the ala (Figure 9.35). Many older patients want to avoid the protracted time (many find it difficult to lie down for an hour or so), inconvenience or expense of a bilobed flap and prefer to try secondary intention to an unsightly graft. In a small series by the author of 10 cases, the majority healed well and only one had minor ala retraction, which was of no concern to the patient. A secondary intention excision is usually smaller than a bilobed defect. A modified improvement to this

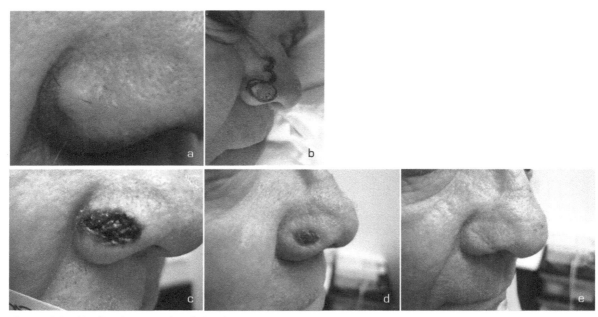

Figure 9.35 Healing by secondary intention

a A nodular BCC on the convex surface of the right alar, interestingly with two hairs growing out of it. The skin was thick, sebaceous and adherent/not easily mobilised. Compare the alar groove now and 2 months postoperatively (**e**).

b The original plan was for a bilobed flap but at excision the site would not stop bleeding in sheets. He had had pre-operative assessment and denied any anticoagulation but, finally, on specific interrogation, admitted to 25 years of high dose fish oil daily. An extensive operation was impossible, and it was felt this would lead to ala retraction and the patient elected for plan B, healing by secondary intention.

c 1 week later. This defect could have been even smaller as the Burow's triangle (to prevent dog-ear) had been excised for the bilobed flap.

d 3 weeks post-op.

e 2 months post-op. Good cosmesis. No ala retraction. In addition, this is in effect slow Mohs and allows the patient time to think about their options (e.g. ceasing the fish oil and proceeding to a flap).

is to purse-string suture the ellipse, thus reducing the central defect to heal faster.

Technique

1 Smear the nostrils with chloramphenicol, local anaesthetic or a maxillary block.
2 Margins for slow Mohs are for 1-mm visual clearance, thus less than the 4-mm for a non-Mohs excision.
3 Mark and orientate the lesion for slow Mohs.
4 Haemostasis is with bipolar cautery.
5 Monosyn 5/0 subcutaneous sutures can be used to narrow the ends to form a smaller defect and duplicate the natural groove/lines but, in doing so, the ala rim must be observed so that it is not pulled or elevated in any way.
6 Chloramphenicol is placed in the defect base.
7 Then an alginate such as Kaltostat is trimmed to fit the defect.
8 A non-stick dressing is applied to cover wide of the defect.
9 Gauze folded to make a pad is then strapped over this with Fixomull tape.

Inform the patient of the risk of ala retraction and poor cosmesis and the option to proceed with a flap or graft.

The result of the Mohs pathology may dictate further surgery.

Lip

Every practitioner knows the sensory cortical representation of the lips and they assume the same importance in society for both beauty and function. Lip surgery requires the best cosmetic result possible with meticulous apposition of vermilion border and is complicated by the labial artery (Figure 9.36).

Note that the upper lip includes the skin below the nose and the lower lip includes the skin down to the horizontal skin (chin) crease. The vermilion border is the mucocutaneous junction between the skin and the dry mucosa or vermilion of the lip. It is all-important to precisely align and reconstruct any disruption to this border.

ANATOMY

Musculature

The basic muscle of the lip is the striated orbicularis oris, which forms a sphincter around the mouth. Some of the fibres run horizontally in the lower lip to form the protrusion of the vermilion. Although most run longitudinally, some fibres are anterior caudal to force the lips against the teeth. The philtral columns are where these longitudinal (horizontal) fibres intersect with vertical fibres. Three other muscle groups work in concert with the orbicularis oris:

- The labial elevators: zygomaticus major and minor and levator labii superioris alaeque nasi, levator anguli oris and the risorius.
- The labial depressors: depressor labii inferioris, depressor angulii oris or triangularis and the mantalis, which also forces the lower lip against the gum by drawing the lip upwards.
- Buccal muscle: forms most of the cheek and forces the cheek against the teeth.

Vasculature

The facial artery ascends from the neck over the mid body of the mandible just anterior to the insertion of the masseter muscle and branches into an inferior and a superior labial artery, which course beneath the orbicularis oris and anastomose with the contralateral vessel. The facial artery then ascends in the nasolabial groove as the angular artery, forming branches to the nasal ala and anastomosing with the dorsal nasal artery. The facial and labial arteries communicate with the subdermal plexus through a dense population of musculocutaneous perforators. A high variability was found in cadaveric dissections, and measurements showed that it is difficult to determine the position of these vessels in surgical reconstruction or when planning cosmetic procedures [21]:

- The **labial arteries** are consistently located between the obicularis oris and the mucosal surface of the lip near the free edge of the lip. Some surgeons ligate the relevant vessel on either side of the lesion prior to excision.
- The **superior labial artery** was a single vessel in all cases and usually found within 10 mm of the free margin of the upper lip [22]. At the oral commissure the vessel was superior to the vermilion border in 94% of the dissections. At the midline the vessel was within the vermilion border in 75% of dissections. The vessel was found within the orbicularis oris in 19% of dissections and between the mucosa and the orbicularis oris in 81% of dissections.
- The **inferior labial artery** was a single vessel in all dissections. Its course was variable in position relative to the vermilion border and to its take-off from the facial artery some 2.6 cm lateral and 1.5 cm inferior to the oral commissure. In the central portion of the lip the vessel was found within the orbicularis oris in 13% of dissections and between the mucosa and the orbicularis oris in 87% of dissections where it runs in the posterior of the lower lip, just under the mucosa, at the level of the (anterior) vermilion border.

Nerves

The infraorbital branch of the trigeminal nerve supplies sensation to the upper lip while the mental branch supplies the lower lip. The facial nerve provides motor innervation. Injury to the facial nerve motor innervation is rare as supply is from the deep aspect.

PRINCIPLES OF LIP SURGERY

- Cosmesis: ensure meticulous alignment of the vermilion border. Retain normal contours especially with respect to the philtra and cupid's bow.
- Undermining is difficult in the philtral area and is done superficial to the muscle.
- Ligation of the labial artery may be necessary. Some surgeons do this prophylactically.
- Damage to subdermal hair follicles in the upper and lower lip should be avoided in males.
- Layered anatomic closure is important to avoid dead space.
- Muscle and mucosa can be 'cobbled'.
- Use braided absorbable sutures deep but 5/0, 6/0 nylon for the mucosal surface/skin.
- Make incisions at junctions of natural boundaries (e.g. vermilion border, nasolabial fold, horizontal chin crease).

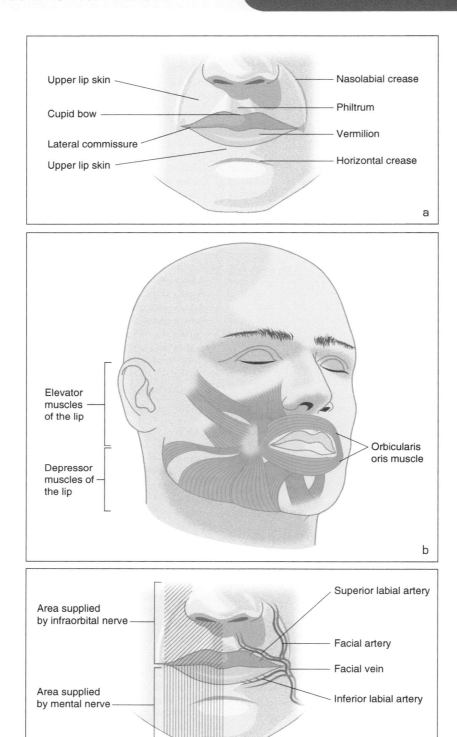

Figure 9.36 Lip

a Topical anatomy of the lip. **b** Basic musculature of the lip. The orbicularis oris muscle provides the bulk musculature of the lip proper. **c** Vascular and nerve supply to the lip and perioral area.

Adapted from Roenigk R, Roenigk H (eds). Dermatologic Surgery, 2nd edn. New York: Marcel Dekker Inc, 1989; Figs 1, 2, 3.

- Consider inter-oral incisions: mucosal advancement flap red (to red never to white skin).
- Mark vermilion border with sutures before excising so as to ensure exact match. Marking pens often wipe off.
- Nerve blocks are best. Local infiltration can then be used for haemostasis.
- Excisions may be wider than 45° rather than the usual ellipse of 30°, which allows for shorter, 'fatter' ellipses that may not have to intrude or cross the vermilion border and come together well (Figure 9.37).

- One-third of the lip can be excised as a wedge; larger defects require flaps (Figure 9.38).
- Wedge resections of the lip should cross the vermilion border at 90° if possible. Do not extend below the horizontal chin crease.
- Nasolabial fold and the cheek are generous harvest areas.
- Defects of the commissure require special consideration.
- Stabilising the lip during surgery is mandatory via an assistant, tension ligatures, chalazion clamps and dental rolls (Figure 9.39).

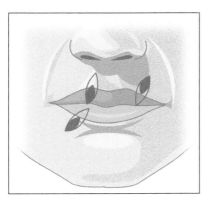

Figure 9.37 Compromise of the standard 30° angles of fusiform incision may be indicated (darker areas) to avoid crossing the vermilion border
Adapted from Roenigk R, Roenigk H (eds). Dermatologic Surgery, 2nd edn. New York: Marcel Dekker Inc, 1989; Fig 6.

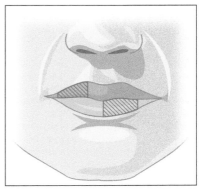

Figure 9.38 Defects up to one-third of the upper or lower lip (shaded areas) can be closed primarily after a wedge excision; larger defects may require flap closure
Adapted from Roenigk R, Roenigk H (eds). Dermatologic Surgery, 2nd edn. New York: Marcel Dekker Inc, 1989; Fig 7.

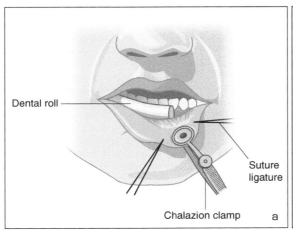

Dental roll

Suture ligature

Chalazion clamp   a

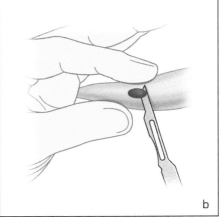

b

Figure 9.39 Stabilising the lip during surgery
a Stabilisation of the lip may be achieved with dental rolls (or rolled gauze) between the lip and gums, suture ligatures temporarily placed or a chalazion clamp. **b** Shave excision of small superficial lip lesions may be allowed to heal by secondary intention.
Adapted from Roenigk R, Roenigk H (eds). Dermatologic Surgery, 2nd edn. New York: Marcel Dekker Inc, 1989; Figs 8, 9.

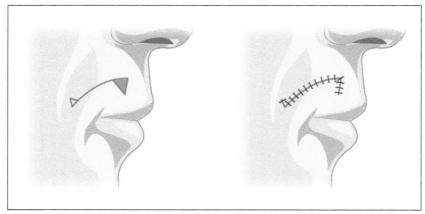

Figure 9.40 Rotation flap with Burow's triangle to reconstruct upper lip defect in an older patient where a portion of the donor area laterally may be hidden in the nasolabial fold and where, because of age, the commissure is lax and maintains its normal position in spite of the primary and secondary motions of the flap
Adapted from Roenigk R, Roenigk H (eds). Dermatologic Surgery, 2nd edn. New York: Marcel Dekker Inc, 1989; Fig 12.

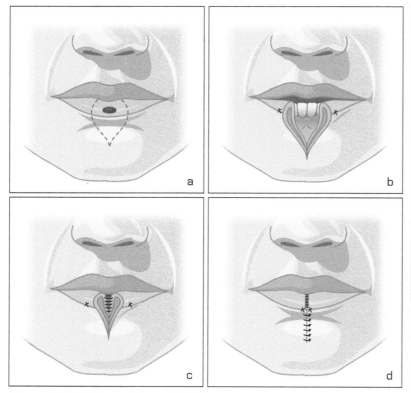

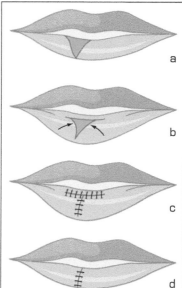

Figure 9.42 A-T closure of a mucosal defect via bilateral advancement/rotation flaps with donor incisions hidden from view
Adapted from Roenigk R, Roenigk H (eds). Dermatologic Surgery, 2nd edn. New York: Marcel Dekker Inc, 1989; Fig 10.

Figure 9.41 Wedge excision of the lip

a Marking the vermilion border. **b** Defect with less mucosal surface removal.
c Closure partially complete with mucosal surface closed and muscle being closed.
d Complete closure.
Adapted from Roenigk R, Roenigk H (eds). Dermatologic Surgery, 2nd edn. New York: Marcel Dekker Inc, 1989; Fig 13.

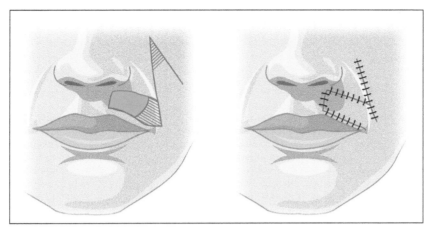

Figure 9.43 Inferioror caudally based nasolabial transposition flap for upper lip defect reconstruction
Adapted from Roenigk R, Roenigk H (eds). Dermatologic Surgery, 2nd edn. New York: Marcel Dekker Inc, 1989; Fig 11.

- Braided absorbable sutures (left long) provide maximum patient comfort intraorally to the mucosal surfaces.

Some common lip procedures are illustrated in Figures 9.40 to 9.44.

A V-Y island flap can provide very good mucosal repairs to the internal lip. See the section under 'Advancement flaps' in the 'Ear' section.

BCCs are the most common cancer of the (white) lip skin. SCC is the most common mucosal lip malignancy and over 90% occur on the lower lip.

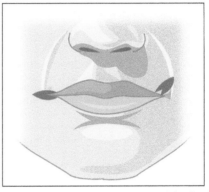

Figure 9.44 M-plasty closure may provide the best results for small lip commissure defects
Adapted from Roenigk R, Roenigk H (eds). Dermatologic Surgery, 2nd edn. New York: Marcel Dekker Inc, 1989; Fig 16.

HINTS AND TIPS

Most patients are unhappy with their lip surgery no matter how well it is done. The diagnosing doctor is often on a hiding to nothing with the patient anguishing if they 'should have seen someone else' whereas, if referred, they are content that 'everything possible has been done'.

Scalp

SUBGALEAL AREA

Most of what is to be undermined with the scalp is located below the strong aponeurosis of the galea, called the subgaleal plane (Figure 9.45). Because it's a fairly bloodless plane it's easily undermined and consists of loose areolar or connective tissue that is devoid of much of the vasculature and nerves that supply the scalp. It makes an ideal dissection plane for defects larger than 1 cm. If defects measure larger than 3 cm they will be likely to require more than a side-to-side closure.

Because the galea is a thick, inelastic, fibrous band of tissue, closure can be very difficult. One must mobilise tissue from areas where the skin is thinner and looser. That's usually referred to as the hatband area.

Other methods that have been used to stretch the galeal area include the buried pulley (or figure eight) stitch or towel clamps.

COMPLICATIONS OF SCALP SURGERY

Bleeding is a lot more common on the scalp due to the convex shape of the calvarium and the fact that blood vessels don't contract as well.

Preserve hair follicles for cosmesis.

Down into bone healing by secondary intention is not always good.

Sometimes it may be appropriate to remove the outer table of the calvarium or (bore) into the space between the two plates to allow the tissue to granulate.

CLOSURE TECHNIQUES

Besides secondary intention, closure techniques for the scalp include simple layered closure, rotation and transposition flaps.

Rotation flaps are greatly helped by back cuts. They help mobilise the flap into position and, if the back cut is closed first, it helps push the flap into position.

HINTS AND TIPS

Back cuts are a great 'trick' to use on scalp closures that are troublesome, especially with a rotation flap.

Double rotation or O-Z flaps can leave a large secondary defect from one of the flaps. Rather than attempting to close it and creating too much tension at the edges of

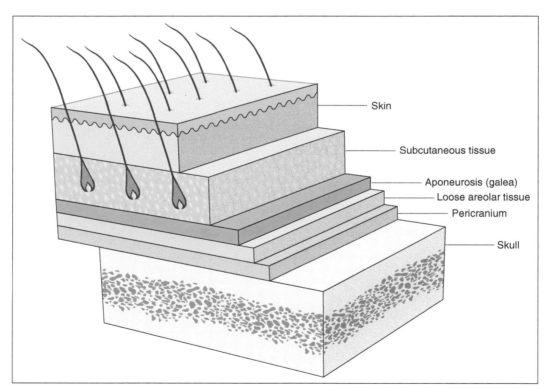

Figure 9.45 Layers of the scalp
Adapted from Larrabee WF, Makielski KH, Henderson JL. Surgical Anatomy of the Face, 2nd edn. Philadelphia: Lippincott Williams & Wilkins, 2004; Fig 11.2.

the flaps, allow the area to heal by secondary intention, by undermining in the more superficial but vascularised plane above the galea. The other option would be putting a graft over the remaining secondary defect, which would probably result in alopecia in this area of the secondary intention healing, but this won't matter if the patient in question is bald.

Additional closure methods include interpolation/axial flaps, full-thickness and split-thickness grafts and free flaps. The latter require microvascular re-anastomosis.

Digits

Most lesions are small and a simple ellipse can be done. Otherwise, a graft using a 12-mm punch makes it very simple.

REFERENCES

[1] Darouiche RO, Wall MJ Jr, Itani KM, et al. Chlorhexidine–alcohol versus povidone–iodine for surgical-site antisepsis. N Engl J Med 2010;362: 18–26.

[2] Radonich MA, Zaher M, Bisaccia E, et al. Auricular reconstruction of helical rim defects: wedge resection revisited. Dermatol Surg 2002;28:62–5.

[3] Krunic AL, Weitzul S, Taylor RS. Chondrocutaneous advancement flap for reconstruction of helical rim defects in dermatologic surgery. Aust J Dermatol 2006;47:296–9.

[4] Majumdar A, Townend J. Helix rim advancement for reconstruction of marginal defects of the pinna. Br J Oral Maxillofac Surg 2000;38:3–7.

[5] Rex J, Ribera M, Bielsa I, et al. Narrow elliptical skin excision and cartilage shaving for treatment of chondrodermatitis nodularis. Dermatol Surg 2006;3:400–4.

[6] Barker LP, Young AW, Sachs W. Chondrodermatitis of the ears: a differential study of nodules of the helix and anthelix. Arch Dermatol 1960;81:53–63.

[7] Jacobs MA, Christenson LJ, Weaver AL, et al. Clinical outcome of cutaneous flaps versus full-thickness skin grafts after Mohs surgery on the nose. Dermatol Surg 2010;36(1):23–30.

[8] Tardy ME Jr, Brown RJ. Surgical anatomy of the nose. New York, NY: Raven Press; 1990. pp. 1–23.

[9] Mulcahy ME, Geoghegan JA, Monk IR, et al. Nasal colonisation by *Staphylococcus aureus* depends upon clumping factor B binding to the squamous epithelial cell envelope protein loricrin. PLoS Pathog 2012; doi: 10.1371/journal.ppat.1003092.

[10] Bode LG, Kluytmans JA, Wertheim HF, et al. Preventing surgical-site infections in nasal carriers of *Staphylococcus aureus*. N Engl J Med 2010;362:9–17.

[11] Ricks M, Cook J. Extranasal applications of the bilobed flap. Dermatol Surg 2005;31(8):941–8.

[12] Moy RL, Grossfeld JS, Baum M, et al. Reconstruction of the nose utilizing a bilobed flap. Int J Dermatol 1994;33:657–60.

[13] Esser JFS. Gestielte lokale Nasenplastik mit zweizipfligen Lappen, Deckung des sekundaren Defektes vom ersten Zipfel durch den Zweiten. Dtsch Zschr Chir 1918;143:385.

[14] Zimany A. The bi-lobed flap. Plast Reconstr Surg 1953;11(6):424–34.

[15] Zitelli JA. The bilobed flap for nasal reconstruction. Arch Dermatol 1989;125(7):957–9.

[16] Dzubow LM. The dynamics of flap movement: effect of pivotal restraint on flap rotation and transposition. J Dermatol Surg Oncol 1987;13:1348–53.

[17] Cho M, Kim DW. Modification of the Zitelli bilobed flap: a comparison of flap dynamics in human cadavers. Arch Facial Plast Surg 2006;8:404–9.

[18] Morgan BL, Samiian MR. Advantages of the bilobed flap for closure of small defects of the face. Plast Reconstr Surg 1973;52:35–7.

[19] Albertini JG, Hansen JP. Trilobed flap reconstruction for distal nasal skin defects. Dermatol Surg 2010;11:1726–35.

[20] Pipitone MA, Gloster HM Jr. Repair of the alar groove with combination partial primary closure and second-intention healing. Dermatol Surg 2005;31(5):608–9.

[21] Torres PA, Galdames IS, Lopez MC, et al. Biometrics study of the upper and lower labial artery in human cadavers. Int J Morphol 2008;26(3):573–6.

[22] Schulte DL, Sherris DA, Kasperbauer JL. The anatomical basis of the Abbé flap. Laryngoscope 2001;111(3):382–6.

Cysts and lipoma

The cyst, the whole cyst and nothing but the cyst.

Surgical axiom

Cysts

EPIDERMOID CYSTS

An epidermoid cyst may also be known as a sebaceous cyst, follicular infundibular cyst, epidermal cyst, epidermal inclusion cyst, keratinous cyst, milia, pilar cyst, wen or steatocystoma.

- **Epidermoid cyst** is now arguably the best term as most originate from the follicular infundibulum. They contain a cheesy keratin and fat and have a central punctum. They are the most common cutaneous cysts and may occur anywhere on the body but most frequently on the face, scalp, neck and trunk.
- **Epidermal inclusion cyst** refers specifically to an epidermoid cyst that is the result of the implantation of epidermal elements deeper in the dermis.
- **Sebaceous cyst** is a term that should be avoided because it implies that the cyst is of sebaceous origin. They are not filled with sebum but keratin.
- **'Infected sebaceous cyst'** is not infected but, rather, it is where keratin has extruded, usually due to it being squeezed, resulting in the surrounding tissues being inflamed (not infected). Antibiotics are not indicated. They settle with time and with not being touched.
- **Milia** are very small, superficial epidermoid cysts. These 1–2 mm lesions can arise spontaneously or can be caused by trauma. A small nick in the epidermis with a no. 11 blade or a 23G needle allows expression of the keratinaceous white kernel or, often, a surprisingly long 'worm' of keratin.

Other epithelial cysts

- **Pilar** or **trichilemmal cyst** (**wen**) occurs predominantly on the scalp, is odourless and has less fat and more keratin than epidermoid cysts. They are very amenable to removal by the minimal excision technique. They do not have a punctum like epidermoid cysts. They are smooth, mobile, asymptomatic swellings, often in the scalp. Overlying hair loss may be noted and multiple cysts may be present.
- **Steatocystoma multiplex** are multiple, small, yellow, cystic nodules (a few millimetres in diameter) that can be found on the trunk, upper arms, axillae and thighs. The multitude of lesions may preclude cyst removal.
- **Favre–Racouchot syndrome (nodular cystic elastosis)** [1, 2] is characterised by multiple lesions, most usually on the periorbital and temporal areas, resulting from profound sun and probably smoking damage [3] that results in severely photo-damaged skin with, atrophy, wrinkles and furrows. The pilosebaceous openings stretch and the orifices fill with keratin material, producing multiple open and closed comedones and cysts with yellowish discolouration, yellowish nodules but with no inflammation, unlike the comedones seen with acne.
- **Dermoid cysts** are congenital cysts with a pungent, rancid odour. They occur in the lines of cleavage around the eyes and on the base of the nose and sublingually. They can extend intracranially, and a CAT scan/MRI is necessary.

TREATMENT

There are many surgical approaches to epidermoid cysts. Although complete surgical excision can ensure removal of the sac and prevent recurrence, this technique is time-consuming and requires suture closure. The minimal excision technique has been proposed as a less invasive and successful intervention and does not require suture closure. The procedure is easy to learn, and most doctors experienced in skin surgery can perform the procedure after three to five teaching sessions. It involves making a 2–3-mm incision, expressing the cyst contents through compression and extracting the cyst wall through the incision. The punch external extrusion excision is a variation.

There are six main techniques: slit incision, normal incision, traditional wide excision, minimal incision, punch biopsy excision and punch external extrusion excision (PEEE).

Slit incision
Refer to Figure 10.1.

Normal incision

Removal of the whole cyst intact
Very often the fibrous capsule (especially of pilar cysts) is thick enough so that the cyst can easily be removed intact via blunt dissection without expression of the contents. Drape, prep and anaesthetise the area with local anaesthetic with adrenaline and bicarb. Anaesthetise the surface, sides and beneath the cyst (if possible) using a long 30G needle. This applies to all techniques. Make a superficial linear incision to expose but not cut into the capsule (i.e. just to expose the cyst superior surface, without cutting into it). Small artery clamps (curved are preferable to follow the curved lateral walls of the cyst) can be inserted, closed, into the centre of the incision between the outer cyst wall and surrounding tissue to do this efficiently and quickly by opening them up to effect this blunt dissection separation. Otherwise an assistant can retract the skin with skin hooks.

This is the preferred method as, if the whole intact cyst is removed, there will be no recurrence (see Figures 10.2 and 10.3).

Note: incision into the cyst does not matter as long as the whole cyst is extracted.

See also the section below, 'Punch external extrusion excision'.

Towel clamp retractor
The towel clamp is a locking clamp with two sharp points separated by 60° [4]. For the excision of epidermoid cysts it can provide a useful, secure/non-slip retractor, especially for the unassisted surgeon [5, 6].

The clamp is locked into the tissue a little away from the distal (to the surgeon) incision end. The security and lack of slippage thus provided allows this end to be moved in any direction to provide excellent retraction either unassisted (non-dominant hand) or assisted.

Traditional wide excision
This method – involving dissection and removal of the cyst completely from the surrounding tissue through an elliptical incision – is considered the gold standard of treatment. This time-consuming endeavour frequently leads to significant scarring in comparison with minimal excision or punch biopsy, but has almost no recurrence when the cyst wall is entirely removed [7]. If the cyst ruptures accidentally during the procedure, remove the remaining contents and wall with a curette. The technique is essentially the same as above. Some surgeons use curved artery clamps to blunt dissect as the curve follows the cyst wall and the blunt instrument is less likely to puncture the cyst wall. In the hands of 'experts' this can be a tour-de-force and very quick, especially for wens.

Minimal incision and punch biopsy excision
These techniques are purported to produce minimal bleeding, have faster healing times and produce less scarring because of the small opening through which the cysts are removed [7]. Though both techniques offer a shorter procedural time, they appear to have a slightly higher rate of recurrence. This was first described by Danna in 1945 [8]. Mehrabi later concluded the punch incision technique, when properly performed, is a satisfactory removal method with a recurrence rate of 8.3% [7]. He analysed and provided data demonstrating that the removal of keratinous and pilar cysts by the punch incision technique is a viable option with an acceptably low recurrence rate and that the removal of keratinous and pilar cysts by the punch incision technique is an alternative to traditional excision methods. It is easy to perform with commonly available instruments, and quick.

Subanalysis revealed a trend showing that inflamed cysts had a lower recurrence rate. Another trend was that cysts removed from the back and ear had the highest recurrence rates (13.8 and 13.0%, respectively) compared to those removed from other locations. Most cysts (54.5%) recurred within the first year after punch incision removal [7].

Recurrence
- 55% recur within the first year
- Ear = 13%
- Back = 14%
- Elsewhere = 8%

Minimal incision technique
This involves a 2–3-mm incision, expression of the cyst contents and extraction of the cyst wall through the incision. Vigorous finger compression and kneading is used to express the cyst contents and loosen the cyst wall from the surrounding tissues to facilitate removal of the sac. The tiny wound can be closed with a single suture, although it is most often left. Expression of the cyst contents through the small opening can cause the sebaceous material to spray across the surgery room. Gauze should be used to cover the area as compression is applied. (splatter shields are also available). Following expulsion of the cyst contents, the loosened capsule is delivered

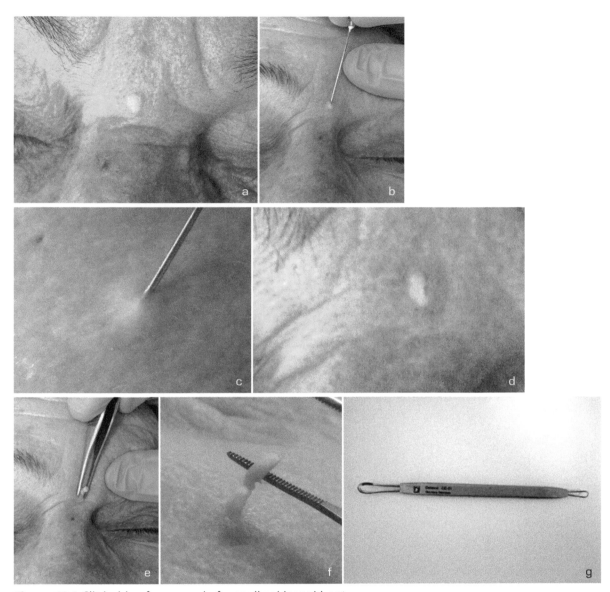

Figure 10.1 Slit incision for removal of a small epidermoid cyst

a A small epidermoid cyst or large milia in a prominent position causing the patient significant embarrassment. **b** A 23G needle is inserted, sideways, edge up, parallel to the cheek skin surface just under the dermis of the cyst and for most of its radius. There is no need for anaesthesia. **c** The cyst surface is lanced by pulling or levering the needle upwards to break the surface. Make sure to go deep enough to access the cyst contents. **d** A definite linear incision should be seen. Failure of keratin to appear usually means the slit has not been deep enough. **e** The contents are best evacuated by pressing either side with plain forceps. This will heal without a trace. **f** Contents can be considerable. With more pressure the cyst contents can be completely extruded. There is always more than one imagines so ensure there is no residium. Sometimes considerable force is needed but firm constant pressure usually yields best results. **g** Specific comedone extractors, such as this, can be a more elegant instrument.

through the small opening. Closure with suture is optional [9].

Punch biopsy excision technique

This was apparently first described by Danna in New Orleans in 1945 [8]. A punch biopsy instrument is used to create the opening into the cyst except that the incision is made using a single-use disposable dermal punch. Expulsion of the cyst contents, with cyst wall, is achieved via lateral pressure [7].

One small randomised study compared traditional wide excision with punch biopsy [8]. They found punch

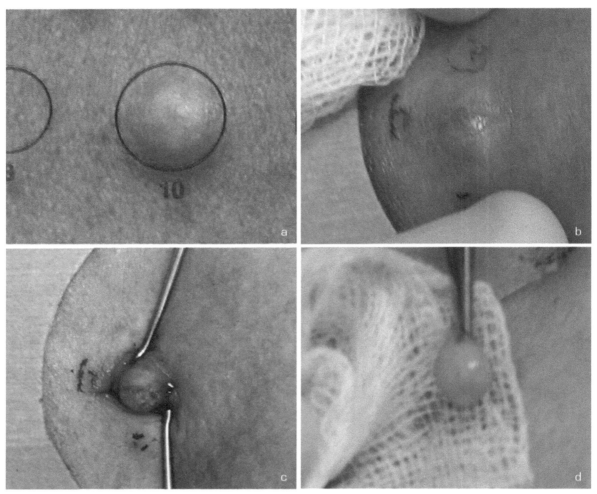

Figure 10.2 Removal of an intact cyst

a A small epidermoid cyst at the base of the neck causing the patient much annoyance. He wanted it removed but was most anxious that it 'wouldn't come back'. A field block is done as a square around the circumference of the cyst. **b** A very shallow epidermal/upper dermal straight incision is made across the radius of the cyst to expose the shiny cyst wall – here pulled apart by thumb and index finger. **c** Retracting the incision edges reveals the cyst walls and adhesions, which can then be dissected off. **d** The cyst in toto is 'delivered' and the patient can be reassured it will not come back. Dissecting out a cyst in toto ensures that there is no recurrence. If any part of the cyst wall is left it will invariably recur.

biopsy to be less time-consuming and to offer superior cosmetic results. However, cysts larger than 2 cm took longer with the punch biopsy technique. Of the 31 patients randomised to the punch biopsy technique, there was 1 recurrence in the 16 months of follow-up compared with none in the wide excision arm.

Study results indicated [7]:

- recurrence rate = 8%
- less pain
- better cosmesis (small scar)
- less bruising.

Technique

1 Prep skin and anaesthetise with 1% lignocaine with adrenaline ring block.

2 Single-use, disposable 3-, 4- and 5-mm dermal punch biopsy; 4-mm most used. Twist as if performing a biopsy.

3 Make a round incision in cyst middle (over the punctum if identified).

4 Apply lateral pressure at the base of the cyst to express and deliver the contents of the cyst, including part of the cyst wall.

5 The greyish cyst wall can then be identified.

6 Tease out remnants through the punch opening.

7 Carefully inspect the wound to ensure complete removal of the capsule to prevent recurrence. Wound closure usually requires only one or two sutures.

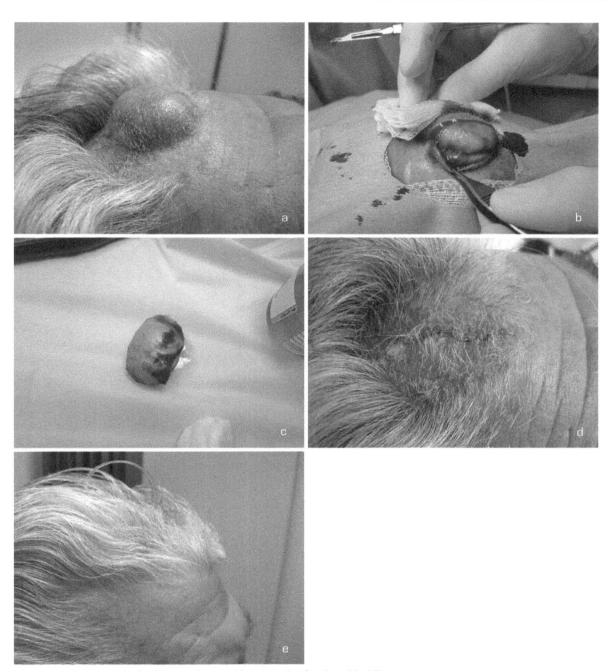

Figure 10.3 Removal of a large epidermoid cyst in the forehead hairline

a The site has been clipped, not shaved. **b** A very narrow ellipse facilitated exposure, retraction of the skin and dissection. A straight incision was considered but the ellipse removed some of the stretched skin so as to minimise any residual loose skin. **c** 'The cyst, the whole cyst and nothing but the cyst.' **d** 8 days later at ROS. Although the patient's hair is silver the blue sutures still make them easier to see to remove. **e** 6 weeks postoperatively. No scar is visible and there is no deformity or loose skin. Skin not only stretches but, as here, can also take up. The patient's (and his family's) only regret was that he had waited so long.

8 The entire extracted cyst wall, as well as the cyst contents, is sent for pathological examination.

Punch external extrusion excision (PEEE)

This is a variation on the previous two techniques, but not all cyst contents are expressed and blunt dissection is used. This may facilitate better identification and removal of the entire sac.

A 4-mm (or larger) punch is used to remove the skin over the punctum or apex.

Technique

1 Once the cyst roof is identified, puncture it and expel enough of the contents to deflate it somewhat.

2 Initial dissection of the top rim of the cyst sac may have to be done with scissors as the cyst wall is most adherent here. But once this first 1 mm or so is free, blunt dissection is then possible and preferable.

3 Secure the edge of the opening and carry out blunt dissection. Curved artery clamps are ideal for most smaller to medium-sized lesions but larger curved clamps or even the needle holder is used for wens and such. Insert the closed end of the clamp curving around the cyst and then open it, breaking down the adhesions.

4 The deflated cyst allows purchase of the rim with the needle holder or such and facilitates manoeuvring the sac to make dissection easier. Continuous traction finally frees the half-filled cyst, which is then delivered effectively in toto (only the 'lid' having also been removed).

5 The punch hole, as with normal biopsies, can be left to heal.

This technique has the advantages of ensuring complete removal and therefore preventing recurrences, being one stage, quick and without the expense and bother of sutures.

Resume incision with expression of the contents

1 Cover the incision with a gauze to prevent the contents spurting.

2 Over the centre of the cyst, to include the punctum, make a small linear incision, an elliptical excision or a 4–8 mm punch (biopsy). A number 11 blade to stab or a 4-mm punch biopsy twisted in is most often used. The punch has the advantage of removing the punctum.

3 Insert a small (straight) artery clamp into the cyst and open/spread the tips.

4 Remove it and express the contents of the cyst by evenly, gradually increasing finger/thumb pressure or by bilateral squeezing. The artery clamp can be reinserted, if needed, to assist with passage of the sebaceous material.

Note: the contents are foul-smelling.

5 After complete expression all attempts should be made to remove the entire sac:

A The clamp is reintroduced into the cyst and the sac at the base is grasped and pulled/teased out.

or

B Grasp the edge of the cyst with forceps and separate the cyst via blunt dissection.

Complications: the sac may break, and several pieces may need to be removed. If the intact sac cannot be removed/identified, use a curette against the inner wall and move it back and forth to dislodge the capsule from the surrounding tissue. If any remnants remain recurrence can occur.

6 Most small incisions do not require suture closure. Punch excisions >4 mm usually do need a suture.

7 Dress with a gauze pad.

Instruct the patient to maintain direct pressure (using the gauze pad supplied) on the site for 1–2 hours (longer if bleeding is suspected) or apply a pressure bandage if possible.

Comparison of techniques

Any technique that does not provide visual confirmation of complete removal of the cyst/sac is fraught with the potential for recurrence. In a randomised study comparing punch incision to elliptical excision, epidermal inclusion cysts measuring 1–2 cm that are located on the face or in an area of cosmetic concern were best treated with punch incision. The mean lengths of the wounds in the punch incision and elliptical excision groups were 0.73 and 2.34 cm, respectively. Mean operative time was significantly shorter in the punch group (12.7 minutes) as compared with the surgical group (21.6 minutes). No complication occurred in the punch incision group. There was no significant difference in the recurrence rate [8].

'Infected' (inflamed) cysts

Epidermoid cysts are benign lesions that rarely require intervention but are excised for cosmetic reasons or because they are inflamed or grow so large as to be a problem [10]. Rarely are these cysts truly infected. The inflammation is secondary to cyst wall rupture with leakage of cyst contents, which elicits the inflammatory response [11]. Inflamed cysts should be allowed to settle prior to attempted removal. Excision of an inflamed cyst is not recommended as the inflamed cyst wall is more friable and therefore more difficult to remove completely [12], which may lead to a higher rate of recurrence. Kitamura et al. (1994) [13] suggest primary resection, wound lavage and primary suture without drainage for infected epidermal cysts.

> **NOTE**
> Do not excise inflamed cysts; let them settle.

RECOMMENDATIONS

- For small cysts (3–4 cm) that have never become inflamed or ruptured: normal straight incision minimal excision technique is recommended because it's likely that the entire capsule can be dissected out and the whole cyst removed with minimal scarring and faster healing time. Also, for cysts on the face, this method produces a better cosmetic result because of the significantly smaller scar.
- For large lesions >5 cm: traditional wide excision is faster than the minimal or punch techniques.
- Ruptured, previously expressed or recurrent: wide excision may be best. In these scenarios, it is extremely time-consuming and often impossible to remove the entire capsule using the minimal excision technique.

EQUIPMENT

Anaesthesia
- Non-sterile gloves
- Mask, glasses; shield may be circumspect
- Site prep
- Gauze squares
- 5-mL syringe
- 23G draw-up needle
- 30G 30-mm needle
- Lignocaine with adrenaline; bicarb

Sterile tray for the procedure
- Sterile gloves
- Fenestrated disposable drape
- Three small mosquito curved clamps
- No. 11 blade/4-mm punch
- Needle holder for suturing (if needed)
- Iris scissors
- Adson forceps
- Sterile gauze swabs
- Skin hooks
- Curved and straight artery clamps
- Suture materials (if needed)
- Splatter control shield (if desired)

Non-sterile technique
As noted elsewhere, non-sterile gloves do not seem to result in more infections than sterile gloves for such skin surgery.

COMPLICATIONS AND DIFFICULTIES

- Content spurt: the cyst contents can burst across the room with no or even with the most gentle pressure. Strong pressure can also precipitate this without warning. Hold gauze loosely over the site to prevent this. Protective splatter masks and eye protection are available.
- Cyst wall can't be extruded: the most common cause is that not enough pressure is applied. Very often great pressure with thumbs is needed and can be quite exhausting.
- Adhesions from previous rupture: previously ruptured or inflamed cysts may have significant fibrous adhesions. Scarring may preclude removal with the minimal excision technique and a wide excision will be needed. Most of these can be avoided by a careful history and examination to ensure mobility. Caution: wide excisions always take longer than estimated.
- Cyst wall breakage: pressure, kneading and careful blunt dissection minimises this complication. If breakage occurs, inspection and curettage to try and remove the entire capsule should be done.
- Bleeding: control the bleeding, especially to prevent a residual haematoma, by direct pressure applied to the site with gauze and possible cautery.
- Haematoma: major bleeding is rare. Haematomas can be avoided by having the patient apply firm pressure, with a gauze pad, to the surgical site after the procedure for 2–4 hours if oozing or bleeding is suspected or applying a pressure bandage if possible. The old surgical axiom that bleeding occurs at 6 and 48 hours may need to be remembered for those patients who seem to bleed or are on anticoagulants. Direct pressure can also express any clot that forms via the original incision.
- Incorrect diagnosis: what appears a typical cyst may be solid when cut into. Remove a solid cyst by a formal surgical excision and send for histological evaluation.

PATHOLOGY

Because malignancy is rarely associated with a cyst it is not necessary to send all epidermoid cyst walls for histological evaluation, but any lesion that appears atypical or one that is associated with a palpable irregularity in the cyst wall should be sent for histological analysis.

If a solid tumour is discovered at the time of the procedure, obtain a biopsy. Incisional biopsy can be performed for very large lesions, and excisional biopsy for the smaller lesions. Pilar tumours of the scalp are often confused with epidermoid cysts and may require wide excision because they can erode into the skull.

Lipoma

The techniques are essentially the same as for cysts. The punch biopsy technique takes more time but offers a smaller scar and better cosmetic result (Figure 10.4). It is then a question as to whether the patient wants this and the extra costs involved for the extra time. It is also somewhat alarming to the patient with the amount of pressure that is needed to extrude the fat. Quite large lipoma can be removed via an 8–12-mm punch biopsy hole but then require a great deal of pressure and extensive exploration and breaking down, inserting and twisting the punch biopsy or scalpel to the far margins of the lipoma.

WARNING

If the diagnosis is in doubt, an ultrasound, CT scan or even an MRI will help diagnose and define. The traps are those lipoma on the back that may go deep into the muscle and are not amenable to this technique but need to be followed with full exploration to be excised, usually in a hospital. If in doubt get radiological help.

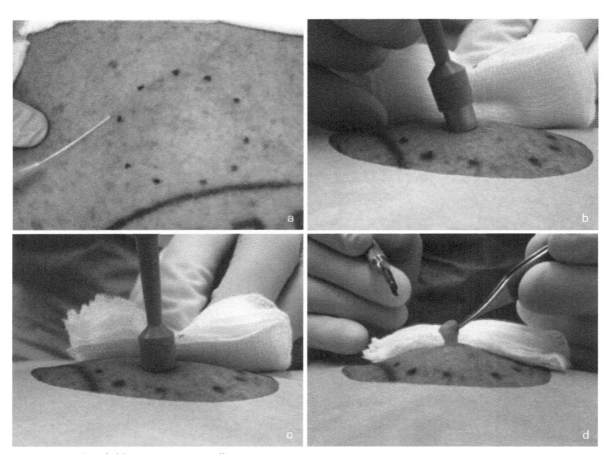

Figure 10.4 Punch biopsy to remove a lipoma

a A relatively small lipoma on L scapula. But lipomata can occur elsewhere. A field block is done by inserting a 25G 32-mm needle with lignocaine and adrenaline at 9 o'clock and injecting to 12 o'clock, then to 6 o'clock by pulling back but without withdrawing the needle. This is then repeated from the opposite side (3 to 12 o'clock, pull back, don't take the needle out but inject to 6 o'clock). This reduces the injections to two. In the end a square of anaesthesia encloses the lipoma. **b** An 8-mm punch is placed in the centre. **c** And twisted to the hilt/shoulder. **d** The plug of skin and attached fat is withdrawn.

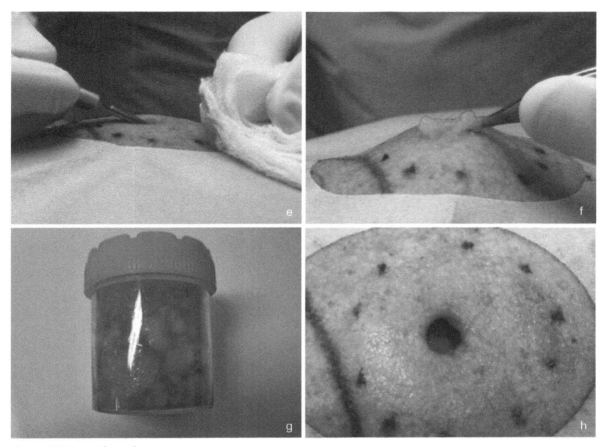

Figure 10.4 continued

e Pushing and squeezing around the lipoma circumference extrudes more fat but then the organised septa have to be broken down with the punch or the scalpel. The septa may be extremely tough. Be brave: keep making sweeps with a scalpel to the marked margins if this is the case. **f** This is continued plus the squeezing until all fat has been cleaned out. Pulling, twisting and levering the fat out with artery forceps may also be necessary. **g** The jars are sent to pathology – in this case two such full jars. **h** Close with an 'X' stitch or interrupteds.

REFERENCES

[1] Favre M. Sur une affection kystique des appareils pilosebacés localisée à certaines régions de la face. Bull Soc Fr Dermatol Syph 1932;39:93–6.

[2] Favre M, Racouchot J. [Nodular cutaneous elasteidosis with cysts and comedones]. Ann Dermatol Syphiligr (Paris) 1951;78(6):681–702.

[3] Keough GC, Laws RA, Elston DM. Favre–Racouchot syndrome: a case for smokers' comedones. Arch Dermatol 1997;133(6):796–7.

[4] Liu CM, McKenna J, Griess A. Surgical pearl: the use of towel clamps to reapproximate wound edges under tension. J Am Acad Dermatol 2004;50:273–4.

[5] Chen HH, Chen JS, Changchien CR, et al. Hemorrhoidectomy with self-retaining retraction. Dis Colon Rectum 1996;39:1058–9.

[6] Link MJ, Converse LD, Lanier WL. A new technique for single-person fascia lata harvest. Neurosurgery 2008;63(4 Suppl. 2):359–61, discussion 361.

[7] Mehrabi D, Leonhardt JM, Brodell RT. Removal of keratinous and pilar cysts with the punch incision technique: analysis of surgical outcomes. Dermatol Surg 2002;28:673–7.

[8] Lee H-E, Yang C-H, Chen C-H, et al. Comparison of the surgical outcomes of punch incision and elliptical excision in treating epidermal inclusion cysts: a prospective, randomized study. Dermatol Surg 2006;32(4):520–5.

[9] Zuber TJ. Minimal excision technique for epidermoid (sebaceous) cysts. Am Fam Physician 2002;65:1409–12, 1417–18, 1420.

[10] GP Notebook. Sebaceous cyst. Stratford-on-Avon, Warwickshire, UK: Oxbridge Solutions Limited; 2003. Available: <www.gpnotebook.co.uk>; [accessed 23 February 2013].

[11] Diven DG, Dozier SE, Meyer DJ, et al. Bacteriology of inflamed and uninflamed epidermal inclusion cysts. Arch Dermatol 1998;134:49–51.

[12] Goldstein BG, Goldstein AO. Benign neoplasms of the skin. Waltham, Mass: UpToDate; 1995. updated 21 November 2005.

[13] Kitamura K, Takahashi T, Yamaguchi T, et al. Primary resection of infectious epidermal cyst. J Am Coll Surg 1994;179:607.

Grafts 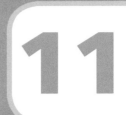 11

Grafts are done too often … Given the superior aesthetic results of flaps, grafts should be done at the last resort, after all possible flaps have been considered and rejected.

Daniel Buchen, Skin Flaps in Facial Surgery, *p 81*

A graft is a portion of skin that has been completely separated from its vascular supply. They have been performed for over 3000 years, when buttock skin was used in India to reconstruct noses. Grafts are becoming less frequently performed (Figure 11.1) as the training and procedural execution of flaps improves. As a Mayo Clinic study concluded: 'For defects on the nose where flap and graft repair may both be technically possible, a flap may be more likely to result in superior cosmetic outcome' [1].

Grafts should be limited to where no other repair is possible. Grafts, however, can be the only way to close certain defects and the method of choice. Their main uses are for burn victims, the lower leg, parts of the ears, tight skin (scalp/fingers) and some nasal ala.

TYPES

There are two types of skin grafts: 1) full thickness (FTSG), which comprises epidermis and dermis, including hair and glands but not fat, and 2) split-thickness (STSG), which comprises epidermis only and may be sheet, mesh, patch or strips.

Full thickness autografts account for the vast majority of grafts performed but, on the elderly, lower limbs where the skin is thin and compromised and cosmesis is not important, STSGs can provide healing and closure where flaps may pose technical problems and potential complications.

> **NOTE**
>
> The thinner the graft, the greater the take.
>
> The thicker the graft, the better the appearance.

DONOR ORIGIN

Donor origin may be
1 autograft: skin from the same individual
2 composite: skin and another tissue (e.g. cartilage)
3 homograft: skin from another person
4 xeno-/heterograft: skin from a different species (e.g. pig to human).

GRAFT SURVIVAL

A skin graft has to be placed on a vascular bed recipient site with sufficient blood supply to ensure its survival. Grafts will not survive where there is no perichondrium/ostium (i.e. bare cartilage or bone or on tendon). Bare cartilage and bone never granulate. (A flap with its own blood supply is then needed.) The dermis or fascia provides more blood vessels than fat, and these are preferred recipient beds. It is possible that a gap of 5 mm on one margin of a skin graft can be supplied if there is good collateral circulation.

> **WARNING**
>
> Do not place a graft on bare cartilage, bone or tendon.

Graft survival depends on re-establishing the graft/detached skin's blood supply via the recipient site which includes three stages: 1) imbibition, 2) inosculation and 3) neovascularisation.

Knowledge of these processes is clinically helpful in monitoring the success or otherwise of the graft:
1 **Imbibition (first 24–48 hours)** – is an ischaemic, critical time wherein the graft is nourished via passive diffusion and sustained by the plasma exudate from the site bed. The graft becomes

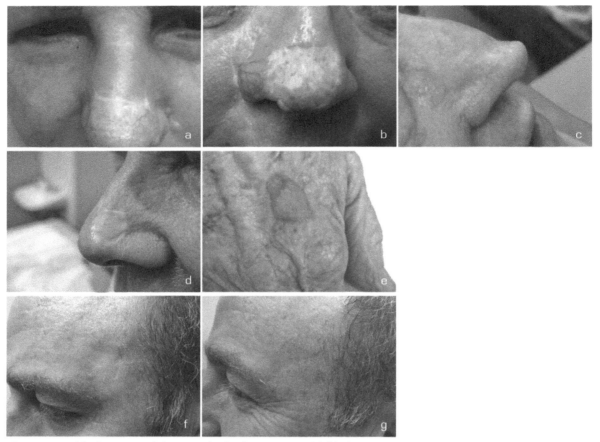

Figure 11.1 Maybe some of these grafts (a–c) were unavoidable but they are certainly not a good look
d A bilobed flap may have been possible here with a much better match. **e** And why would a graft be done here? **f** Or here? This patient requested a scar revision/excision of this unnecessary graft, which he had endured for some 5 years. He was an outdoor worker with no affectations as to his looks, which nevertheless shows how deeply most people feel about their appearance. There was obviously more than enough loose skin to have done a flap originally, as this graft revision demonstrates (**g**). However, revising was difficult because of the reduced available skin, however, two years later the patient was extremely happy with the improvement.

progressively swollen and oedematous and may increase its weight by up to 40%. Granulation tissue then starts to grow into the graft.

2 **Inosculation (48 hours to 10 days)** – is the revascularisation stage where the recipient bed vessels link with those in the dermis of the graft. (This phase requires a healthy vascular base, which is why cartilage and bone do not support grafts.)

3 **Neovascularisation (day 4 and day 7)** – capillary ingrowth from the wound periphery and base occurs to restore full circulation to the graft.

4 Lymphatic flow is concurrent with blood vasculature re-establishment usually by day 7 and witnesses the regression of oedema, swelling and bulk.

5 Nerve supply is invariably interrupted and the graft seldom ever feels the same. Some reinnervation begins within 2 months (some claim earlier) but may continue for years and may never be complete. FTSG achieves better innervation.

DELAYED GRAFTING/SLOW MOHS

Refreshing: after 5–6 days dry edges should be scraped such that they bleed to 'refresh' them and then re-suture. Secondary intention healing usually starts around day 5 so it is preferable to do this before then. Traditionally, a Fox curette has been used but the sharper disposable curettes or a scalpel blade can be used.

PROS AND CONS
A (thinner) STSG:

- resists infection better
- takes more easily
- allows the donor area to recover quickly but often with more problems/pain than recipient site
- is less likely to cause keloid formation in the donor area.

  But an STSG also:

- is more fragile
- provides a worse colour match – smooth, shiny, pale white or abnormally pigmented
- contracts more
- wears worse
- is more difficult to sew in place
- does not grow with the patient
- provides less sensation than an FTSG
- is hairless
- is thinner; hence the graft will look worse.

SPECIAL CONSIDERATIONS
- Nose – appearance is most important.
- Shin – take is most important.

SITE PREPARATION
Skin grafts rarely take when placed on bone, cartilage or tendon without the presence of periosteum, perichondrium or paratenon. Meticulous haemostasis of the recipient bed is also key in preventing haematoma formation between the graft and wound bed. Haemostasis is typically achieved via precise electrocoagulation. Infection also compromises graft survival; therefore, careful preparation of the recipient bed is necessary. A recipient bed that contains a bacteria concentration greater than 10^5 organisms per gram of tissue will not support a skin graft.

FULL THICKNESS SKIN GRAFT (FTSG)

Technique
1. Not on tendon, cartilage, bare bone, fat.
2. Template – consider oversizing to allow for immediate contraction.
3. Excise tumour.
4. Harvest graft (into saline if delays).
5. Close donor site.
6. Debride **all** fat until only white dermis remains.
7. Attach graft. The graft is now the first and last in order, which allows bed observation to ensure haemostasis.

8. Stab or needle – make drain holes.
9. Button sutures (through the ear/nose).
10. Dressing: firm dressing.
11. Don't disturb for as long as possible.
12. If looking black or 'terrible', leave alone! Most come good or heal by secondary intention.

> **NOTE**
> Flaps leave some fat. Grafts leave none.

Complications
The most common complication is bleeding under the graft. This can be best avoided by meticulous haemostasis with as long an observation as possible and then stabbing/lancing the graft with slits to allow any such sub-graft fluid to escape rather than separate the graft from its bed.

Recipient sites
- Ears – superior helical rim
- Nasal ala
- Nasal tip – perhaps
- Fingers – punch technique
- Scalp
- Thick skin

Harvest/donor sites
The obligation is to find a donor site where the skin colour, texture and sebaceous qualities best match the recipient site. Selection is based on:

1. skin colour
2. texture
3. dermal thickness
4. vascularity
5. potential donor site morbidity.
   Potential sites:

- Supraclavicular fossa
- Upper eyelid
- Postauricular
- Preauricular – good for nose but ensure no hair
- Ear concha – best for nose (and heals by secondary intention).
- Toe – plantar aspect 4th toe – good for fingerprint sites
- Hypothenar eminence – good for fingerprint sites
- Nasolabial
- Medial arm (especially the elderly) – good for fingers (not fingerprint)
- Upper thigh

FTSGs taken from supraclavicular or pre- or post-auricular areas provide a suitable colour match for defects of the face.

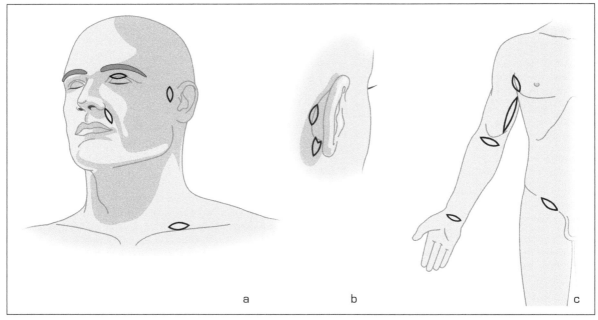

Figure 11.2 Available donor sites for full-thickness skin grafts

a–c Preauricular and nasolabial fold donor sites are more easily used in women than men whose beard hair follicles can be transplanted. In men, displacement of the sideburn can occur in the preauricular donor site. Adapted from Robinson JK, Arndt KA, Le Boit PE et al. Atlas of Cutaneous Surgery. Philadelphia: Saunders 1996; Fig 14-1.

Other donor sites of course are used but the cosmetic results are often poor (e.g. the nose and the inner canthus). In these sites a flap or secondary intention healing invariably provides a better result.

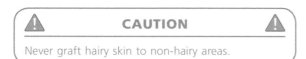

> ⚠️ **CAUTION** ⚠️
>
> Never graft hairy skin to non-hairy areas.

Limitations

Although they give a better cosmetic result than STSGs, FTSGs are limited to relatively small, uncontaminated wounds. Their survival depends on establishing a nourishing blood supply. To achieve this, the recipient site must be well vascularised and no fluid can accumulate between the graft and the bed to optimise its 'take'.

Cosmesis is the other limitation. An ugly or deforming graft on the tip of the nose is to be avoided if at all possible.

Again, the ear concha provides both the best colour match and also the best tissue type match for noses. No matter how blasé or rough-and-ready the patient may affect to be, they all resent and are embarrassed by such

a poor or obvious result. The side of the nose and temple, however, are difficult for patients to see and they are much more tolerant of a graft in these and other invisible sites. The essential surgical priority, however, is to excise the cancer with adequate margins and this may not then allow for a flap.

Pre-op technique
- Medications
  - Anticoagulants, aspirin, NSAIDs, fish-oil, vitamin E, alcohol and some herbs promote bleeding.
  - Cease if possible: aspirin 14 days before, alcohol, vitamin E, NSAIDs 5 days before and warfarin 3–5 days before.
  - Don't resume for 5 days (warfarin in 1 day).
- Exercise
  - Inform the patient that exercise disturbs the graft and can cause a haematoma and thus should be minimised for 2 weeks.
- Potential infection
  - Meticulous prep.
  - Cover diabetics with oral antibiotics.
- Topical antibiotics
  - Consider instillation into nares for nasal grafts.

Procedure

1 Excision of lesion: the skin cancer is excised ensuring appropriate margins (4 mm for BCC/SCC, 5–10 mm for melanoma)

   A Secure complete haemostasis of the bed (bipolar electrocautery best).

   B Make a template by pressing non-stick Melolin™/Cutilin™ or the suture cardboard insert onto the excision site and getting an impression from the bloody border or ink the edge and transfer the ink.

   C Score this template outline with the scalpel to later identify the exact graft outline for trimming.

 WARNING

Always ensure adequate margins are taken or Mohs surgery done to completely excise the cancer. Cosmesis is always secondary to cure.

2 Harvest

   A Excise the FTSG with a scalpel at the subdermal level of the superficial fat.

   B Take a slightly oversize (10–20%) harvest to compensate for immediate graft dermal elastin contraction. This is usually a simple ellipse (and the graft trimmed later as per the template impression).

   C Some transfer this graft to a saline bath but this destroys the fibrin and impairs 'take'.

   D The quicker the transfer, the better.

3 Close

   A Close the donor site (interrupted nylon sutures). This is done now to allow longer observation of the recipient site to ensure the all-important haemostasis (to prevent sub-graft haematoma that impairs take).

4 De-fat: the residual adipose tissue is usually removed with sharp, curved iris scissors as the fat is poorly vascularised and prevents direct contact between the graft dermis and the wound bed

   A This is often done by stretching the ellipse on a gauze square over one gloved index finger, fat side up, while securing it by its ends with the thumb and index or middle finger or artery clamps and using the curved iris scissors to denude all the yellow fat down to the shiny, white dermis.

   B Some surgeons now place this graft into normal saline while the donor site is sutured closed. Others feel this removes the fibrin, which helps the graft take. Avoid saline if possible

but do not let the graft desiccate – moisten with local anaesthetic or saline rather than bathe it.

5 Donate

   A The graft site can be undermined but also can be left. If undermining is done take care to ensure the subdermal plexus is not compromised as the graft edges as well as the base need a good blood supply.

   B Now is the best time to slit the graft by stabbing with the scalpel blade or an 18G needle. This is to provide drain holes for any sub-graft fluid, which may lift the graft, to escape. In the heat of battle this is often forgotten. Basting sutures are usually central so avoid the very centre. Fluid is most likely, however, to accumulate in the centre of flat or concave grafts, so peri-central drains are optimal or where the donor site has more of a hollow. The number of slits or holes varies from a minimum of one to as many as the site area dictates.

   C Trim the graft to shape using the template 20% larger than the site but with the exact graft size scored as in step 1. It is preferable to now err on the side of making the graft very *slightly* smaller than the donor site as it will stretch. Having a graft that is too big that overlaps the donor site edges or having one too small so it stretches to leave a potential sub-graft space is to be avoided. An oversized graft can cause trapdooring.

   D The most important factor for graft survival is securing it to 'adhere' to the donor site.

      i Securing sutures: on the nose or ear place button sutures in the centre of the graft where it is most likely to lift, to pass right through to the nasal cavity or the external ear to return and tie off (centrally).

      ii Basting sutures: where the site is too thick to pass sutures through to the other side, sutures that bind the centre of the graft to the centre of the donor site can be done in two ways using absorbable sutures:

         a Buried suture: a 6/0 monofilament suture is passed through the dermis of the underside of the graft in a small bite, then through the donor bed at the corresponding site and tied off with the suture ends coming out the side of the graft, thus allowing access. This suture is then allowed to absorb.

         b A similar small bite suture goes from the external centre of the graft, loops down, through and up from the graft donor site bed, then back up to exit superficially close to the origin and is tied off. This can be absorbable or, as it is accessible, non-absorbable.

  iii Or, it can be secured by two adjoining anchoring sutures and a central basting suture to be trimmed in situ.

E Sew the graft edges into the excised deficit.

  i Secure one side of the graft with two adjoining sutures as above.

  ii Secure the centre with a basting suture as above.

  iii Place opposing sutures (12 and 6 o'clock, 3 and 9 o'clock etc) until the graft is secure with sutures 3–4 mm apart (closer if needed).

  iv For the greatest graft security, the suture should *enter the graft first* and not the donor site skin as this pins the graft down, whereas entering the surrounding skin first pushes the graft up.

  v Some surgeons use nylon; others use rapid absorbing sutures.

  vi Meticulously appose the epidermal edges.

  vii Make sutures deep (in the reticular dermis). Superficial sutures risk dead space, scarring and pin-cushioning.

F Finally, leave four opposing sutures, 90° apart (e.g. 12, 3, 6 and 9 o'clock), long so that they

can be tied over a pressure pad bolster dressing. Leave these until last; otherwise, they get in the way. These bolster sutures can also be done later away from the graft margins in the surrounding skin so that they are independent of the graft and don't get in the way.

G Make small slits in graft to allow sub-graft fluids to escape, if not previously done.

H Trim any excess.

Dressings

1 Some surgeons apply chloramphenicol ointment to the graft surface; otherwise, use white soft paraffin (Vaseline).

2 Cut a non-stick dressing (Cutilin, Melolin) and/or a petroleum gauze to fit as per the template/deficit.

3 Place a mould cut to the size of the graft on top of this. The author has found Allevyn™ thin non-stick dressings cut to size to apply uniform pressure exactly to the graft very suitable when secured by the bolster sutures. A sterilised make-up sponge can also be used. These can also be sutured in place.

4 Push the graft gently but firmly down on the floor by this mould to optimise 'take'.

5 Bolsters are usually fashioned from dental rolls or gauze pads cut to shape and applied to secure the graft from shearing forces and disturbance (Figure 11.3). They are not necessary if the graft is secure

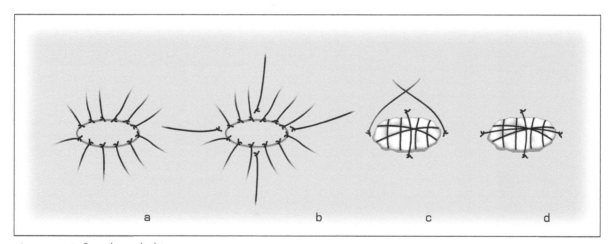

Figure 11.3 Securing a bolster

a Sutures for the bolster are placed into the graft and wound margin like a regular interrupted suture, but one tail is left long enough to tie over the dressing. A haemostat should be available to temporarily hold all ends together. **b** Some surgeons also place four sutures into the skin away from the graft. **c** At least four pairs should be used, and each should be tied to its corresponding suture on the other side of the bolster. Always tie the sutures that are 180° away from each other rather than going in sequence. **d** If the surgeon chooses to use tie-over sutures distant from the graft, these are tied last. Adapted from Robinson JK, Arndt KA, Le Boit PE et al. Atlas of Cutaneous Surgery. Philadelphia: Saunders 1996; Fig 13-9.

and the patient can reliably avoid disturbing the site. Bolsters are used in areas where a pressure dressing is difficult.

6 Apply an overall pressure dressing of gauze or waterproof squares and strap it down. AcquaPlast® is a perforated firm sheet that softens in hot water. It can be cut to size and moulded over convex or irregular surfaces to harden and be sutured in place through its perforations and skin edges. At present it does not seem to be available in Australia.

7 Leave bolsters in place for 7 days.

8 Remove the sutures at 7 days or later, depending on the site.

9 If there are concerns as to bleeding inspect at 4 days and, if necessary, insert needle into graft to allow fluid to escape. At this stage an 18G needle should be used.

Haematoma stages

Haematomas lift the graft off the bed and prevent take. They are best avoided by site observation and meticulous haemostasis, slitting the graft to provide drain holes and applying basting sutures and bolster pressure dressings. Intervention, as follows, should only be done if and when bleeding/haematoma is obvious and definite and then early.

- **Stage 1: accumulation**
  - The wound becomes swollen and is warm and fluctuant. Aspiration with an 18G needle may be all that is necessary to allow release of the accumulated blood together with slitting the graft or puncturing for drain holes.
  - If ongoing bleeding is suspected the whole graft should be opened and explored, the bleeding site(s) found and haemostasis established. The wound should then be irrigated with normal saline and observed until haemostasis is guaranteed. The graft can now be re-sutured as hopefully it is still viable.
- **Stage 2: clots**
  - Clots form quite quickly and the site becomes more spongy than fluctuant. The skin may have a purple hue. A small clot may be left to resorb but evacuation by pressure is usually preferable.
- **Stage 3: organisation**
  - Clots organise into adhesive, harder, rubber-like structures and the wound feels firm. These adhesive clots are hard to evacuate by squeezing or even exploration and instrument-aided removal. It is now better not to do anything but wait for clot lysis. This is avoided by earlier intervention.

- **Stage 4: lysis**
  - Between 7 and 10 days the wound again feels fluctuant. This is because fibrinolysis is liquifying the clot(s) to be resorbed. Aspiration with an 18G needle or pressure is now possible.

Post-op

- The graft is fragile and vulnerable for several weeks.
- Above all, leave alone no matter how 'bad' it looks. Grafts often look bad at 2 weeks; the dermis takes but the epidermis may look dusky.
- Advise patients that grafts do not look normal for many months.
- Minimise exercise for 2 weeks.
- Avoid the sun.
- Appearance at ROS will vary greatly.
- Do not debride any eschar but closely observe.
- Debride only if and when necrosis is definite – many dark areas improve and heal.

HINTS AND TIPS

Do not express concern or dismay if the graft looks bad as the patient will not know and will only get upset. In any event, it will invariably heal well by secondary intention.

ROS

- Ear: 7–10 days
- Nose: 7 days
- Fingers: 2 weeks
- Lower leg: alternate sutures out at 2 weeks, rest at 3 weeks

Grafts not taking

These are black, with lifting eschar.

Repair

Let it heal by secondary intention.

Special sites

- **Digits**: if the lesion is small enough (<4 mm) a 10–12 mm punch biopsy can be used to both excise the lesion and take the graft from the medial upper arm. Obtaining haemostasis of the digit is the practical problem. A tubular gauze dressing applies excellent pressure and splinting also minimises disturbance.
- **Ears and nose**: a central 'button' suture right through the ear or nose and back fastens the graft to the floor.

SPLIT SKIN GRAFT (STSG)

STSGs are epidermal with the donor skin, usually from the buttock or thigh, being stretched and then harvested with a harvesting (Humby/Watson) knife. They have very low metabolic demand and thus usually heal very well. Their down side is that they are so thin they 'fall into' the excision deficit they cover, and so there is always a contour deformity – a depression with altered looking skin. They are now done very occasionally.

However, they are very useful on the lower leg where the skin is tight and there is none to mobilise. They are even more useful where the skin is also old and friable, a not uncommon combination. Here cosmesis is secondary to healing. A modification of the standard technique is detailed below wherein a mould is cut and seated on a bed of tulle gras to hold the graft, which is pressed to the bed to provide greater security and take.

Although grafts are used too frequently and STSGs do not give the best cosmetic result, they do have a place in lower legs in the elderly and those with compromised circulation. An O-Z or other flaps may give a good result, but they are technically more difficult and may leave a central deficit necessitating 6 weeks or so to close by secondary intention with the risk of infection and a chronic ulcer. Another site is the anterior and posterior surfaces of the ear where the skin is naturally thin with little subcutaneous tissue. The appearance of an STSG in these ear sites may be preferable to any other repair. If cosmesis is not the concern, the cancer can be excised with the correct margins and an STSG inserted, which invariably takes with fewer postoperative complications.

Contractions

Generally, an STSG will result in greater long-term contraction than an FTSG that will, due to the greater content of elastin fibres, initially contract more. An FTSG is better for small deficits.

If there is any delay in donation, some surgeons oversize the graft by 10–20% before it is placed in the wound because it will contract before it is sewn into the site bed.

Avoid STSGs where there is a free edge, such as the nasal alar and lower eyelid, as long-term contractions will deform the free edge.

Types

1 **Sheets** cover the wound completely. This, in effect, is the only technique to be recommended here. The aim is to acquire a good technique to provide a sheet of graft to cover the deficit.
2 **Mesh sheets** are cut and expanded to make a mesh graft. Meshing, scoring or punching holes in an STSG allows it to be expanded to cover a larger area.
3 **Patches (stamp grafts)** are: (a) more resistant to infection because the exudate easily drains from under them; (b) small enough to fit into the concavities of an irregular wound; (c) easier to take.

However, they: (a) cannot be expanded into a mesh patch; (b) do not require any less skin; (c) take longer to heal; (d) are uglier than single sheet grafts, so they are particularly contraindicated on the face. They are useful if a wound is very irregular or there is serious oozing or infection is not completely controlled. They are very much better than nothing, but to be avoided if possible.

4 **Strips** are used for wounds that will only be completely covered if sheets of skin are used. In all other kinds of STSG, including mesh grafts, the epidermis has to grow across gaps. This it does easily but the cosmetic result will not be so good.

Indications

Lower limb cancers with compromised conditions (elderly, venous stasis, friable skin) where cosmesis is not a major concern.

Anterior and posterior surfaces of the ear (but simple ellipses or flaps can mostly be done).

Instruments

Electric or compressed air dermatomes are used in high throughput situations. Occasional users are more likely to use a hand-held roller blade, which is recommended. Razor blades, cutthroat razors and scalpel blades have also been used but don't provide the uniform thickness of a dedicated instrument.

The most common harvesting knives are the Humby and its modification, the Watson (Cobbett and Braithwaite).

Harvesting hand-held knives

These are blades with a roller and a calibration device to cut skin grafts of different thicknesses. In truth their result is similar to that of a cheese or ham slicer. There are some four models to choose from, namely the original 19.8-cm wide Humby with four holes and the later, modified 15.8-cm wide Watson, Braithwaite and Cobbett with three holes (Figure 11.4). All provide adequate width samples for skin surgery as very few lesions are >4 cm, especially on the lower leg where STSGs are recommended. A Weck blade can be used for small grafts. Aesculap have a 'silver' razor blade graft knife that is half the price but limits the size. These stainless steel knife handles are used in conjunction with the sterile skin graft blades for harvesting grafts. The knives have an in-built adjustable guard that limits the maximal thickness of the graft harvested depending on the properties of the skin at the donor site. The blades can be re-sterilised and used several times.

Technique

The exact thickness of the graft depends upon:

- the blade setting
- the contact angle between the blade and skin while harvesting (angle of attack)

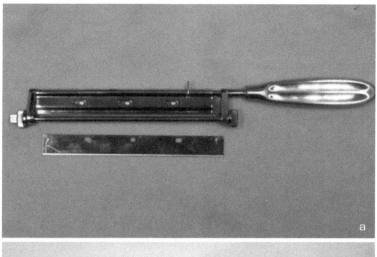

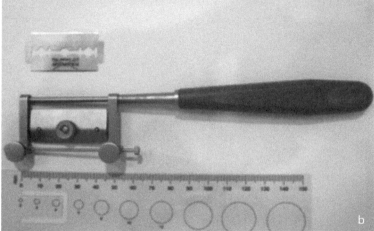

Figure 11.4 Harvesting hand held knives

a The Watson skin graft knife or 'handle' with the stainless steel blade below. The Watson, Braithwaite and Cobbett handles or knives are modifications of the Humby with a slightly shorter blade of 158 mm and three holes, with the one blade fitting all three. The original Humby has 4 holes and the blade is somewhat longer at 196 mm. **b** The silver razor blade knife (Aesculap).

- the pressure applied by the operator onto the knife while harvesting
- the efficiency in stretching the donor site to a uniform tension
- the donor area
- the age of the patient.

Selection of skin thickness

The usable thickness of thigh skin graft varies from a minimum of 0.25 mm to a maximum of 0.55 mm in most cases, though in elderly patients or steroid-damaged skin a thinner graft needs to be taken [2].

Although a number of papers have suggested ways to select the gauge, the simplest method is to wind the roller down to the thinnest setting. In practice, being able to vary the thickness of a graft is not important, and a graft of average or even varying thickness is enough for most purposes.

Another way to determine the appropriate gauge is simply to look at it at eye level such that there is the thickness of a razor blade gap. Yet another is to insert a scalpel blade as a feeler-gauge. A standard number 15 scalpel blade, which is 0.39 mm thick, is a good guide to surgeons who harvest skin grafts infrequently. The skin graft knife is adjusted to a setting just wide enough to permit the scalpel blade to fit snugly between the roller guard and the skin graft blade [3]. This is recommended until it is known if the thinnest gauge of the instrument is reliable.

The skin on the anterior and lateral aspects of the thigh is most easily accessed and used (posterior is difficult for the patient to access to treat and medial may rub). To facilitate harvesting, take it from the same limb as the excision. This thigh skin is classed as intermediate thickness for the purposes of skin grafting; an optimum harvest is 0.35 mm thick [2]. This would include the full thickness of the epidermis and the papillary layer of the dermis in the graft and part of the reticular layer with full preservation of the adnexal structures. This provides a durable, relatively cosmetic

graft and would also permit good regeneration of the donor site.

Donor sites
Refer to Figure 11.5.

- Upper thigh (anterior, lateral); posterior is too hard for the patient to dress and medial rubs

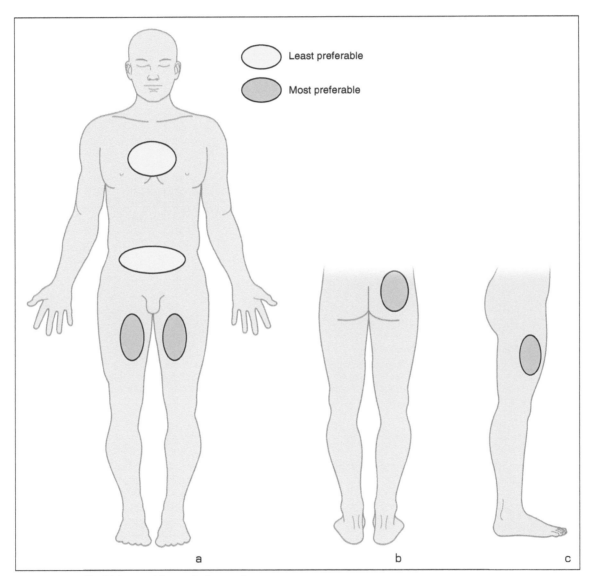

Figure 11.5 Split-thickness skin graft donor sites

a Optimal areas for patient wound care are identified by pink shading. **b, c** When cosmesis of the donor site is a concern, buttock skin should be harvested. These sites are preferable because of the ability to get a firm, flat area. This makes it easier to harvest the STSG.

Adapted from Robinson JK, Arndt KA, Le Boit PE, Wintroub BU (eds). Atlas of cutaneous surgery. Philadelphia: WB Saunders, 1996; (Fig 13.2a).

- Buttocks
- Upper arms (inner)

STSGs are commonly harvested from the thigh, buttocks, abdominal wall or scalp.

Tensioning and stretching the skin

The key is to present the surgeon with a flat, tense area providing a constant resistance and a uniform sheet of graft split skin. There are a number of methods to stretch and tension the skin. Originally, blocks of wood were used to press down and away from the donor site. These can be placed both above and below the donor site. Tongue depressors are sometimes used. An assistant can also stretch the skin above and below with thumb and index finger. Perhaps the best way, which provides the operator with some feedback, is for the assistant to stretch the starting end while the operator stretches the end closer to where he is slicing or the surgeon secures the starting end while the assistant places a tongue depressor immediately above the blade and drags the edge, flattening and stretching the skin immediately in front of the sawing knife.

The area is marked as a rectangle somewhat larger than the donor site and a field block performed. The donor skin is prepped, which is then wiped off with saline.

Lubricating the harvest area

Normal saline, rather than lubricating cream, is used immediately before harvesting to hydrate and lubricate the skin. Sterile 5-mL ampoules are readily available.

Harvesting the STSG skin

Refer to Figure 11.6 to see the sequence of steps for excising the lesion, harvesting the graft, applying it to the recipient site and dressing the wounds.

1 Hold the knife at the start of the drawn rectangle.
2 The assistant stretches the skin both sideways and away from the knife with either the hands or a tongue depressor. At the same time the operator either stretches the far end if the assistant is stretching behind the knife or crosses hands to stabilise the skin immediately behind the knife if the assistant is dragging the tongue depressor in front.
3 When a flat, tense field is secured, saw the knife at a 45° angle into the skin and continue this sawing, back-and-forth action to the marked lateral edges and towards the operator's other hand, trying to ensure a rectangular, complete harvest.
4 At the finish, turn the knife down and remove it, if possible, and cut the attached end with a scalpel.

Transferring the graft

Place the STSG on some tulle gras/paraffin gauze/Cuticerin™ or a non-stick dressing.

> ### Important
>
> **Ensure the skin graft (external) surface is face down on the tulle gras** as this is to be turned over so that it is uppermost in the recipient site (i.e. the graft is placed internal epidermis up, skin surface down, on the tulle, then later turned over, skin/external surface up, into recipient site). Dedicated carriers for the graft are available but these excisions are usually small enough for the surgeon to use the open hand.
>
> Thin skin graft surfaces can look the same when harvested. Applying skin grafts inside out is not unknown.

Applying the graft to the recipient site

The lesion should have already been excised and haemostasis secured. The most common complication is a subgraft haematoma preventing attachment and therefore healing.

The site should be clean. STSGs usually heal on any surface. Over the tibia, where many of these lesions are, there is frequently little fat and hence little blood supply. Don't worry; the STSG will still heal.

1 Place the graft on the site (tulle up) to get a bloody outline impression of the recipient site.
2 Cut the graft to this outline and fit it into the site.
3 Sew the graft and tulle to the edges, alternating opposite sides. Suture from the graft first to the fixed excision site edges. Ensure eversion of the epidermal edges. 6/0 and 5/0 nylon are usual though absorbable sutures can also be used.
4 Get a mould of Allevyn thin or sterilised make-up sponge and again make an imprint of the site and cut to fit (see Figure 11.7).

Dressings

Fulgurate the **donor site** to secure haemostasis. Theoretically, no antibiotic is needed but the size of the site seems to make these wounds more susceptible to infection and a smear of chloramphenicol may be used.

The STSG donor site epidermis regenerates by secondary epithelialisation from the wound edges and from immigration of dermal cells originating in the shafts of hair follicles as well as adnexal structures remaining in the dermis. Although the dermis never regenerates, the same site may be harvested again for subsequent grafts as only a portion is removed in an STSG. STSG donor sites generally heal within 7 days and can be dressed in various ways.

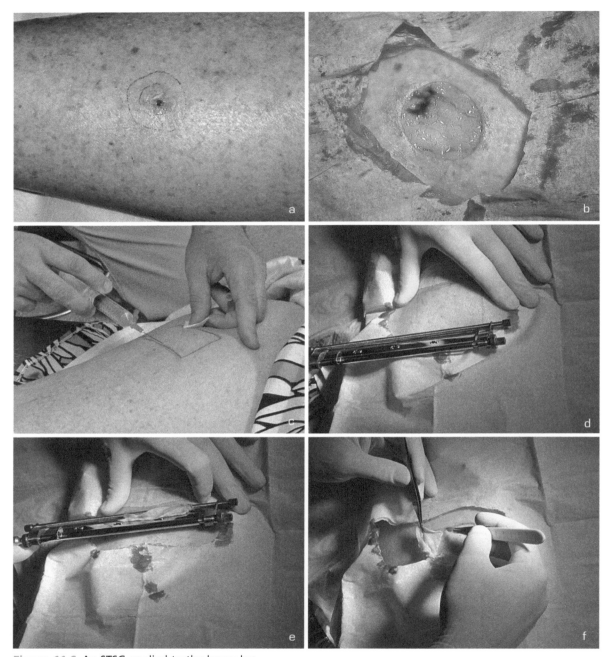

Figure 11.6 An STSG applied to the lower leg

a SCC lower leg. **b** Excised. **c** Donor site is the thigh; marked and field blocking. **d** Donor site harvested using a Humby knife. Assistant holds and stretches the skin both top and bottom. Use the harvesting knife on the thinnest/most wound down setting. **e** Direction of shave doesn't matter: proximal-distal or distal-proximal. **f** WARNING: ensure the split skin is transferred to a paraffin gauze correctly orientated. It is easy to make a mistake and, although it may not seem so, it can be difficult to identify which is the superficial external surface and which is the cut internal epidermal surface of a very thin graft. Thinness of the donor split skin is immaterial.

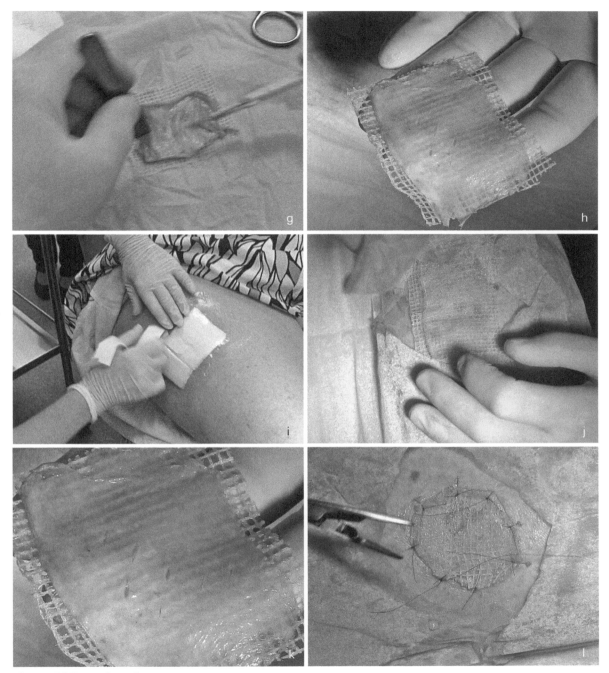

Figure 11.6 continued

g Place the harvest skin on paraffin gauze. Make sure it is surface side up. The paraffin gauze will be the external surface dressing of this STSG; hence the surface of the graft should be placed down on the gauze, which is later turned over to be placed on the graft site. **h** Perhaps the simplest explanation is to imagine your palm is the paraffin gauze and that ultimately you will be placing your palm over and down on the graft site with the paraffin gauze uppermost. **i** The harvest site is cauterised/fulgurated to achieve haemostasis. Alginate dressings have proven satisfactory (Kaltostat gauze squares). A transparent waterproof is then placed over this. The harvest site can cause more problems than the graft site (as it is a large open area, meticulous sterility should be observed). **j** Harvest graft is put on paraffin gauze and applied to the recipient site to get a bloody impression outline template. **k** Cut around the outside of this impression. It is better to initially have a graft slightly too big that can be trimmed than one too small that has to be stretched, which potentially causes a space under it. Don't panic if you cut too small as slits in the graft will allow it to expand and seat into the bed and also provide drains for any exudate. **l** The graft cut to fit is sutured into place. Suture from the opposite side (e.g. 12 then 6 o'clock) and from the graft to the fixed edge.

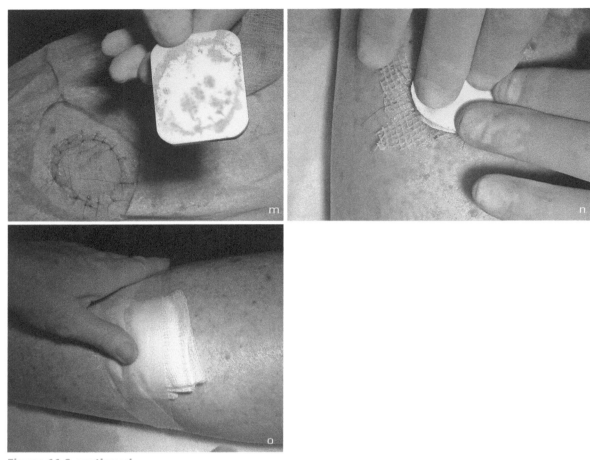

Figure 11.6 continued

m A sterilised make-up sponge or an Allevyn non-adhesive dressing is pressed onto the graft and cut to shape. This will form a compression mould pressing the skin graft onto the site bed. **n** Another layer of paraffin gauze is laid over the graft and the cut and fitted mould pressed into the site. This mould can also be sutured into place. **o** Pressure cotton gauze and paper adhesive bandage. Conforming bandages are applied to both sites.

(Above surgery by Dr Bill Ansiline.)

A Kaltostat® dressing has been traditionally used but clear waterproofs are also used if the patient is phlegmatic and can cope with looking at a raw site; alternatively, gauze squares can be placed on top and strapped firmly down and secured with paper strapping. An occlusive, semipermeable, polyurethane dressing such as OpSite™/Tegaderm™ can be applied to the donor site and has the advantage of significantly reducing pain at the donor site in many patients while keeping the wound moist and thereby enabling it to heal faster. Should the serous fluid production preclude the use of an OpSite dressing, materials such as Xeroform™ (Kendall) or Acticoat™ (Smith & Nephew) may be applied to the donor site and left in place until healed. A conforming bandage is used for 2 days.

These sites can be more problematical than the graft site and need close attention. Review at 2–3 days. The donor site can take 2–3 weeks to heal and be red for 6 months to a year. The donor site is not without impaired cosmesis as hypertrophic scar formation or changes in skin pigmentation can occur upon healing. They usually remain as a distinct pale patch.

It is essential that the **recipient site** dressing:

- is non-adherent so the graft is not peeled off when the dressing is removed
- applies constant 'good' pressure to the graft pushing it onto the bed (? mould)
- allows the egress of sub-graft sero-sanguinous fluid

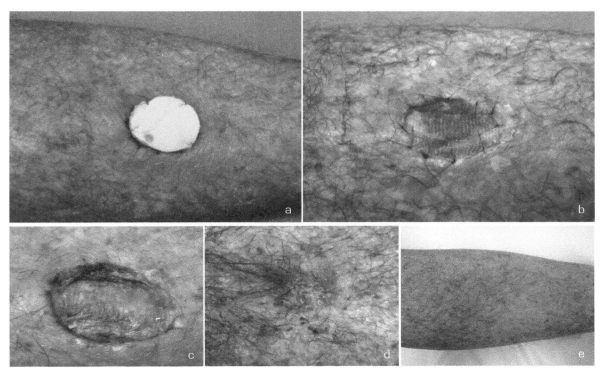

Figure 11.7 Mould application and healing of an STSG

a Anterior tibial surface STSG with mould for large BCC. Here the mould has been sutured onto the graft. The greatest cause of graft failure is bed exudate lifting the donor skin off the bed. Moulds prevent this by providing even pressure and seating the graft into the site bed. **b** 7 days later: mould can be removed. Although grafts are to be avoided wherever possible, the size and position of this BCC made an STSG the only option. **c** 2 weeks later. Don't panic! Leave. **d** 6 months later. **e** 18 months later.

- minimises shearing forces or disturbance to the graft.

A non-stick dressing such as Melolin or Cutilin is cut to the shape of the graft by pressing it onto the wound to get a template or the same is done using Allevyn Thin or similar to apply as a mould. For STSGs a paraffin gauze is usually used rather than the non-adherent dressing and can be secured by a couple of sutures through the mould.

Then sterile gauze or dental rolls are mostly used as a pressure bolster/pad plus a conforming bandage to keep pressure pushing the graft and mould onto the site bed. Gauze net tubing can also be used.

The initial dressing should be left in place for approximately 5 days (3–7 days) unless pain, odour, discharge or another sign of a complication develops. Inspect at 4–5 days. Be careful not to disturb the graft when removing the dressing. Replace a new dressing. A haematoma or seroma encountered at the dressing change should be addressed by making a small incision directly over the collection and expressing the underlying contents in order to minimise disruption of graft adherence, but this can be obviated by placing slits in the graft immediately after suturing it in. After 10–14 days the graft looks like it is healing (i.e. pink and adherent). Sutures can be removed at this stage.

On the ear the dressing can be left off after 2 weeks, but the healed graft site should be kept well moisturised with a petroleum-based ointment for another 2 weeks. The leg takes longer and regular dressings are needed. All should be kept dry. If a scab/eschar forms resist all impulses to debride it. Let it slough off in its own unassisted time.

GRAFTS ON DIGITS

Small lesions on fingers can be quickly and easily grafted using a 12-mm punch, which not only excises the lesion but provides the perfectly sized graft (Figure 11.8).

There is very little loose or available skin on the fingers and grafts are both practically and cosmetically acceptable here.

Grafts: Patient postoperation instructions

Grafts are more delicate than normal wounds and require more care and protection. The whole aim is not to disturb the graft in any way whatsoever to allow it to 'take'.

The first 2 weeks are critical.

- Reduce all activity
  - Any activity can overload the graft circulation and cause damage.
  - Ensure your blood pressure is well controlled.
  - No heavy lifting.
  - Avoid stress, conflict, arguments.
  - Avoid anyone touching the graft area.
- Reduce all exercise and movement
  - The graft has to 'marry' to its bed and any movement will shear it away from this bed and then cause bleeding, which will lift it off and cause the entire graft to die.
  - Blood vessels have to grow from the bed into the graft to nourish it if it is to survive. Any movement breaks these incredibly delicate new blood vessels.
  - No moving the area, no bending.
- Medications
  - Ensure blood pressure is controlled.
  - Cease blood thinners if possible (only under prescribing doctor's permission).
- The next 2 weeks are also risky
  - Continue to avoid all activity that may elevate your blood pressure or pulse rate.
  - Avoid anything other than very mild exercise. No lifting, carting parcels, walking more than short distances. No racing around.
- Avoid pressure/movement while sleeping
  - Grafts on the face and ears are at danger of being sheared while rolling over during sleep. Ensure secure dressings are in place.
  - Ensure 'security strips' are put over the site if and when sutures are removed.
- Specific sites
  - Nose and ears: are not prone to outside interference of movement but rather more likely to be damaged turning in one's sleep. Good secure dressings are the secret.
  - Hands: are most at risk from movement that causes shearing and bleeding. A sling, splinting and absolute adherence to stabilising the affected part is essential. Use the sling to keep the hand to the opposite shoulder above the heart.
  - Legs: standing or walking increases the hydrostatic pressure and can 'blow out' the graft. Minimise standing and walking to absolute essentials. Elevate with heels on cushion above nipples, nothing under calves. Keep contracting calves to avoid deep vein thrombosis.

(Courtesy MoleChex)

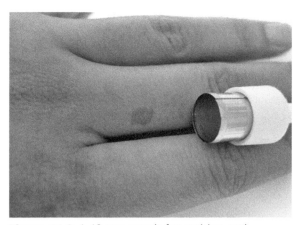

Figure 11.8 A 12-mm punch for excising and harvesting

REFERENCES

[1] Jacobs MA, Christenson LJ, Weaver AL, et al. Clinical outcome of cutaneous flaps versus full-thickness skin grafts after Mohs surgery on the nose. Dermatol Surg 2010;36(1):23–30.

[2] Ostrovisky NV. Selection of the skin graft thickness with regard to the structure of the donor site skin. Acta Chir Plast 1985;27:145–51.

[3] Nnene CO, Abu-Seido H, Isbister ES. Harvesting split skin grafts of appropriate thickness using the hand-held knife. Ann R Coll Surg Engl 2000;82:339–40.

Postoperative care 12

Dressings

Early to bed,
Early to rise,
Work like hell,
And advertise.

Ted Turner on the creation of CNN

Time spent making a clinically correct dressing, but also a neat and elegant one, is not only good medicine but provides (if not advertising) the visible evidence of clinic standards and is most reassuring to patients, their friends and your waiting room. A 'dog's-dinner' dressing is off-putting to patients and potential patients. Dressings may be regarded as a dark art by modern clinicians, but an excellent operation can be made to look inferior by a vulgar dressing. Ears and noses are the most difficult sites and, although staff can be trained to do an excellent job when it comes to ears, for noses and grafts the person who operated best understands how the dressing should go and should not entrust this to anyone else until they have demonstrated their expertise.

Skin surgery usually only deals with acute clean sites and non-contaminated and non-complicated wounds where a waterproof dressing does the job. It is essential to provide the best conditions for optimum healing. This means occlusive dressings left on as long as possible. Today there is a selection of such dressings that come ready packed and ensure waterproof occlusion, such as SurgiClear, OpSite or Tegaderm. Wounds in the scalp and hairy areas, where sticking any dressing is impossible, are best treated with barrier film sprays which, in effect, work the same. Grafts, however, can break down and flaps may have defects, and secondary intention healing may be needed. Diabetic patients are prone to develop ulcers below the knee. These and other chronic, complicated wounds are best treated in a dedicated hospital dressings unit but, if not available, the practitioner or clinic nurse can avail themselves of the latest dressings.

Knowledge of the total spectrum of dressings is provided in this chapter. The main problem is convincing the patient and other health workers not to take them off. The days of 'daily dressings' are over.

THE IDEAL DRESSING

- Is sterile.
- Provides mechanical and bacterial protection.
- Maintains a moist environment.
- Is non-adherent.
- Removes excessive exudate without allowing the wound to dry out.
- Allows gaseous and fluid exchange.
- Is thermal insulating to maintain core temperature at 37°C.
- Is impermeable to microorganisms, minimising contamination from outside.
- Is safe, non-traumatic, non-toxic, non-allergenic.
- Does not damage granulating tissue at dressing change.
- Is easy to use.
- Has patient acceptance as to comfort and pain relief.
- Does not need frequent changing.
- Is available in a range of sizes.
- Is cost effective.

OPTIMUM HEALING

It has been observed that blisters that remain intact ('roofed') heal faster than those that have been debrided or burst. Subsequently, wounds covered with an occlusive dressing (Figure 12.1) were shown to heal 40% faster than those exposed to air. This is thought to occur because of enhanced keratinocyte migration due to moisture, containment of wound fluid with growth factors in it, creation of an electromagnetic current and the

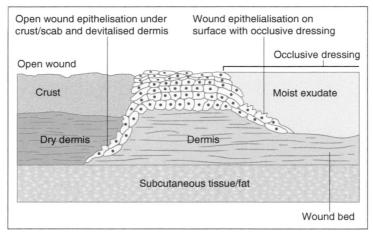

Figure 12.1 Occlusive dressing
Occlusive dressings allow epithelialisation to occur at the wound surface. In open wounds the epithelium migrates beneath a desiccated crust and devitalised dermis.
Adapted from Habif TP, Clinical Dermatology, 4th edn. Philadelphia: Mosby, 2009; p 923.

prevention of infection [1, 2]. Fibroblasts populate the wound after 48–72 hours and their growth is enhanced by low oxygen and high lactate levels, which may explain why occlusive dressings help.

Occlusive dressings

Wounds under occlusive dressings heal 40% faster:

- 4 days minimum
- 7(+) days best.

THE BASIC DRESSING

For skin surgery the fundamental dressing (Figure 12.2) incorporates:

1 surface lubricant – white soft paraffin (Vaseline) or an ointment
2 a non-stick, non-adherent layer
3 a pressure pad cushion layer of folded gauze
4 strong stretch adhesive strapping (Fixomull, Hypafix®).

This is the fundamental dressing for noses and ears as it can be cut and shaped around eyes, nose and ears. It is best used where pressure is needed, as with a graft, and where it won't get wet. Elsewhere, waterproof dressings are best.

NON-ADHERENT DRESSINGS

Non-adherent dressings include Cutilin, Melolin and Telfa, which are made of gauze, lint or cotton absorbent

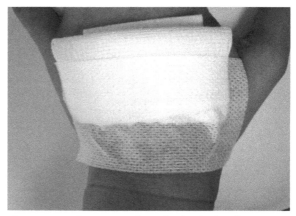

Figure 12.2 Demonstration of a basic dressing
A non-stick sheet is applied immediately next to the skin where the actual incision is best covered with a lubricant. Folded gauze squares provide both a protective cushion and pressure if and when the final stretch adhesive tape is strapped over.

pads covered with a perforated plastic film to prevent adherence. Telfa also contains latex and is potentially allergenic.

For normal postoperative dressings, the distinct advantage of commercial dressings is the convenience of their being waterproof. Although more expensive, they can be applied with greater speed, less trouble, better healing and patient satisfaction. SurgiClear, OpSite Post-op and Tegaderm are frequently used.

ADHERENT DRESSINGS

The most adherent dressings are hydrocolloids, followed by acrylates, polyurethane dressings and silicone dressings [3].

OTHER DRESSINGS

The only other dressings that may occasionally be needed are those for:

- granulating wounds healing by secondary intention
- open slow Mohs wounds (temporary dressings)
- threatened infections/grafts (antimicrobial)
- covers to improve scars
- hairy areas where it is impossible to stick a dressing such as the scalp (barrier films).

Interactive dressings

Interactive dressings help control the microenvironment by combining with the exudate to form a hydrophilic gel or by controlling the flow of exudate from the wound into the dressing (using semi-permeable membranes). They may also stimulate activity in the healing cascade and speed up the healing process.

There are six classes of interactive dressings:

1 Non-absorbing
2 Absorbing:
  A Hydrocolloid
  B Foam
  C Alginate
  D Hydroactive
  E Hydrogel

Non-absorbing, waterproof, transparent island films – no-to-low exudate wounds

These are waterproof commercial substitutes for the classic dressing in Figure 12.2. They are the standard postoperative dressing (Figure 12.3). Each has a thin polyurethane membrane coated with a layer of acrylic adhesive and the following attributes:

- flexible
- transparent
- waterproof
- gas and vapour permeable
- protect from shear, friction, chemicals and microbes
- spread tension forces.

Plain film dressings are available but the island pad is recommended for postoperative dressings. The plain type can be used as a wound binder/support, rather than tape strips, after removal of sutures (ROS) to reduce tension and prevent dehiscence. They should not be used for infected wounds. Their disadvantages are cost and fixed sizes that cannot be trimmed to shape. They can be used on all skin cancer clean surgical wounds (postoperatively) except on the nose, ears and hairy areas.

Hydrocolloids – low-to-moderate exudate wounds

Hydrocolloids are complex dressings containing polymers held in suspension plus methylcellulose, pectin, gelatin, polyisobutylene and adhesives. They slowly absorb wound fluids changing their physical state to become a covering, soft gel that sits on the wound. They promote autolysis to aid the removal of slough.

Initially changed daily, when the exudate has diminished they may be left on for 7 days.

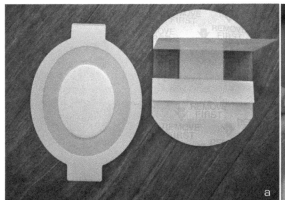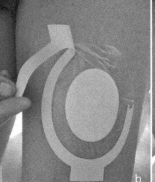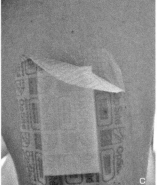

Figure 12.3 Two popular waterproof island dressings
a Tegaderm (left) and OpSite (right). **b** Tagaderm has a paper peel-off peripheral strip. **c** OpSite has a double layer and the entire printed top peels off. Newer, similar dressings such as SurgiClear do the same job but are considerably cheaper.

- Presentation: pad, sheet or filler form for occlusive use.
- Indications: small, solitary non-draining ulcers or light-to-moderate exudate wounds; after debridement; granulating wounds.
- Advantages:
  - flexible
  - waterproof
  - impermeable to bacteria and other contaminants
  - promote autolysis, angiogenesis and granulation
  - self-adhesive and mould well
  - limited-to-moderate absorption
  - create moist environment
  - may be left in place for up to 7 days
  - may be worn in the shower
  - no secondary dressing needed
  - thin transparent brands are available
  - powder, which forms the gel, available for deeper wounds and can be covered with a wafer.

Superficial surgical wounds

According to trial results, faster healing in comparison with the control treatment supported the use of a hydrocolloid wound dressing for the treatment of superficial surgical wounds (shave excisions etc). The hydrocolloid wound dressing (Avery H2460) induced significantly ($p < 0.05$) faster healing (median = 8.5 days) in comparison with the control treatment (median = 10 days). Histological investigations showed no significant differences between the two groups for the investigated parameters [4].

Foams/polyurethane pads – medium-to-high exudate

These are soft, non-adherent hydrophobic or -philic dressings.

- Indications: non-infected, draining granular wounds or light-to-medium-to-high exuding wounds. Mould for grafts. They have many of the properties of the ideal dressing.
- Advantages:
  - non-adherent
  - won't injure surrounding skin
  - allow passage and absorption of exudate into the dressing
  - absorbent
  - repel contaminants
  - may be used under compression
  - cushion wound surface
  - maintain moist wound environment
  - highly conforming
  - gas permeable
  - thermal insulating
  - non-residual.

They come with or without adhesive borders. Good for granulating wounds healing by secondary intention and can be left on for up to 7 days.

Calcium alginates – medium-to-high exudate

Alginates are derived from seaweed and are highly absorbable and biodegradable. They are used for non-infected, exuding wounds. They should not be used on dry wounds but may be used as a temporary dressing for an open slow Mohs excision site. They form a gel that absorbs the exudate while maintaining a moist environment at the interface with the wound. Alginate dressings can be changed by washing the saturated dressing away with saline solution. As a result, newly formed tissue is said not to be disturbed.

Advantages:

- highly absorbent
- combine with exudate to form a gel
- maintain a moist surface
- easily removed
- haemostatic.

Algin, which is obtained from seaweed, can be converted into alginic acid, which is insoluble, and then into soluble salts such as sodium alginate or insoluble salts such as calcium alginate. The use of calcium and sodium alginate materials made into wool or gauze in surgery and in the dressing of wounds has been well known for many years having, for example, been reported in surgery annals as early as 1947. UK-based research in the 1960s and 1970s showed that alginates (e.g. Sorbsan) produce the ideal warm, moist environment for healing wounds, including long-standing infected ulcers. More recently, various alginate wound dressing products have become commercially available, mainly in the form of calcium alginate fibres that can be processed into a non-woven fabric, cut to size, packaged and sterilised.

Kaltostat is a calcium alginate fibre produced by a special wet-spinning process from a variety of seaweed species. Supplied as non-woven wound dressings for the treatment of exudating wounds, the product is said to encourage the formation of a controlled ion-active gel over the wound site, which reacts with the sodium ions in the exudate or blood to aid wound healing. Use in oozing open wounds or slow Mohs.

Hydroactive – medium-to-high exudate

These are highly absorbent, multilayered polymer dressings with a surface adhesive and a waterproof outer layer similar to hydrocolloids. However, instead of forming a gel with the exudate, the exudate is trapped within the dressing itself.

Properties:

- highly absorbent
- waterproof
- expandable
- non-residual
- semi-permeable.

Hydroactive dressings are indicated for highly exuding wounds including leg ulcers, pressure wounds and minor burns. They are especially useful over joins such as elbows, knees, fingers and toes because they can expand and contract. They are contraindicated for dry or lightly exuding wounds.

Hydrogels – dry or sloughing wounds

Hydrogels are complex organic polymers with a cross-linked hydrophilic matrix impregnated into gauze. This type of pad allows transmission of water, vapour and CO_2 but discourages dehydration. As they are 30–90% water they have taken the place of the classic 'wet dressing' and are suitable for all stages of wound healing except infected or heavily exuding wounds. They re-hydrate and absorb. They swell but do not dissolve and are available as gels or sheets.

- Indications: full thickness wounds with moderate drainage; dry necrotic wounds; burns including sunburn, scalds and other partial thickness burns. The gels have been used in chicken pox and shingles.
- Advantages:
  - soothing with marked pain reduction
  - conform to the wound
  - fill in dead spaces
  - highly absorbent
  - can be used on infected wounds.
    Disadvantages: difficult to keep in place; encourage gram negative organisms.

Hypertonic dressings for hypergranulation – 'proud flesh'

Hypergranulation was traditionally treated with topical silver nitrate or copper sulfate ('blue-stone'). These were frequently hard to source and there were no 'instructions'. Thankfully, an alternative and less toxic method is the application of hypertonic saline.

Hypertonic saline dressings are available as Mesalt® and Curasalt™ and are changed daily and held on the hypergranulating wound by a secondary dressing and a compression bandage.

Adhesive silicon gel sheets for scar treatment

Silicone dressings are inert flexible sheets or gels that are useful for flattening scar tissue, increasing elasticity and reducing discolouration. They are expensive and patients sometimes wonder if their scar wouldn't have healed just as well without them.

Self-adhesiveness and durability mean that application is simple and the gel sheet can be washed and used several times (e.g. Cica-Care™, Smith & Nephew).

Resorbing matrices

Matrix is a primary dressing that transforms into a soft, conformable gel, allowing contact with the entire wound bed. It consists of 45% regenerating cellulose and 55% type I collagen.

The persisting inflammatory phase in chronic wounds contributes to exudate with high concentrations of matrix metalloproteases (MMPs). Overabundant MMPs result in degradation of extracellular matrix proteins and inactivation of growth factors. The cellulose/collagen combination binds more MMPs than oxidised regenerated cellulose or collagen alone.

Barrier films

Barrier films form a membranous cover that reduces the amount of moisture lost by the skin. They are protective polymers in a quick-drying solvent. They often reduce pain and are obviously ideal for scalps and areas where dressings cannot stick.

Antimicrobials

Silver has been used for decades as an antimicrobial dressing. It is thought to interfere with bacterial ion transport, bind to bacterial DNA inhibiting replication, interact with the cell membrane and form insoluble and metabolically ineffective compounds. In any case, it seems to work! Broad spectrum antimicrobial action, bacterial toxin management and odour control are claimed by the manufacturer for Actisorb® Silver 220.

Acticoat™ is a newer product available in a non-absorbable and also a calcium alginate absorbable form and has demonstrated improved antimicrobial performance over existing silver-based products.

> **Summary: dressings for skin surgery**
>
> Postoperative: waterproof plain or island film dressings; non-stick film, gauze, adhesive strapping
> Graft donor sites: alginates, foam, film
> Slow Mohs: alginates
> Shave excisions: hydrocolloids
> Ulcers/exudates: dry – hydrogels; light to moderate exudate – hydrocolloids, foams, alginates
> Hairy areas: spray

DRESSINGS FOR SPECIAL SITES

The fundamental dressing is comprised of a non-stick base, a gauze if more pressure is wanted and Fixomull/Hypafix trimmed to shape.

Nose

Chloramphenicol ointment, which has already been smeared in the nares preoperatively, is again used first on the wound. Then a non-stick dressing (Telfa etc) is applied, followed by a gauze pad and, finally, some Fixomull, all cut to shape (Figure 12.4). Simply trimming the Fixomull to follow the contours, while medically not necessary, greatly reassures the patient.

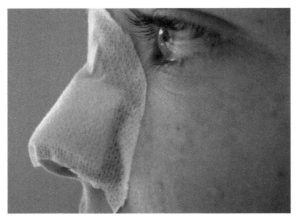

Figure 12.4 **Nose dressing**

Ears

Ears are the most difficult sites to dress. Ear surgeons use an array of bulky plastic and foam protectors but these are not necessary for skin cancer excisions. Furthermore, pressure dressings were found to lead to an increased incidence of bruising, erythema and dehiscence [5].

Although not universally applicable, the trapdoor ear dressing is often the easiest and most useful dressing as it minimises bulk and unwanted pressure [6] (Figure 12.5).

Fingers

Please refer Figure 12.6.

RETENTION TAPES: STRAPPING

Retention tapes are permeable and flexible, allowing exudate to flow through. They are not waterproof but may be washed and will dry and remain in place. Removal can be painlessly achieved using a proprietary or citrus oil. They can be cut to form economical steristrips suitable post ROS to apply to a healed wound as they are not sterile. They are most useful for designer dressings for the nose, ears and around the eyes (e.g. Fixomull, Hypafix).

These will not adhere if touched with the fingers. Either apply with forceps or as illustrated (Figure 12.7).

Better strip adherence

Clean the skin with acetone (often found as nail polish remover). Paint with Tinct Benz Co until it dries tacky. Smith & Nephew Skin-Prep, in sachets like alcohol swabs, also works with the added benefit of guaranteed sterility.

Fixomull strips

Tape strips are not recommended in place of sutures as they do not guarantee security and can peel off, leading to dehiscence. They may be used to reduce tension in sutured wounds but are mostly used after ROS when the wound has healed but may need protecting or further

security. The face, nose and ears are especially vulnerable as sutures are removed early and the patient may roll over in bed smearing the wound open. When the wound is healed and sealed sterile tapes, which are expensive, are not necessary, Fixomull cut into strips does an excellent, if not superior, job as its glue seems stronger and it stretches forming a dumbbell-like strip with broader ends and applying tension across the wound (Figure 12.8). Sterile strips won't stick if touched other than by forceps whereas Fixomull strips are inexpensive and will stick. Hence, patients can be given a supply of these.

RETENTION CONFORMING BANDAGES

Lightweight conforming bandages have, to a large extent, taken over from the crepe bandage for holding dressings in place and for applying sufficient pressure to aid haemostasis and prevent haematoma formation. They are especially useful on the forehead, lower arm and leg.

WHEN TO TAKE A DRESSING DOWN

Wound infection and excessive bleeding, not staining, are reasons to take a dressing down. Most are taken off incorrectly as the wound exudates have growth factors that promote healing.

Dressings are mostly removed prematurely due to patient alarm or staff misconceptions. As emphasised, a waterproof dressing that allows the wound to bathe in its own sweat and exudate has been found to be most beneficial to wound healing. Most patients who want their dressing changed do so because either they or, more often, their family are alarmed at the blood staining emerging through the dressing. However, when it is taken off, although there is some coagulated blood, the wound is looking good. If the patient cannot be reassured, there is

---

 NOTE

No daily dressings!

Wound infection is indicated by:

- pain and increasing or new pain are the first indications
- inflammation (usually greater than 1 cm from the wound edges)
- temperature
- malaise
- bleeding – fresh oozing blood escaping from under the dressing
- haematoma (may be able to be palpated through the dressing)
- discharge – any suspicion of a purulent discharge must be investigated (and cultured).

Apart from that, leave it on!

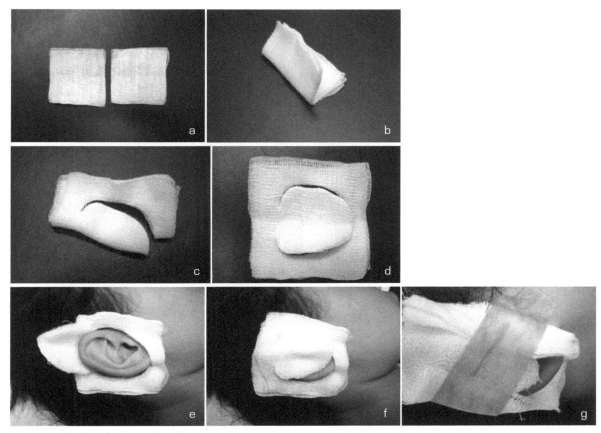

Figure 12.5 Trapdoor ear dressing

This is a fast, easy and controllable dressing. **a** Take two 4 × 4 gauze squares. **b** Fold them over to create a solid spine. **c** Cut an incomplete semicircle (from the folded side) with a diameter somewhat less than half the diameter of the patient's ear. When this is opened, it provides a hole for the ear that is smaller than the actual ear due to its free posterior margin. **d** The opened dressing now has a tongue. **e** Slip the dressing over the ear. As it is smaller, it snuggles under the posterior margin of the ear. **f** Push the tongue into the ear's internal surfaces. A non-stick dressing, white soft paraffin (Vaseline) or chloramphenicol ointment moulds this as needed. **g** Fold the anterior and posterior edges of the gauze back over the helix and tragus (for demonstration purposes this is deliberately done here with a different coloured tape). Folding over the gauze superiorly and inferiorly is also possible, and the dressing can then be made neater than most other ear dressings by trimming and strapping.

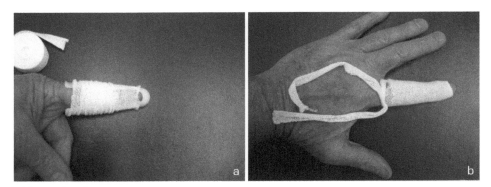

Figure 12.6 Finger dressing

a Tubular gauze is supplied in rolls with a plastic over-slip guide. Push about 4 times the length of the finger onto the guide, which is then put over the finger. Hold the web end of the gauze as the guide is withdrawn, turned and pushed down again and repeat prn. **b** There are themes and variations: taking the guide off the finger before twisting closes the fingertip; cutting the remainder longitudinally provides ties to go around the wrist to hold the dressing in place.

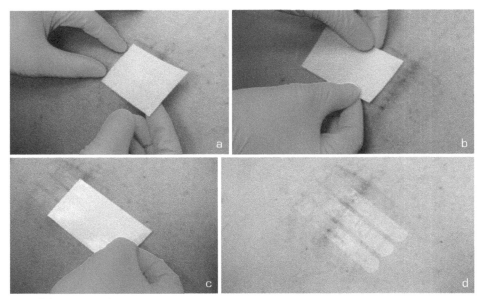

Figure 12.7 Applying tape strips

a The tapes are on a backing board that breaks away to expose bare short ends. Here the tapes are on top with the bare ends being pressed onto the skin. Measure the lesion so that the tapes are equal either side. The wound has been prepped with compound tincture of benzoin (Tinct Benz Co) which, when dry, becomes tacky and makes the tapes adhere better. **b** Flip the backing board over 180° so that the tapes are underneath. Push the board towards the wound until it is possible to grab enough bare board to pull rather than push. **c** Sufficient tapeless board can be pulled such that the tapes are applied to the skin with the neat spacing they present on the board. Use the non-pulling hand to press on the ends that are already on the skin to donate extra security. Pull the board as far as possible. There is then usually another break where the backing has to again be removed. Do not touch the sticky tape surfaces or they will not adhere. **d** The final tapes are neat and secure. They are of most use on facial, nose and ear wounds where the patient may roll over during sleep and shear open a wound that has just had the sutures removed.

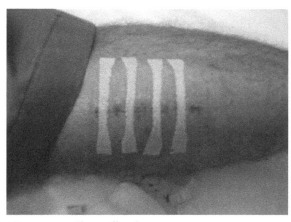

Figure 12.8 Fixomull strips

Fixomull is cut into strips then stretched across the wound when sutures are removed. The wider 'dumbbell' ends give greater purchase and the stretching gives closing tension across the wound. They are considerably cheaper than the sterilised commercial versions and arguably better.

no alternative but to remove the dressing, but this does not prevent the clinician gently expressing the observation that it should have been kept on, as recommended, as this ensures the best result.

Wound infection risk

1.5% with no antibiotic prophylaxis.
Sites:

- Below knee = 70%
- Thigh = 2%
- Head = 1%
- Trunk < 1%

ADHESIVE DRESSING REMOVAL

Sticky tape is difficult and painful to remove and can leave a tacky residue.

The author's preference is to use solvent ether, after protracted practical experience where my father used to quickly rip the Elastoplast off my innumerable wounds. Other products such as Zoff work but are not as good. Smith & Nephew have both a flask and rip sachets (like an alcohol swab) called 'Remove', which are good.

The best technique is to elevate the adhesive plaster and swab the leading edge while applying traction.

Healing and postoperative care

No wound will heal when one salve is tried after another.

Seneca (4 BC–AD 65), Moral Epistles to Lucilius

WOUND CLASSIFICATION

Thickness

- Superficial: these wounds only involve the epidermis and dermis down to the dermal papillae.
- Partial thickness: with these wounds the epidermis and some parts of the dermis and adnexa remain in the wound bed and contraction is minimal if only the superficial part of the dermis is removed. Partial thickness wounds are caused by shave excisions, curettage, electrodesiccation, dermabrasion, chemical peels and CO_2 lasers.
- Full thickness: these occur where the epidermis and dermis (skin and subcutaneous tissue) are lost along with hair follicles and sweat ducts (adnexa). They heal by contraction of myofibroblasts, which is responsible for a 40% reduction in the size of the wound with granulation tissue formation (fibroblasts and neovascularisation), and then re-epithelialisation from the wound edges. Myofibroblasts are modified fibroblasts that resemble smooth muscle cells and contain large quantities of contractile proteins [7].
- Deep: these wounds penetrate into cavities or organs with laceration of blood vessels and nerves.

Age

- Fresh: <8 hours
- Old: >8 hours

Morphology

- Abrasion, excoriation
- Incision
- Crushed
- Contused
- Lacerated
- Slicing
- Stabbing
- Bullet
- Explosive
- Bite
- Poisoned

Multiple structure involvement

- Simple: one tissue or organ
- Combined: mixed tissue and organs

CLASSIFICATION OF HEALING

Primary intention

Primary intention healing occurs by approximating the wound edges. In skin surgery this usually follows a scalpel excision and suturing (elsewhere, staples, glue or tape can be used). Wounds can be closed directly by flaps or grafts.

Sharp wounds from scalpels heal faster than destructive or ablative wounds.

Secondary intention

The wound is left open to granulate and close over from remaining dermal adnexa (hair follicles) or from the wound borders (e.g. abrasions, split-thickness donor sites).

Tertiary intention

This is delayed primary closure (e.g. slow Mohs, skin grafts, after infection and debridement).

PHASES OF HEALING

The overall wound healing sequence is as follows:

1 Immediate: vasospasm and local blood coagulation
2 15 min–14 days: wound contraction
3 15 min–3 days: inflammation; revascularisation
4 12–48 hours: epithelialisation
5 3 days–7 weeks: scar (collagen, matrix)
6 6–18 months: nerve repair

Healing is a continuous event of three overlapping phases:

1 haemostasis/inflammation
2 proliferation
3 remodelling.

Haemostasis

Vasoconstriction/spasm with visible blanching is followed by platelets aggregating in the first 15 minutes, which adhere to damaged endothelium and promote thrombocyte clumping to plug the wound. Platelets contain and release multiple growth factors that stimulate endothelial proliferation, migration and tube formation. The healing cascade of chemical mediators and cells is thus initiated with haemostasis the first step with the development of a fibrin clot and coagulation.

Inflammatory phase

Initial blood and fluid leakage with blocking of the lymphatics results in rubor, tumour and colour or redness, swelling and heat (i.e. there is erythema, heat, swelling and pain). This happens in the first 1–2 days and may last 2 weeks and should not be mistaken for an infection. Along with neutrophilia it is the inflammatory response during which leucocytes invade within 6 hours, maximise at 24–72 hours and then start to disappear. Wound debridement/phagocytosis is performed initially by the leucocytes and then by macrophages (days 3–4).

Angiogenesis is initiated immediately upon wounding and is mediated throughout the entire wound healing process. Capillary buds sprout from venules to form capillary loops to connect to the bloodstream and form a plexus. Angiogenesis is stimulated by inflammation, hypoxia and growth factors. New capillaries proliferate to form granulation tissue in the wound bed, which is evident by day 4. This process is sustained until the terminal stages of healing.

Proliferative phase

This consists of fibroplasia, matrix deposition, neovascularisation and re-epithelialisation:

- 15 min–14 days: contraction occurs in the direction of the relaxed skin tension lines (RSTL). The depth of the wound determines the degree of contraction.
- 12–48 h: re-epithelialisation is performed by keratinocytes. Proliferation and migration are from the epithelial cells at the edges of the wound and from any appendageal structures remaining in the wound bed. The rate of re-epithelialisation is directly related to the moistness of the wound.
- 48–72 h: fibroblasts populate the wound after and their growth is enhanced by low oxygen and high lactate levels (which may explain why occlusive dressings help).
- 48 h–7 weeks: growth factor via macrophages.
- 72 h–3 weeks: collagen deposition by fibroblasts.
- Days 3–4: granulation tissue is a sign of healing in progress.
- Days 4–7: further granulation.
- Days 7–9: re-establishment of basement membrane essential for the re-establishment of normal skin.

Remodelling phase

Remodelling occurs throughout the entire process of wound repair, initially with the deposition of matrix materials with the fibrin clot containing much fibronectin and granulation tissue containing type III collagen and blood vessels, which maximises at 2–3 weeks. Subsequent changes in new collagen synthesis and lysis of old collagen sees type I collagen with few blood vessels forming the scar. Scarring is part of the normal process of healing and, in most instances, occurs below the skin surface with cross-linking of collagen connective tissue replacement donating tensile strength. Scar tissue is pale, contracted and firm and has no blood supply.

The tensile strength of the collagen or scar increases to 40% at 1 month and continues to strengthen for a year but is never more than 80% of its pre-injury strength [8]. See Figure 12.9 in the section 'Wound strength'.

Over a year the dermis returns to stable, pre-injury type I collagen:

- Days 4–14: re-approximation by wound edge contraction due to myofibroblasts.
- Weeks: remodelling increases strength (up to 20% of normal dermis). Extracellular matrix is laid down by fibroblasts.
- Weeks: increased strength (up to 50% of normal dermis).
- Months: increased strength (80% of normal dermis).
- Weeks to months: decreased induration; regression of macrophages and T lymphocyte inflammatory process.
- Weeks to months: decreased redness – regression of endothelial cells.

Hypertrophic scars are the result of excessive fibroblast proliferation confined to the wound site.

Keloid formation is the result of further fibroblastic exuberance and can result when scar production extends beyond the area of the original wound.

Atrophic scars result from insufficient healing.

Nerve injury and repair

Three degrees of nerve injury

1 A transient interruption of nerve conduction without loss of axonal continuity (i.e. neuropraxia, conduction block)
2 Transection of axons but with preservation of the endoneurium during Wallerian degeneration (i.e. axonotmesis)
3 Complete disruption of the nerve fibre with loss of the normal architecture

Response and repair

- 12–48 hours: Wallerian degeneration of the distal and part proximal axon
- 48–72 hours: axons disintegrate and disappear

Four phases of regeneration

1 The neuron recovers, axonal growth commences and the axons reach the injured zone.
2 Axons must traverse the scar tissue, which causes delays.
3 Axons propagate beyond the site of injury to reach the peripheral target.
4 Functional recovery with restoration of normal patterns of conduction.

The duration of the regenerative process varies and may require 6–18 months, depending on the length of the nerve and the site of the lesion.

For skin surgery the main complaint is loss of or altered sensation. The usual advice is to reassure patients that it will take at least 6 months to regain former sensation and may take as long as 18 months. It is a moot point whether, for small areas of nerve injury, the patient has not just adapted during this time. Motor injuries should be referred immediately.

OPTIMISING HEALING

The most important factor for optimising healing is to provide the best substrate for epithelial/epidermal migration. This means a clean wound with no necrotic debris or denatured protein and maintenance of a moist environment.

Formation of an eschar or scab means the new epidermal cells must slowly digest it, delaying healing.

The new epidermis, even after epithelialisation is complete, is fragile and bruises and blisters easily due to weak attachment to the dermis. Melanocyte function also can lag behind repopulation such that hypo- or hyperpigmentation occurs, especially if exposed to UVR, chemicals (diazepam) or hormones (oestrogen). Full thickness wounds may not re-pigment.

Good technique, handling tissues gently without excessive tension and ensuring a good blood supply are covered elsewhere but other factors come into consideration:

1 Wound size: healing time is proportional to the log of the wound area (and why some large wounds heal faster than expected). Wound size lags for the first 2–3 weeks, then accelerates.

2 Wound shape: healing time is proportional to the diameter of the largest circle that can fit within the wound. Thus, a circular excision of 12-mm diameter will take longer to heal than a 40-mm long ellipse where the greatest diameter is only 10 mm.

3 Site of wound: the face heals most quickly and the lower leg most slowly.

4 Cleaning: hydrogen peroxide is sometimes recommended to clean wounds but it significantly decreases the tensile strength (TS) of nylon, polyglactin, polydioxanone and absorbable sutures. After the nylon sutures are exposed to hydrogen peroxide, they retain only 35–40% of their TS. White soft paraffin (Vaseline), the medium for most topical antibiotics, does not affect suture TS.

WOUND STRENGTH

The healing wound has minimal TS (Table 12.1). The deposition and remodelling of collagen gradually increases the TS of the wound. The wound regains some 7–10% at 1 week, then may weaken to 3–5% of its original strength at 10 days to achieve some 20% at 2 weeks which, of course, is when most sutures are removed. The TS is 15% at 3 weeks and progressively increases to a final strength of 80% after several months (Figure 12.9). It never regains its previous normal strength.

TABLE 12.1 Tensile strength of wounds

Days	Months	Wound tensile strength (TS), % of normal
7		10
10		3–5
14		20
30	1	30–40
60	2	60
90	3	80
150	5	85
180	6	85

Note: strength recovery is variable and suggested patient advice is: 20% at 2 weeks, 30% at 30 days, 60% at 60 days and 90% at 90 days.

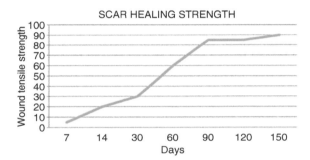

Figure 12.9 Scar healing strength
Note: TS may decrease from day 7 to day 10.

REMOVAL OF SUTURES (ROS)

Traditional recommendations

- Scalp: 7–10 days
- Limbs: 10–14 days
- Below knee: up to 21 days
- Joints: 14 days
- Body: 7–10 days

ROS after skin cancer surgery

Skin cancer surgery leaves a larger defect than lacerations or other operations and, despite best techniques and minimisation of wound edge tension, there is some wound tension. It is the author's experience that sutures should be kept in longer than the traditional recommendations, which are based on wounds without tension:

- Scalp: 14+ days
- Ears: (5) 7–9 days

- Face: (4) 5–8 days
- Limbs: 14 days
- Below knee: alternate sutures at 15 days, remainder at 21 days
- Joints: alternate sutures at 15 days, remainder at 21 days
- Body: 15 days

The figures in brackets above are where there is absolutely no wound tension and, even then, support strips are advisable after ROS. Wounds, especially on the face, should have tape strips applied as rolling over when asleep may shear open the wound.

The wound, of course, must be monitored, any infected sutures removed and inflammation managed.

HINTS AND TIPS

Always secure wounds after ROS with tape strips. Patients may roll over in their sleep and shear open the wound.

Suture removal scissors, which have a curved hook on one blade, are a revelation and to be recommended. They come in two main sizes and both are needed.

Infected wounds

Sutures promote infection. Remove alternate sutures or as many as possible in the infected area. At worst, all may have to be removed and the wound drained and healed by secondary intention.

Who should remove sutures

In many clinics nurses remove sutures as this is considered a free service. However, sutures in delicate areas such as the nose, lips, ears and face, especially with complex flaps, are best removed by the surgeon. A simple ellipse may just as well be done by a nurse.

SCAR MINIMISATION

After sutures are removed, the edges of a healing incision are pulled in different directions by the taut, surrounding skin, causing scar tissue to thicken and spread. Placing the incision where there will be the least pull across it will minimise scarring. Support strapping to minimise pull across the incision will help thereafter, but this has to remain in place as the sub-tissues mature and re-mould, which takes months. Ongoing support to the closed wound by distributing and therefore reducing the tension across the total surface area minimises scar formation.

- Minimise wound tension at the operation.
- Reduce wound tension postoperatively.
  - Tape strips (Steri-strip or similar) across the incision line.

  - Cover the strips with a film dressing (for 7–10 days and then change) for 4–5 months.
- **Vitamin E** has been used commonly for many years and applied topically to reduce scars but a double blind study found that, in 90% of cases, topical vitamin E either had no effect on or actually worsened the cosmetic appearance of scars. 33% of patients treated in the study developed a contact dermatitis to the vitamin E [9].
- Massaging with various lubricants (Bio-Oil®, aloe) is advised but robust evidence is lacking.
- Paper tape (Micropore™ etc) is usually applied for 4 weeks to any scar postoperatively. Any effect may be due to increased support, greater patient awareness (less movement) and perhaps a reduction of surface oxygen.
- Silicon gels (Dermatix®) and sheets also help. Their effect seems to result from a combination of occlusion and hydration, rather than from an effect of the silicone.

Previous studies for hypertrophic/keloid scars reported that, in patients treated with silicone occlusive sheeting with pressure worn 24 h/d for up to 12 months, 34% showed excellent improvement, 37.5% showed moderate improvement and 28% demonstrated no or slight improvement. Of patients treated with semipermeable, semiocclusive, non-silicone-based dressings for 8 weeks, 60% experienced flattening of keloids, 71% had reduced pain, 78% had reduced tenderness, 80% had reduced pruritus, 87.5% had reduced erythema and 90% were satisfied with the treatment. Cordran® tape is a clear surgical tape that contains flurandrenolide, a steroid that is uniformly distributed across the tape, and it has been shown to soften and flatten keloids over time.

IMPAIRMENT TO WOUND HEALING

The balance between infection and inflammation is relatively fragile. A certain amount of inflammation is necessary. If this is insufficient, the wound will heal badly and could become infected. If there is excessive inflammation, healing is also compromised. Commensal bacteria of the skin affect this process. Lipoteichoic acid from *Staphylococcus epidermidis* inhibits the inflammation triggered by the activation of TLR3 receptors, which play an essential role in cutaneous inflammation [10]. Other factors that impair healing include the following:

1 Surgical technique: poor technique with excessive tension and impaired blood supply delays healing.
2 Wound type: wound healing is delayed if there is necrotic debris present that has to be digested while the epidermis migrates under a dry denatured collagen crust. Thus, slower healing to that caused by a scalpel occurs with cryosurgery, electrosurgery, laser surgery, hot scalpel and acid peel.

3 Temperature: at a certain point, the lower the temperature the slower the healing.

4 Exposure: wounds under occlusive dressings heal 40% faster than exposed, dry wounds.

5 Infection: frank infection will delay healing but there is often colonisation by resident flora, which does not impair healing. The diagnosis of infection is made when there is pain and pus and the redness extends >3 mm with systemic symptoms of fever and feeling unwell. Culture of the wound is mandatory. Herpes simplex is a recognised complication of dermabrasion. *Candida* is often overlooked and should be thought of when a wound does not respond to topical antibiotics.

6 Drugs:

  A Systemic

    i Steroids inhibit wound healing and delay the development of TS if taken before or in the first 3 days of healing due to monocyte migration inhibition. Prolonged systemic steroid treatment makes the skin thin and easily torn, and it is advisable to use non-cutting taper needles to suture.

    ii Aspirin and NSAIDs have been reported to impede healing in animal experiments but this has not been extrapolated to humans. They are, however, antiplatelets and the increased bleeding can cause haematoma formation, especially under grafts.

    iii Colchicine has also been implicated.

  B Topical

    i Steroid ointments, especially the fluorinated ones, inhibit wound healing. 1% hydrocortisone does not.

    ii Mupirocin (Bactroban®) and white soft paraffin (Vaseline) have no effect. There is statistical but not clinical evidence that a single dose of topical chloramphenicol to high risk sutured wounds produces a moderate absolute reduction in infection rate [11]. Three small studies found that a petrolatum-based ointment advanced wound healing as well as topical antibiotics [12–14].

7 Antiseptics and vitamin E: it would seem advisable to avoid all antiseptics. 1% povidone–iodine, 3% hydrogen peroxide and 0.5% chlorhexidine are toxic to fibroblasts and keratinocytes and may delay granulation. Vitamin E has also been found to inhibit healing.

8 Contact dermatitis: allergic reactions to tapes and dressings are not uncommon. Allergic reactions to topical antibiotics, especially neomycin, should be borne in mind.

Nostril antibiotic ointment

Decolonising of nasal carriers of *Staphylococcus aureus*, by treatment with mupirocin nasal ointment and chlorhexidine soap, reduces the risk of *S. aureus* infection [15].

Given the increasing resistance of *S. aureus* to mupirocin, the author now coats the nares/nostrils with chloramphenicol ointment preoperatively.

Below the knee and diabetics also have a higher postoperative infection rate that may influence the surgeon's decisions.

---

9 Haemostatic solutions: Monsel's solution (ferric sulfate), 30% aluminium chloride and silver nitrate produce tissue necrosis and delay re-epithelialisation.

10 Systemic factors: malnutrition and vitamin deficiencies delay healing as do severe illness and neuropathies. Diabetes delays healing. Venous stasis and arteriosclerosis, peripheral vascular disease.

11 Age: may impair healing probably via impaired metalloproteinases. Malnutrition, impaired circulation, medications or inability to care for the wound must also be considered.

12 Miscellaneous: **radiotherapy** alters the skin and delays healing. As a personal observation, PDT for cancer (BCC) treatment (not actinic keratosis) also seems to alter the skin, making it more friable 'like blotting paper', as does severe or repeated **cryosurgery**.

13 Smoking: in one study smoking was claimed to not interfere with healing but, as it is a known contributor to platelet aggregation, peripheral vascular disease and venous thrombosis, it is certainly no help. The Australian National Preventive Health Agency advises that 'in one month there is a better blood flow which improves the skin' ('Stop smoking start repairing' poster 2011). Further, cigarette smoking has a deleterious effect on the survival of reconstructive flaps and grafts. Smoking results in vasoconstriction, increased blood viscosity, hypoxia and increased platelet aggregation, which promotes microvascular thrombosis. Patients who smoke more than 1 pack of cigarettes per day have a 3-fold risk of necrosis of flaps and full-thickness grafts when compared with persons who have never smoked, low level smokers (<1 pack/d) and ex-smokers. When necrosis does occur, the median area involved tends to be greater in smokers (approximately 3-fold) than in patients who never smoked. Many of the

adverse effects of cigarette smoking on the microvasculature are reversible; benefits in flap and graft survival may be realised by stopping (or decreasing) smoking for at least 2 days before surgery and for 1 week after surgery. Treatment with parenteral pentoxifylline and topical nitroglycerin has been shown to improve skin flap survival in animal models [16–18].

Natural healing

Despite the public's enthusiasm for extrinsic healing balms, oils and potions and the commercial promotions of such, wounds heal best if the body itself is allowed to heal them. Millions of years of evolution of the endogenous healing and growth factors liberated by the body into the wound site should not be interfered with and rendered less potent by any such external assaults. Hypoxia, moisturisation and inflammation are all that is proven.

Influence of preoperative skin appearance

A prospective dermatological unit study showed that patients whose lesion preoperatively had a crusted or ulcerated skin surface were significantly more likely to develop clinical wound infections than patients whose lesion had a normal or scaly surface. The risk of infection was significantly increased ($p < 0.05$) for crusted and ulcerated skin surfaces compared with intact surfaces, and for ulcerated surfaces compared with scaly surfaces. It was not affected by perioperative topical antibiotics, site of the lesion, closure technique or surgeon experience. *S. aureus* was the causative organism in 18 out of 20 infections. Patient age was a significant risk factor, and older patients were more likely to have lesions with a broken surface. The overall risk of infection was 3.5% (3/81) for intact surfaces, 12% (5/42) for scaly lesions, 18% (6/33) for crusted lesions and 33% (6/18) for ulcerated lesions [19].

RECOMMENDATIONS

Assessment of the patient

The following may persuade consideration of the use of systemic and/or topical prophylaxis:

- poor patient hygiene (unkempt, lives alone)
- skin appearance (crusted or ulcerated)
- systemic illness – diabetes, compromised immune status (immunosuppressives, high WCC, age, obesity, malnutrition, renal failure)

- smoking may not impede skin healing much but it would seem to do so in major surgery
- dirty areas (lower limbs, groin, axilla, external genitalia)
- site (lower leg – not only 'dirty' but poor blood supply, poor and tight skin)
- type of operation (graft/flap).

Surgical technique

The following will minimise postoperative infection:

- meticulous hand washing for more than 2 minutes
- meticulous site preparation with alcohol–chlorhexidine mix allowed to dry
- good technique (asepsis, no haematoma, no dead space, no wound tension, no compromised blood supply)
- nasal chloramphenicol for nose and perinasal operations
- topical antibiotic in diabetics and for operations below the knee
- air-conditioning, minimising stress (reduction of surgeon sweat)
- waterproof/occlusive dressings – undisturbed; pressure dressings lower limbs
- written postoperative instructions (no stretching, elevation of lower limbs).

AFTERCARE

Pain relief

Most patients state they experience very little pain even with extensive flap surgery on the face, nose and ears. Any pain seems controlled by paracetamol. In the author's experience, even for wedge resections of the ear, trilobed flaps of the nose and large O-S flaps on the back, all the patients need is paracetamol. The need for increased analgesia may raise the question of wound infection. Aspirin and NSAIDs should be avoided because of their bleeding effect.

Digesic was often the next choice but these contain dextropropoxyphene, a potent cardiotoxic agent, and the Committee on Safety of Medicines of the UK determined that the risk of deliberate and accidental overdose was unacceptably high and the product should be withdrawn from the UK market. In Febuary 2011 the FDA similarly recommended discontinuation of marketing of these products.

The use of codeine 10 mg or 15 mg let alone 30 mg would seem overprescribing for normal post-operative recovery. The constipating effect alone is enough to revert to plain paracetamol and reassurance, but some colleagues issue a prescription 'just in case' the patient does get severe pain and have found that such patients only needed one or two doses.

Rest

Keeping mobile to prevent deep venous thrombosis (DVT) is preferable. Wounds on the lower leg can be a problem but a sensible patient can walk 'flat-footed', not bending their foot, and most cope doing so.

Elevation

It is important to elevate wounds below the heart, especially those on the lower leg. Advise patients to put the heels only on a support with nothing under compressing the calves.

No stretching of the wound

Wounds on the back can be put under tension by stretching to put shoes on or with physical work. An 'elbows in' policy should be advised. Wounds across joints usually require some 'aide mémoire' or restriction/splinting.

Bleeding

Bleeding traditionally was said to occur at 6 and 48 hours. Whether this is so, it is still a useful warning to the patient to take care. Instruct patients how to apply pressure. For wounds on the back, sitting with a cushion against the wound is good. Elevate legs, and pressure dressings there and on the forehead should be used.

Patients on anticoagulants are at greater risk, but prevention is better than having to re-open a wound, and obtaining secure haemostasis is the key.

Advise patients that some blood will stain through the dressing but that this is normal and *not to take the dressing off*.

Numbness

Nerve blocks can numb the mouth. Warn patients not to take hot drinks until back to normal.

Alcohol

Alcohol promotes bleeding and careless behaviour. Warn the patient not to drink immediately after an operation.

Infection

Instruct the patient to report any excessive pain, discomfort, temperature or malaise.

Dressings

Wounds heal better occluded – at least for 4 days. Encourage patients to leave a waterproof dressing on, despite 'staining'. The exudate contains growth and healing factors. Uncovered wounds have more scab formation, more infection and worse scarring.

SECONDARY INTENTION HEALING

Secondary intention healing can, and frequently does, lead to excellent cosmetic results. It has 'fallen off the radar' because it is not rebatable. Hence, grafts and flaps are more frequently done where there is no need and with poorer cosmetic results. The technique of making the excision and ellipse align along the relaxed skin tension lines or in a natural wrinkle/line and then slightly closing this with absorbable sutures, such as Monosyn, closes the deficit somewhat, which speeds healing. This would seem to help promote healing and perhaps cosmesis. In this way such surgery is rebatable.

The main thing the surgeon has to learn is patience to let the wound heal. Nevertheless, many of these wounds heal more quickly than may be expected and most are remarkably pain free and do not necessitate the second daily dressing often recommended.

After haemostasis is secured, a floor of chloramphenicol covered with an anti-stick dressing (Telfa/Melolin/Cutilin) and then a gauze held on with Fixomull can be recommended. If the wound is slightly oozing, Kaltostat may be substituted for the non-stick dressing until the wound stops oozing. Second daily dressings may be needed initially then bi-weekly, more to check for infection and to reassure the patient but also to guard against hypergranulation. Suture spitting is not unknown but, as these are absorbable, just cut it off flush.

Flaps that don't quite close, such as on the scalp or lower leg where the skin is tight, can also be left to heal this way. Venous stasis of the lower leg, however, is a concern in such cases and the complication of a venous ulcer, especially with diabetics, is ever present. With venous stasis a split-thickness skin graft is probably the better option.

Figure 12.10 prioritises the areas on the face as to excellent, satisfactory and variable results from secondary intention healing. Secondary intention healing is often more likely to be itchy.

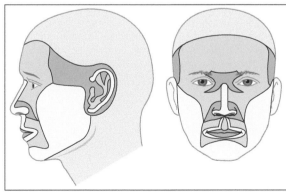

Figure 12.10 Cosmetic results of healing by secondary intention

Dark pink areas show excellent cosmetic results; mid-pink areas show satisfactory healing; pale pink areas show variable cosmetic results.

Adapted from Eedy DJ, Breathnach SM, Walker NPJ. Surgical Dermatology. Oxford: Blackwell Science, 1996; Fig 13.1.

Complications

Don't worry about the bleeding during the operation, worry about the bleeding that occurs when you are not there.

Surgical axiom

Complication rates for cutaneous surgery:

- Overall: 4.4%
- Mohs surgery: 1.6%
- Below the knee: 11%

It is a reasonable practice to inspect the wound at 6 weeks or 3 months and to implement follow-up plans and recalls as dictated by the lesion.

The most important step in follow-up visit(s) is to examine the rest of the skin. Melanoma patients have a high risk of a second tumour. A patient who has had one non-melanoma skin cancer has a 67% chance of developing another. A patient who has had three skin cancers will nearly always develop another.

The most common complications are:

1. infection
2. sutures too tight – wound edge tension
3. bleeding (haematoma, seroma)
4. dehiscence
5. ugly/widened scar.

COMPLICATIONS OF SKIN SURGERY

Patient factors

Personality/anxiety

One of the greatest drawbacks to cutaneous surgery is that patients are able to talk and their garrulousness is directly proportional to their nervousness. A patient who talks during facial surgery can make life difficult for the surgeon. An assistant with the 'gift of the gab' who can relax the patient with a patter that doesn't invite a reply is invaluable.

Free arms

Inform patients that the drape is sterile and not to 'help' secure it, put their hands on it or, during facial surgery, scratch their face.

Cough/sneeze

A cough or a sneeze can cause quite violent head movements. An unexpected cough without any warning has seen a lovely temporal flap unravel. Any unexpected movement can, of course, cause problems. If the patient has developed a cough, ask them to warn you if they want to cough.

Anticoagulants

No therapeutic anticoagulation should be ceased, but it is now considered that people who have no cardiovascular risks need not be taking aspirin.

Epilepsy

Operating on a patient having an epileptic fit is somewhat more difficult than usual. The surgeon is well advised to include this in the preoperative assessment.

Needle phobia (belonephobia, trypanophobia)

Needle phobia is estimated to affect 3.5–10% of the population [20, 21]. Approximately 80% of affected patients report strong needle fear in a first-degree relative [22]. Adolescents and adults may recognise that their fear is unreasonable [23]. Most patients fear injections but some people have a real phobia with significant and dramatic signs and symptoms [23]. No one, even the most phlegmatic, can admit to not having some concerns about an injection into their nose, lip or the sole of the foot. The practitioner must be aware of this initial complication as it can significantly delay an operation or even abort it. There are techniques to relax the patient and deliver the most painless injection possible.

The onset of the vasovagal response may be immediate (2–3 seconds) following the needle-stick. However, one study of 84 blood donors who fainted found that 16.7% experienced syncope 5–30 minutes after the phlebotomy [24], and another series of 64 blood donors who fainted found that 14% fainted after leaving the phlebotomy site and returning to work, sometimes several hours later [25].

Intervention

Individuals with belonephobia require reassurance about the prevalence of needle fear, explanation of the inherited and involuntary nature of belonephobia and clarification of methods available to counter reactions. The majority of belonephobia victims believe that the problem is 'all in their head'; thus, compounded anxiety can be relieved by giving their problem an illness label and a physiological explanation [22].

Medications may be useful for some individuals. Topical anaesthetic creams (e.g. EMLA cream [lignocaine 2.5% and prilocaine 2.5%]) can numb injection sites. Rapid-acting benzodiazepines, such as diazepam (Valium®) or lorazepam (Ativan®), have an onset of action of 5–15 minutes and may be useful for some patients [22].

A counselling referral can be advantageous. Desensitisation therapy warrants a motivated patient; however, it may decondition the autonomic symptoms and fear experienced by those with mild needle phobia and may extinguish associated blood–injury fears [22]. Cognitive–behavioural therapy focuses on patterns of maladaptive thinking and the beliefs that underlie such thinking (National Alliance on Mental Illness 2003 [26]).

Technique

Perhaps the best approach is, if the injection has to be in an obviously painful area or the patient admits to a great dislike of needles at the preoperation assessment: 5–10 mg of oral diazepam 2 hours beforehand, hide the needle, use the smallest gauge, use bicarbonate, keep up a barrage of questions that the patient has to answer to distract their attention, have soothing music, pinch up the site, identify a pore, place the needle, hold for a moment increasing the pressure but not penetration, then introduce slowly and inject slowly. Nerve blocks may be the better option. Veterinary surgeons have another technique, mostly for larger injections and larger patients, where they flick the animal, which reflexively contracts the muscle that then physiologically relaxes into the refractory phase, and that is when the vet injects into this relaxed muscle.

Infection

Surgical site infections (SSI) have been defined by The Australian Commission on Safety and Quality in Health Care (http://www.safetyandquality.gov.au/). Superficial incisional infections must meet the following criteria.

Infection involves only skin and subcutaneous tissue of this incision and occurs within 30 days after the operative procedure and exhibits **at least one** of the following from the superficial incision and exhibits either 1 and/or 2:

1 Purulent discharge (NOT stitch abscess).
2 Organisms isolated from an aseptically collected culture of fluid or tissue.

   Note: a positive wound swab (in contrast to wound aspirate) without other significant evidence of infection is not adequate for diagnosis of infection.

3 Displays at the site of incision any of the following signs and symptoms of infection:

   A pain or tenderness
   B localised swelling
   C redness or heat.

In contrast, the US CDC defines SSI as 'any surgical wound that produces pus (suppurates) within 30 days of the procedure even in the absence of a positive culture'. The Australian Council on Healthcare Standards (ACHS) threshold for the acceptable infection rate associated with clean surgical procedures is given as 1.4–4.1% [27].

Clean surgery

Clean surgery is defined as elective incisions carried out on non-inflamed tissues under strict aseptic technique and with no entry into the gastrointestinal, respiratory or genitourinary tracts.

It may be claimed that bleeding is the most common complication, but the author's experience is that, for skin surgery, it is infection. Bleeding after all can mostly be prevented with good technique but, although surgical site preparation with alcohol and chlorhexidine and aseptic technique reduces skin bacterial counts, wound infection can never be completely eliminated. Some 5% of apparently healthy people are carriers of *S. aureus* and most wound infections originate from the patient's skin and are introduced during surgery. Carriage increases this to 15% in the axilla and 25% in the groin and perineum. The commonest pathogen to cause skin wound infections is *S. aureus*, then *Streptococcus pyogenes* and *Pseudomonas* (ear).

Further, postoperatively the patient can promote autoinfection. The elderly, the diabetic and the unkempt are more susceptible, and there are those patients who simply choose to ignore all advice and instructions and take down their dressings immediately, get the wound wet and introduce postoperative infection.

An Australian prospective study of infection associated with skin surgery

Infection rates for skin surgery:

- Non-diabetics: 2.0%
- Diabetics: 4.2%
- Diabetics have a 66% higher risk for infection.

For non-diabetics and diabetics:

- Leg wounds = 4 times more likely to become infected
- Flaps/grafts = 3.5 times more likely to develop wound infections
- Other complications (bleeding, dehiscence, edge necrosis, contact dermatitis, wound depression/elevation, hypertrophic scar/keloid, granuloma, deep scar) = 1.8% [28]

Antibiotic prophylaxis may be considered in light of this information.

Systemic and topical antibiotic prophylaxis

Infection occurs after surgery in 1.5–20% of cases but good quality trials as to the effect of topical antibiotic prophylaxis are lacking [11].

The American Heart, Orthopedic and Dental Associations now feel antibiotic prophylaxis (even with endocarditis) is not warranted. However, it is considered circumspect with:

- below knee
- large flaps
- diabetics.

Regimen:

Give 1 hour before operation:

- dicloxacillin 2 g
- cephalexin 2 g
- roxithromycin 300 mg.

See also the section 'Wound infection prevention – surgical site infection (SSI)' in Chapter 7, 'Operating'.

Prevention of infection

Meticulous site preparation and aseptic technique followed by an occlusive waterproof dressing that is left on until ROS are mandatory but a dedicated operating theatre and adequate sterilisation and hygiene are also advised. Skin surgery infection rates are accepted to be between 5% and 10% but most studies report lower rates (0.7–2.29%) [29–31].

It would seem reasonable for the practitioner to aim for 2% in healthy, clean patients. If wound infection rates are higher than this, or there is an unusual spate of infections, the practitioner must scrutinise every step of procedures, as infections are usually due to a lapse in aseptic technique and a lowered host immune defence and poor hygiene/wound care.

- Preoperative measures:
  - identify patients at risk – single, unkempt, poor nutrition, anticoagulants including herbs
  - treat intercurrent skin infections
  - give prophylactic antibiotics for diabetes.
  - perinasal operations – consider smearing antibiotic ointment in nostrils.
- Surgical site prep: preoperative cleansing of the patient's skin with chlorhexidine–alcohol is superior to cleansing with povidone–iodine for preventing SSI after clean-contaminated surgery [32].
- Infected wound closure: the incidence of SSIs in relation to the different types of closure techniques used is given in Table 12.2.

Increased risk of infection

Poor technique
- Poor asepsis
- Interference with blood supply

TABLE 12.2 Incidence of SSIs following closure/ delayed closure of an infected wound

Opening and re-closure times	Reinfection rate
Opening and re-closure at once	50%
Opening and re-closure after 2 days	20%
Opening and re-closure after 4 days	5%
Opening and re-closure after 9 days	10%

Note: all wounds were closed under antibiotic cover.
Adapted from *The Scandinavian handbook of plastic surgery*.
Malmoe: Studenterliteraturen, 2005.

- Excessive and rough tissue handling, especially of wound edges
- Poor closure
- Gaps: obvious portals of entry for bacteria
- Excessive electrocautery: can cause necrosis, which causes an immune reaction [33]
- Dead spaces: blood and serous fluids collect and provide an ideal bacterial growth medium
- Incorrect sutures: highly allergenic sutures can cause inflammation that promotes infection; braided sutures may harbour more bacteria than monofilament; sutures too large for the wound provide larger portals of entry via their puncture sites
- Sites: nose, axilla, mouth, ears and genitalia have a higher bacterial count; below the knee, wedge excisions of the lip and ear and skin grafts may carry increased infection risks [34]
- Inflamed or infected sites
- Patient: age, diabetes, malnourishment, immunocompromised, obesity
- Smoking: has deleterious sequelae but one study found that smokers do not seem to get more infections [35]

Diagnosis

Infection is diagnosed when the patient complains of malaise, increasing wound pain with the wound inflamed and more tender than it should be, swelling, induration, possibly visible pus and lymphangitis. Infection usually manifests from days 4–8 (postoperative).

Treatment

There are recommendations for systemic antibiotic prophylaxis and there should be no need for routine wound topical antibiotic. One exception, however, is the instillation of chloramphenicol ointment into the patient's nares for nasal operations [15]. A wound swab culture and sensitivity should be considered based on the practitioner's experience and, depending on the appearance of the infection and cellulitis/lymphangitis, a wound swab (culture and sensitivity) should be considered. Most infections due to *S. aureus* are treated with cephalosporin or penicillinase resistant penicillin (dicloxacillin). *Pseudomonas* (ears) is treated with ciprofloxacin. Treatment should be started immediately after the swab is taken and adjusted if sensitivitiy dictates.

Bleeding

Operative

See Chapter 4, 'Haemostasis'.

Surgeons were not able to predict a patient's anticoagulant status based on intraoperative observations [36]. Although the use of aspirin, warfarin and NSAIDs may be associated with increased intraoperative bleeding in dermatological surgery, whether this results in poorer outcomes is not clear [37]. Cases of thromboembolic stroke after temporary discontinuation of warfarin and aspirin prior to cutaneous surgery have been reported [38, 39].

Therapeutic anticoagulation should not be stopped. If there is a potential problem, patients are best treated in hospital with full support and resuscitation facilities.

Severe bleeding complications

- Aspirin: 1.3%
- Warfarin: 5.7%

Warfarin accounts for 7-fold moderate-to-severe complications compared to control. Aspirin and NSAIDs account for 2-fold [40].

Clopidogrel is associated with significantly increased risk of severe postoperative wound complications whereas the risk for severe complications after skin surgery does not increase in patients on aspirin or warfarin. Severe complications were significantly more likely with larger defects [41].

Postoperative

It used to be said that postoperative bleeding occurs mostly at 6 or 48 hours. What this probably means is that the vasoconstrictive effect of adrenaline has worn off and rebound bleeding is noticed at 6 hours or that bleeding hasn't stopped and it's 48 hours before the patient complains or it is noticed that BP is falling and PR increased. In any event, the risk of postoperative bleeding is greatest during the first 48 hours.

Rest, elevation, pressure and cold packs are important during this first 48 hours.

Advise patients to lie down, elevate the site and apply direct pressure constantly for a minimum of 15 minutes if they suspect bleeding.

Rest

All activity should be reduced and patients need specific instructions to do so. Any activity that stretches the wound is to be avoided. No bending and lift only light objects. No twisting limbs or body. Avoid activity that increases heart rate, hence BP.

Elevation

Avoid bending over after facial surgery. A figure-of-eight bandage for lower arm lesions to keep hand to shoulder is helpful for those patients on anticoagulants.

Advise patients with leg operations to put their feet up above their nipple line, resting on the heels. Do not compress calf muscles (DVT).

Pressure dressings

Conforming bandages are a great help, especially around the forehead, arms and legs.

Surgifix/tube for scalp, fingers and lower legs is excellent.

Backs may present a problem but advising the patient to watch TV with a cushion against the wound is advice seemingly followed.

Hydrostatic pressure

From the heart to the ankle is a long drop with a large pressure gradient, especially in the elderly with incompetent venous valves or those on anticoagulants. Even when the wound looks super-dry, ensure a pressure dressing before the patient stands up.

Secondary bleeding

This is most likely oozing that builds up until the patient notices it. An opaque cover over the intact original dressing is the best treatment.

Alcohol

Alcohol is a vasodilator and 2 days abstinence is good advice.

Trauma

Situations such as sport where the wound may be subjected to trauma should be avoided.

Patients who turn and twist in their sleep may need tape strips and extra insurance.

Summary: postoperative prevention of bleeding

- Pressure bandages – foreheads, forearms but especially lower legs. Cushions into backs.
- Rest, elevate (legs resting on heels, nothing under calves). Don't lift, stretch, stoop or bend for 3 days. Then slowly mobilise but avoid overactivity for 1 week.
- Be aware of possible rebound when vasoconstriction of adrenaline wears off.
- Remember hydrostatic pressure: any wound below the heart will have increased pressure to bleed the lower it is.
- The first 24 hours is regarded as when most bleeding occurs. Urge extra rest.
- Drains: often forgotten but of use, especially with coagulopathies, where bleeding continues as a slow ooze. Insert a Penrose drain into the wound; withdraw after 48 hours.
- Analgesics but not NSAIDs.
- Leave dressings on. Instruct patients to come back if worried.

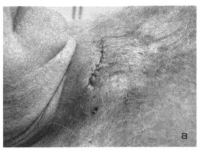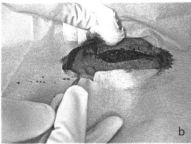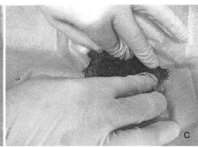

Figure 12.11 A classic haematoma
a Due to its position and the risk of tracheal compression, it was evacuated immediately. The sutures were cut (**b**) and the clot evacuated by compressing the edges (**c**). The offending vein was identified, ligated and the wound closed.

Bruising or ecchymosis

Ecchymosis and **bruising** are the same thing. Some consider ecchymosis as the deposition of blood manifesting while it is still red and bruising as the change in colour to green and yellow due to haemoglobin being degraded to bilirubin. Although both may be alarming to the patient, they clear with time. Warn the patient of the likelihood of a 'black eye' with any periorbital surgery as bruising is most common there.

Undue or excessive bruising usually indicates a venous bleeder. Consideration should then be given to re-opening the wound to tie it off.

Haematomas

Continued bleeding and haematomas are rare in dermatological surgery but are always a potential risk in those patients on anticoagulants. Periorbital haematomas are an emergency as are those in the neck if they compress the trachea.

The most problematic feature of a haematoma is that the wound itself seldom bleeds externally, which can delay the patient seeking attention. New throbbing pain is the most usual symptom that provokes the patient to see the doctor.

Haematomas promote infection, necrosis and dehiscence and should be evacuated if possible.

Haematoma stages

Stage 1: accumulation

The wound becomes swollen and is warm and fluctuant. ROS may be all that is necessary to allow release of the accumulated blood and the wound or part thereof left open. If ongoing bleeding is suspected, the entire wound should be opened and explored, the bleeding site(s) found and haemostasis established. The wound should then be irrigated with normal saline and observed until haemostasis is guaranteed.

The wound can then be resutured or left open. There is no 'hard-and-fast' rule but infection would mandate leaving it open with antibiotic cover to heal by secondary intention.

If the haematoma is easily expressed, local anaesthetic may not be necessary. Further exploration, breaking up of clots and resuturing, however, may require it.

Stage 2: clots

Clots form quite quickly with the site becoming more spongy than fluctuant. The skin may have a purple hue. A small clot may be left to resorb but evacuation by squeezing is usually preferable.

Stage 3: organisation

Clots organise into adhesive, harder, rubber-like structures and the wound feels firm. These adhesive clots are difficult to evacuate by squeezing or exploration and instrument-aided removal. It is better not to do anything but wait for clot lysis.

Stage 4: lysis

Between 7 and 10 days the wound again feels fluctuant. This is because fibrinolysis is liquefying the clot(s) to be resorbed. Aspiration with an 18G needle is possible rather than opening the wound. Resorption can take many months.

Seromas

A seroma is the accumulation of serous fluid and is often mistaken for a haematoma. Drainage with a large bore needle makes the diagnosis. Ensure drainage is complete and, although it should be sterile, send a specimen for culture and sensitivity if it is cloudy. These are exudates into dead spaces and can be prevented by careful closure to avoid any dead space.

Wound burst, dehiscence and epidermolysis

Wound burst and **dehiscence** are the same thing when the wound separates along the suture line. Some practitioners, however, use wound burst to refer to when separation occurs at ROS or shortly thereafter and dehiscence for separation sometime after ROS. The usual cause of wound burst is premature removal and there are no complications such as haematoma or infection and/or wounds under tension. ROS schedules are recommended; however, there is little to be gained and much to lose by not leaving sutures in if there is any suggestion of separation. Removing alternate sutures may be the best option or leaving them all in if there is no infection.

Epidermolysis is separation of only the epidermal edges and manifests as an erythematous healing ridge.

Dehiscence is a separation or splitting of all layers of a wound along natural or surgical suture lines, usually as a complication during wound healing or secondary to poor technique (sutures too close to margins and pull through). Risk factors include diabetes, advanced age, obesity, steroids, malnutrition and trauma in the postsurgical period and complications such as infection, haematoma and necrosis are present.

Dehiscence usually occurs after and within 2 weeks of ROS and implies some pathological process such as infection. Thus, the cause must be addressed first and the wound cleaned, debrided and any infection treated. If infected, the wound is not re-sutured immediately but the infection is allowed to heal and/or any oedema is allowed to regress. Healing may be by secondary intention or the wound edges refreshed and then re-sutured when the infection has subsided.

As wound strength is only some 3–10% of its original strength at ROS and only 35% at 1 month, dehiscence is a real prospect to be prevented. This can be done by using tape strips and with patient advice and education.

Preventive technique

Use deep sutures of polydioxanone (PDS II/Monoslow) for back wounds and anywhere else where the wound is so wide as to predict too great a tension if only skin or superficial sutures are used.

Re-suturing

If the wound separates at ROS, re-suture immediately.

If dehiscence occurs within the first 6 days after ROS, the wound can be re-sutured if no infection is present and any necrotic tissue cut out.

Freshening the edges is **not** recommended as healing fibroblastic activity will have already started and this should be allowed to continue undisturbed.

Tape strips alone cannot be relied on for closure unsecured by sutures as they often peel off too soon and dehiscence may result. Wound edge eversion is not as good as with sutures.

Tape strips on the site cleaned with acetone or made stickier with Tinct Benz Co or Skin-Prep may be used on patients who refuse re-suturing. Tape strips are best reserved to secure wounds, especially facial and ears, after ROS. Acetone degreases the skin and facilitates better adhesion of wound closure tapes [42].

Refreshing

After 6 days, scrape dry edges such that they bleed to 'refresh' them and then re-suture.

Secondary intention healing usually starts around day 5 so it is preferable to do this before then. Traditionally, a Fox curette has been used but the newer, sharper disposable curettes or a scalpel blade can be used.

Clinical studies

Not much has been written on skin wound dehiscence but, in a study on chest wounds that had dehisced, some were debrided and re-sutured while others were allowed to heal by secondary intention [43]. Those with direct wound closure required an average of 12.2 days of treatment versus 29.7 days for healing by secondary intention. The average number of medical treatments was 3.7 in the direct closure group versus 9.4 for second intention. Moreover, many of the direct closure wounds were closed in the face of positive wound cultures, and most resulted in prompt healing despite the presence of infection.

A randomised clinical trial comparing closure of skin wounds after insertion of hormone implants with Steri-Strips or 3-0 Dexon II found that significantly more bleeding occurred in the Steri-Strip-treated group, causing the authors to recommend use of suturing [44]. Another study found that the use of Steri-Strips resulted in slightly wider scar widths than use of sutures [45]. However, most studies evaluating closure with Steri-Strips have found them to result in 'cosmetically satisfactory' surgical wounds with low complication rates [46, 47].

Necrosis

Necrosis is the end result of tissue ischaemia from any cause but usually results from poor surgical technique such as incorrect undermining of the subdermal plexus or from a complication such as wound tension, crush injury, infection or haematoma. As covered in the section, 'Impairment to wound healing', cigarette smoking also has a deleterious effect on the survival of reconstructive flaps and grafts.

Flap and graft necrosis ranges from 1.9% to 10.4%.

Treatment

Treatment of necrosis is conservative (Figure 12.12). The necrotic area should be allowed to fully demarcate. Debridement prior to this time may injure viable tissue and should be avoided, except in cases of haematoma and infection. When the eschar begins to easily separate from the wound bed, careful sharp debridement may be performed, and the wound may be allowed to heal by secondary intention granulation. If the eschar is left on to drop off by itself the results may even be better.

The wound should be cleansed frequently. Allowing water to run over it in the shower and dabbing dry with a disposable soft paper towel is sufficient if there is no infection. Covering with white soft paraffin (Vaseline) or such to keep it moist is recommended.

These wounds are at higher risk for infection, and the need for topical and systemic antibiotics should be considered. If necessary, scar revision may be performed at a later date.

Reaction to sutures

Sutures are a foreign body and elicit reactions to varying degrees. Nylon, the workhorse of cutaneous surgery, thankfully causes little reaction in most patients but will do so if left in long enough and if combined with tension, let alone infection.

Contributing factors:

- The longer the suture is in situ, the greater the reactivity
- For every increase in calibre, there is a 2- to 3-fold increase in reactivity
- Synthetic sutures are less reactive
- Monofilament sutures are less reactive than braided
- Sites (chest, back, extremities, sebaceous face)
- Males
- Age
- Surgeon inexperience

As this is an easily avoided complication, the practitioner should be critical of brands and different materials and choose those found to give least problems.

Studies in mice have demonstrated increased adherence of bacteria to braided subcutaneous sutures when compared with monofilament sutures [48].

Suture tracks – 'tension and time'

Suture tracks or 'train lines' or 'snake bites' (Figure 12.13) are the puncture holes often joined by transverse scars that are caused by sutures being tied too tightly (tension) or being left in too long (time).

If a wound is oedematous or likely to be so, polybutester (Dyloc/Novafil) sutures are unique in that they stretch and hence don't cause this complication. They then recoil to take up the slack as the oedema lessens.

In general, take care to gently approximate the wound edges but not pull the sutures too tight. Some surgeons leave the first throw loose and secure the knot with the second and third throws. Gentility, a word not used much in scientific or medical literature, is the best technique.

Dermabrasion may improve established tracks.

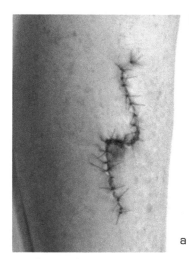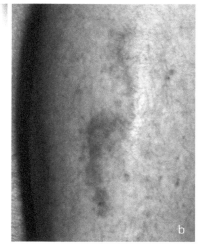

Figure 12.12 Threatened necrosis

a Threatened because the horizontal incision cut across blood vessels and too much tension at mid-tip (pre-tibial).
b Alternate sutures removed immediately; the rest ASAP. No other treatment. 3 months later; all healed. If this had necrosed, it should have been allowed to heal by secondary intention.

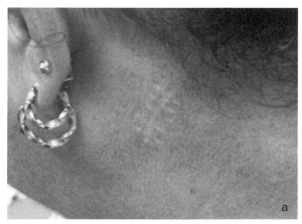
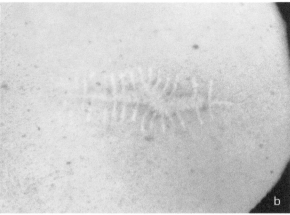

Figure 12.13 Suture tracks
a This excision was obviously too short, resulting in too much tension. **b** The cause of this amazing result would seem most likely to be 'surgeon inexperience'.

Suture spitting

Spitting refers to where deep sutures emerge through the skin. Usually these are subcutaneous sutures that have been placed too high in the dermis. This is the body's normal rejection of any foreign body, as with a splinter. It usually occurs around 8 weeks post-op but sometimes up to several months later.

Signs

Spits usually present as non-inflamed papules followed by extrusion or 'spitting' of the suture. Inflammation can occur but this is usually secondary to patient squeezing.

Treatment

Warn patients that this may occur and cause inflammation (otherwise they may see another doctor and be prescribed unnecessary antibiotics). Use magnification/loupe and pull the suture(s) up as much as possible and cut off flush. The remnant will then retreat under the skin and eventually be resorbed. Most absorbable sutures depend on hydrolysis for their absorption and hence don't dissolve when exposed to the air.

Poor cosmesis – trapdooring, pin-cushioning

Wound assessment

Assessment of how the final wound will look is best done at 6 months. By then wounds have settled and give the best indication of the long-term result.

Most poor cosmesis can be prevented by careful planning as to incision placement, gentle tissue handling, lack of wound tension and everted edges correctly matched and closed using the smallest sutures with optimum removal time and occlusive dressings.

Subcuticular 'invisible mending' suturing should be mastered and offered, especially to women, on exposed areas.

Dermabrasion and scar revision can be done later if necessary, usually 4–6 weeks after surgery.

Flaps can also present problems where the flap is donated. This is especially the case with bilobed flaps of the distal nose:

- Pin-cushioning is where the donated flap elevates (Figure 12.14a).
- Trapdooring is where the donated flap is depressed (Figure 12.14b).

The section on 'Bilobed flap' under 'Nose' in Chapter 9 fully describes how to avoid or minimise these complications.

Shortfall in a flap invariably causes too much tension with poor cosmetic results.

The mediastinum is notorious for hypertrophic scars and gentility and postoperative care (silica gel/Dermatix) mandatory.

The shoulders are prone to scar spread and deep sutures are recommended.

Ears are prominent unless covered by hair. Helical defects and deformities are noticable.

Hypergranulation – 'proud flesh'

Hypergranulation is an overabundance of granulation tissue, which is an impediment to normal wound healing as it prevents the migration of the epithelium across the surface of a wound to close it.

Hypergranulation was traditionally treated with topical silver nitrate or copper sulfate ('blue-stone'). These were frequently hard to source and there were no 'instructions'. Thankfully, an alternative and less toxic method is the application of hypertonic saline.

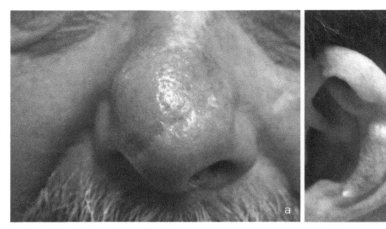

Figure 12.14 Pincushioning and trapdooring
a This was done by a competent plastic surgeon. It is difficult to always get a great result. **b** The patient is adamant this was done 'by a specialist'. This need not occur – see the section 'Ear' in Chapter 9.

Hypertonic saline dressings are available (Mesalt and Curasalt) and are changed daily. When held on the hypergranulating wound by a secondary (usually foam) dressing and some external compression applied they have been shown to be successful. However, they are not always a magic bullet.

In the case in Figure 12.15 the proud flesh had to be anaesthetised and the lesion **fulgurated**. Then and only then was there real progress.

Scars – spread, contraction

Despite the best planned and performed operations poor scarring can result, and this should be explained and documented in the patient consent form.

Scar care

Correct advice as to wound care is essential, viz:

1 Waterproof dressing/don't get wet.
2 Don't remove this dressing.
3 Avoid stretching.
4 Cover with Micropore for 4 weeks.
5 Use silica gel sheets/Dermatix if raised or high risk areas (mediastinum).
6 Rub/massage with a moisturiser or a non-oxidising vitamin C cream.

Scar spread

Scar spread (Figure 12.16) is a problem on the back, shoulders and across joints.

This may be minimised or even prevented by deep sutures of polydioxanone (PDS II/Monoslow) to pull the wound together. Polydioxanone sutures last 180 days.

Another technique is to use nylon deep sutures, which last 14 years or so. In a small series the author has used this technique with good results for large wounds on the back or those in areas of stretch (the small of the back)

with no complaints from patients as to irritation or a feeling that something is there. Elsewhere, deep sutures of Monosyn or Maxon seem to give enough support to prevent spread. However, no matter the best prophylaxis, the back is notorious for wound spread ('burst') and can do so a year or more later without provocation.

To summarise, deep sutures are recommended for all wounds on the back and shoulders and anywhere else where the width of the wound, tension and activity suggest. The minimum is PDS II (Monoplus, Monoslow), which has a 6-month life, but some surgeons are using nylon, which has a 14-year life. Although there is no hard and fast evidence this technique has been documented in text books since the 1980s [49], and firsthand experience with both has been good so far. No patients with deep nylon sutures have complained of any wound irritation. Even if it doesn't work and, despite all efforts, scar spread still occurs, the surgeon at least knows that everything possible has been done.

Scar contraction

Contraction commences approximately a week after wounding, when fibroblasts have differentiated into myofibroblasts [50]. In full thickness wounds, contraction peaks at 5–15 days post wounding [51]. Contraction can last for several weeks [52] and continues even after the wound is completely re-epithelialised [53]. A large wound can become 40–80% smaller after contraction [54, 55]. Wounds can contract at a speed of up to 0.75 mm per day, depending on how loose the tissue in the wounded area is [51]. Contraction usually does not occur symmetrically; rather, most wounds have an 'axis of contraction', which allows for greater organisation and alignment of the cells with collagen [50].

If linear scars contract it is usually up to 30% of their length, maximum. The most obvious effect of this is around the eyes. Horizontal incisions below the eyelid

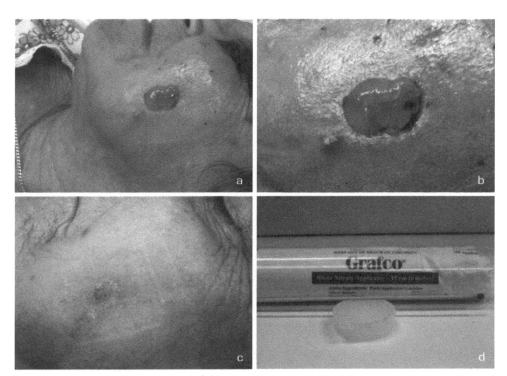

Figure 12.15 **Hypergranulation treated with fulguration**

a Surprisingly vigorous reaction to a shave biopsy. **b** Hypertonic dressings applied but with not much improvement. The lesion was friable, spongiform and bled easily to the touch. **c** Finally, 21 weeks later after regular hypertonic dressings had not made much improvement, fulguration (twice) was tried and resulted in improvement and complete healing. **d** Silver nitrate applicators (75% AgNO₃) can also be used. The area turns white, then grey, and necrotic tissue sloughs off in some 2 weeks, usually followed by normal healing although reapplication is sometimes needed.

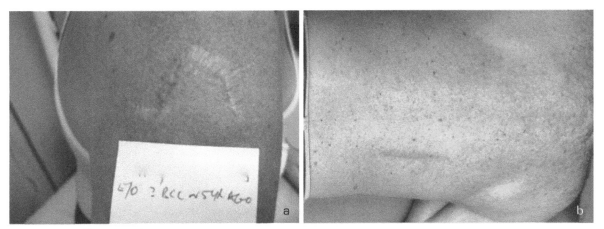

Figure 12.16 **Scar spread**

a Scar spread on a most obvious site; the shoulders are notorious for such a complication. Why was such a complex (flap) operation done when an ellipse could have been done and why, on an attractive young woman, were deep and subcuticular sutures not offered? The patient was 'pretty sure' it was a BCC and 'not very large' and was willing to pay to get good cosmesis. **b** This 100-mm scar closed a 30-mm (+) deficit (melanoma >10 mm). The patient was a self-employed carpenter and also a sailor. Despite advice, he pursued both immediately. He has deep 3/0 nylon sutures. He has felt no irritation. This photo was taken 6 years post-op.

can pull it down into an ectropion, and above the eyebrow can lead to abnormal looking raised eyebrows, especially laterally. These can be avoided by using a vertical ellipse or A-to-T technique.

Scar contracture on the nose can be disfiguring, even bending the nose to one side, but can also close the nasal flap or reduce the diameter of the nares, making breathing more difficult.

Scars should also be avoided over joints as contractures can reduce the range of movement. If unavoidable, the middle of an O-S flap running vertically along the limb acts as a hinge that allows extension.

Keloid/hypertrophic scars

Keloids only occur in humans. Both dominant and recessive modes of inheritance have been described. They are benign dermal fibrotic variations of the normal healing process wherein there is excess proliferation of collagen, elastin, extracellular matrix proteins and proteoglycans, presumably from a prolonged inflammatory process that seems to be the trigger. Keloid and hypertrophic scars also develop secondary to wounds as a result of trauma – insect bites, ear piercing, lacerations, tattoos, vaccinations and burns. Hypertrophic scars are more common in burns and scalds.

- Age: mostly occur between 10 and 30 years and are rare in the young and elderly but with a currently increasing incidence with coronary artery bypass operations and such.
- Race: keloids are more frequent in Polynesian and Chinese than Indian and Malaysian people. 16% of black Africans have been quoted as having keloids. Whites are least affected.
- Sex: keloids and hypertrophic scars affect both sexes equally in all age groups except that in young females the prevalence may be higher, probably due to the greater incidence of earlobe piercing in this group.

There are practical differences between hypertrophic scars and keloids (Table 12.3).

Ultrastructural histological differences between hypertrophic and keloid scars relate primarily to orientation of collagen bundles in the substratum of the skin surface. Hypertrophic scars have parallel flat bundles of arranged collagen sheets, whereas keloids have disarrayed collagen sheets rather than discrete bundles.

Hypertrophic scars and keloids also may be immunochemically and biochemically differentiated. Keloids demonstrate a greater tissue concentration of immunoglobulin G (IgG) relative to hypertrophic scars and normal skin. When compared to uninjured skin, relative concentrations of the collagen metabolic enzymes collagenase and proline hydroxylase are 3–4 times higher in hypertrophic scars and 15–20 times higher in keloids.

Keloids and hypertrophic scars have proven an enigma and a problem as to both predictability and treatment.

TABLE 12.3 Distinguishing hypertrophic scars and keloids

Hypertrophic scars	Keloids
Occur soon after surgery	Slowly develop over months
Usually regress	Continued growth
Restricted to incision margins	Exceed surgical margins
Usually over joints/highly mobile areas	Usually where no movement of skin
Amenable to therapy	Often recur after therapy in a worse form
Wide and flat	Often dome-shaped or pedunculated
Usually asymptomatic	Painful, burning and initially itchy

They only occur in humans and occur in 5–15% of wounds. They are more common with pigmented skin.

Aetiology

- Genetic basis: the ratio is 10:1 in dark-skinned compared to white-skinned populations in scar development. This may be due to an abnormality of melanocyte stimulating hormone.
- Skin and tissue tension: increased tension at the skin will cause the scar to widen as the body reacts to the forces trying to separate the wound. Tension at the cellular level will also cause changes in enzyme activity and an increased collagen production, which is why some people develop more pronounced scarring.
- Endocrine factors: increased hormonal activity. Keloids enlarge during pregnancy and regress with menopause. Abnormal function of the pituitary, thyroid, parathyroid and hypothalamus may also be implicated.

Prevention

Every patient must be warned as to this potential complication. Certain sites (Figure 12.17), the mediastinum and ear lobes especially, are much more prone to develop keloids. Postoperative silica gel or Dermatix® is recommended.

Wounds should be closed with minimal tension, placed in wrinkles/RSTL and not cross cosmetic boundaries.

Treatment

Numerous methods have been described for the treatment and prevention of keloids, with the optimal management strategy yet to be found. No matter what

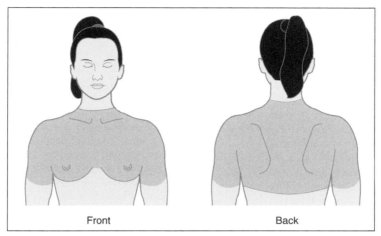

Front	Back

Figure 12.17 Keloid/hypertrophic scar prone sites

The upper back, anterior central chest, upper arms, shoulders and breasts are all keloid prone sites. Avoid unnecessary procedures in these sites, particularly in predisposed individuals.

Adapted from Lawrence CM, An Introduction to Dermatological Surgery, 2nd edn. London: Churchill Livingstone, 2002; Fig 7.2.

treatment is used, it is essential to explain the difficulty in obtaining a resolution and the distinct likelihood of recurrence and side effects (hypopigmentation etc).

Many experimental treatments exist from onion extract to vitamin E but the following are mainly used. None can be guaranteed to achieve complete lasting resolution.

Topical

Moisturisers, vitamin E, steroid ointment, imiquimod, retinoids, occlusive/compression dressings, silicon sheeting and cryotherapy have all been used.

- Vitamin E cream/oil has no demonstrated benefit and may actually retard wound healing.
- Moisturisers will help keep the scar soft.
- Bio-Oil is a specialist skincare product that may help improve the appearance of scars, stretch marks and uneven skin tone.
- Occlusive dressings are usually silicone gel sheets. The silicone does not enter the skin so it is thought that the increased pressure, temperature, hydration and reduced oxygenation of the scar may increase collagenase activity. Although paper tape should be routinely applied to all wounds for 4 weeks or so, the cost of silicone gel sheets and the obligation to wear occlusive dressings 24 hours a day for up to a year for something that may never occur makes the uptake and use of these limited to those who have had a past history or who are cosmetically conscious. A patient who has developed hypertrophic or keloid scars is more willing to so comply. There are a number of products with some success in reducing the appearance of these types of scars.

- Cica-Care gel sheet is a soft, self-adhesive, semi-occlusive sheet made from medical grade silicone reinforced with a silicone membrane backing.
- Mepiform® is a thin, flexible dressing consisting of a viscose non-woven fabric bonded to a semi-permeable polyurethane membrane. The inner surface of the non-woven fabric is coated with a layer of soft silicone, which facilitates application and retention of the dressing to intact skin, but does not cause epidermal stripping or pain on removal. The dressing is waterproof but permeable to water vapour.
- Dermatix is a transparent, fast-drying silicone gel. It should not be applied to open or fresh wounds, mucous membranes or close to the eyes. The effect seems to result from a combination of occlusion and hydration, rather than from an effect of the silicone.

Previous studies for hypertrophic/keloid scars reported that, in patients treated with silicone occlusive sheeting with pressure worn 24 hours per day for up to 12 months, 34% showed excellent improvement, 37.5% showed moderate improvement and 28% demonstrated no or slight improvement. Of patients treated with semipermeable, semiocclusive, non-silicone-based dressings for 8 weeks, 60% experienced flattening of keloids, 71% had reduced pain, 78% had reduced tenderness, 80% had reduced pruritus, 87.5% had reduced erythema and 90% were satisfied with the treatment. Cordran tape is a clear surgical tape that contains flurandrenolide, a steroid that is uniformly distributed on each square centimetre of the tape, and it has been shown to soften and flatten keloids over time.

Intralesional

Corticosteroid injection (triamcinolone [Kenacort®]) is the most used treatment; it comes as Kenacort-A 10 (10 mg/mL) and Kenacort-A 40 (40 mg/mL).

There are slightly varying regimens (see Figure 12.18):

- Kenacort-A 10: inject a small amount into the mass of the lesion to cause blanching. Review at 4–6 weeks and repeat if flattening. Maximum of three injections. If no response, Kenacort-A 40 diluted to 50% with local anaesthetic can be tried.
- Triamcinolone (Kenacort) 10–40 mg/mL: inject every 2–6 weeks (especially for stubborn keloids that do not respond to intralesional Kenacort, especially post-CABG sternal keloids). The higher dose is more effective with a maximum total dose not exceeding 40 mg. Inject into the papillary dermis where the collagen is produced. Avoid injecting into the subcutaneous fat as this causes fat necrosis.
- Depo-Medrol® 40 mg/mL (normally used by orthopaedists for injecting joints) has been successfully used as its crystals are much less soluble than those of Kenacort. Serious atrophy and telangiectasia are likely but the patient may prefer to have the thick and probably symptomatic keloid replaced with atrophic skin.
- Triamcinolone (0.1 mL, 10 mg/mL) + fluorouracil (5FU) (0.9 mL, 50 mg/mL): inject 1–3 times a week. Injections are painful and high pressure is needed so luer-lock syringes and local anaesthetic are needed. Inject until the scar blanches using a 1.0-cc luer lock syringe and a 25G–30G needle. Repeat at 2-weekly intervals until a good response and then drop out the triamcinolone (to stop potential fat atrophy – try and inject into papillary dermis) and just use fluorouracil (5FU). Takes 10–20 treatments. The sooner started the better. Patients are left with a flat white scar.
- Dermatix or silicone sheeting: apply at night. Fluorouracil (5FU) comes as 500 mg in 10 mL × 10 ampoules.
- Shave + mitomycin: mitomycin C is an antitumour and antibiotic drug that inhibits DNA synthesis; at high doses it inhibits RNA and protein synthesis and is used for chemotherapy to treat breast, lung and prostate cancers. In topical form it has been shown to suppress fibroblast proliferation and decrease fibrosis during the wound healing process.

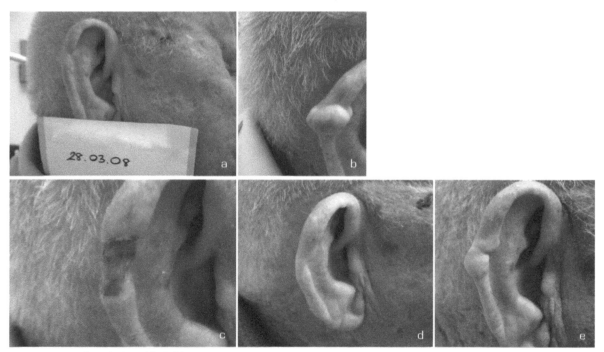

Figure 12.18 Intralesional keloid treatment

a A satisfactory, but not great result after complete excision of a basosquamous carcinoma R helix March 2008 (excision January 2008). **b** 2 years later the patient reported this swelling. Fortnightly Depo-Medrol failed to improve it. **c** The keloid was excised and imiquimod applied to the base in April 2010 and, after some 30 months, it was felt the treatment was successful. **d** However, 30 months later – recurrence. **e** As intralesional steroids had no effect and this had at least lasted 30 months with minimal side effects, the same procedure was repeated.

Thus, topically it has been used to prevent scar tissue formation after various types of surgery. Treatment of the resected bed of shave-removed ear keloids may suppress recurrence. Apply 1 mg/mL to the resected bed for 5 minutes. Repeat 3 weeks later. Of 11 patients (all keloids caused by ear piercing), there was only one recurrence after 12 months [56].

• Shave + imiquimod (Figure 12.18): shave the keloid and apply imiquimod for 7 days, then on alternate days for 3–4 weeks or nightly for 8 weeks with breaks if and when there is a reaction. Imiquimod cream 5% may prove to be a reasonably effective adjuvant therapy for prevention of recurrence in excised earlobe keloids when applied daily for 8 weeks [57]. 5% imiquimod cream [58] is an immune response modifier that is currently approved for the treatment of genital warts, actinic keratoses and superficial BCC. Along with induction and activation of immune mechanisms, there is also a dose-dependent inhibition of human collagen production by INF-α and INF-γ [59, 60]. INF-γ has also been found to decrease both collagen and glycosaminoglycan production [60, 61]. Berman and Kaufman (2002) [58] described excision and surgical repair of the keloid, followed by imiquimod 5% cream applied for 8 weeks. Since publication of this technique, 60 patients have been treated with shave excision without surgical repair. Earlobe keloids were removed by shaving the keloids flat to the earlobe on both sides, and defects left to heal by secondary intention. Patients were instructed to administer imiquimod 5% cream to the excision sites the night of the surgery and for 8 weeks post-surgery. Patients were examined at approximately 4, 8 and 24 weeks post procedure. The most common complication seen was erythema and irritation of the area treated with imiquimod 5% cream. Secondary infection was found and treated in 6 patients. To date there has been one recurrence of an earlobe keloid treated with this method [62].

Other methods

• Cryotherapy: excellent results were obtained in a small series of seven young patients (aged 9–22 years) where scarring followed plastic surgery in six cases and ear piercing in one. The freeze time varied (30–60 seconds) depending on scar size and thickness, the effect of cryotherapy and patient tolerance. With improvement in the clinical state the duration was decreased. Duration was by optical inspection. A freeze-thaw cycle was used with a 1–2-mm spread lateral to the lesion margins. Treatment was always repeated at least 2 weeks after complete healing of that session – about every 6 weeks. The number of sessions needed varied (2–12) [63].

• Wedge excision: wedge resection is simpler than other described techniques for keloid excision and has provided incomparable aesthetic results in thousands of earlobe keloid excisions over 40 years. The technique allows for more complete keloid removal, decreasing the risk of recurrence. Although not appropriate for all cases, it works well with nodular, dumbbell-shaped, and horseshoe-shaped lesions that involve the central lobe and lateral rim. As the footprint of the lesion approaches half the size of the earlobe, the ability to achieve an acceptable cosmetic outcome diminishes. Clinical judgement should prevail regarding the application of this technique, with the benefit of keloid excision outweighing the risk of extensive and unacceptable postoperative deformity. Monthly postoperative injections of intralesional triamcinolone acetonide (40 mg/mL) reduce the likelihood of recurrence [64].

Pigmentation

Damage to the epidermis can cause pigment changes from its melanocytes. The broader the wound, the more likely the pigmentation. Wounds closed primarily can have hypo- or hyperpigmented scar lines but rarely more than that. More extensive wounds such as shave excisions, electrocautery, cryosurgery, laser or dermabrasion may produce more pigmentary changes. The degree of injury to the melanocytes determines hypo- or hyperpigmentation outcomes. Melanocytes are more prone to cold than other cells and hence cryosurgery leads to depigmentation.

Post-excisional pigmentation appears inside the scar and can occur in any surgical scar. If a melanoma has been completely excised, this pigmentation is not caused by the persistence of naevus cells [65].

Nerve damage

Most skin surgery involves cutting minor cutaneous nerves, leading to altered sensation distal to the incision. Warn the patient about this and reassure them that most sensation returns to normal in 12–18 months with regeneration, which can be preceded by itching, crawling sensation or shooting pains. Deep incisions on the forehead often result in scalp numbness.

The real danger areas are the temporal nerve where it crosses the zygomatic arch, the facial nerve where it winds around the mandible in front of the masseter and the accessory nerve at Erb's point on the posterior sternomastoid (see Chapter 2, 'Essential anatomy for skin surgery'). If these are cut they do not regenerate and neurological deficits result:

• cutting the temporal nerve results in depression of the eyebrow and inability to wrinkle the forehead on that side

- transecting the facial nerve leads to a dropped lip and asymmetry of lip movement/drool
- cutting the accessory nerve results in paraesthesia, pain, shoulder drop and difficulty with abduction.

Patients should be referred to a microsurgeon immediately.

> ### HINTS AND TIPS
>
> Examine the patient for any asymmetry or possible previous nerve damage. If there is any asymmetry or differences a photograph will save any possible medicolegal problems.

Ongoing pain or pruritus

'It's itching so it must be healing' is the age-old observation and is normal. Severed small cutaneous nerves can give altered sensation and some pain up to 18 months. Persistent pruritus or pain that exceeds 6 months may warrant investigation as to nerve entrapment from scar formation or even previously unsuspected perineural invasion.

Secondary intention healing is often more likely to be itchy.

Incomplete excision

There is arguably nothing much more unpleasant for the patient (and the doctor too) than to get a report of an incomplete excision. Patients, perhaps unreasonably, often feel this is a reflection of some incompetence by the doctor. To some degree this can be attenuated by explaining the difficulties with infiltrating BCC and those of certain sites such as the nose. Meticulous examination of the lesion margins with a dermatoscope may help. 4-mm margins are mandatory but 5-mm may provide better clearance with only a 3.9% incomplete excision rate [66]. The rate of incomplete excisions for BCCs with 3-mm margins has been reported at 4% [67].

Slow Mohs is arguably the 'way to go' for difficult lesions and excisions.

At least 30–50% of incompletely excised BCCs recur clinically [68–70]. When BCCs recur they are usually deeper and more aggressive, necessitating more extensive surgery especially if flaps were used initially [70].

Treatment
Immediate surgical resection [71].

Recurrent tumours

Recurrent tumours may occur even with apparent histological clearance. This may be because only some 1–2% of the specimen is examined in normal, routine, 'bread-loaf' dermopathological slide specimen examinations or because of an outlying satellite focus or it may, in fact, be a new lesion and not a recurrence.

Perineural invasion, aggressive histological types and ears and lips have a higher recurrence rate.

Margin clearance and recurrence
Correct and adequate margin clearance is necessary to minimise recurrence. Mohs surgery is recommended for high recurrence risk tumours.

Recurrence of BCC and SCC [72]:

- 2-mm margin = 70% clearance, 30% recurrence
- 3-mm = 85% clearance, 15% recurrence
- 4-mm = 98% clearance, 2% recurrence.

With 5-mm margins incomplete excision was limited to 3.9% of cases, and the recurrence rate was 1.7% [66].

Risk of local recurrence
Refer to Tables 12.4 and 12.5.

Delayed healing or closure

Some wounds are impossible to close but will heal well by secondary intention rather than an unsightly (and unnecessary) graft. The lower leg is such a site where both O-S and ROM flaps can leave a central defect. Learning how to manage and monitor this secondary intention healing is necessary. It is important to recognise the difference between normal granulation tissue and exuberant hypergranulation 'proud-flesh' and the difference between a normal discoloured exudate and infection. Above all, patience and patient reassurance are needed.

Contact dermatitis and hypersensitivity

Contact dermatitis is usually recognised by the characteristic shape of the erythematous area forming a contact shadow image of the dressing. It must be differentiated from wound infection and suture reaction, both of which cause erythema around the wound. Vesicles and pruritus further support the diagnosis of a sensitivity reaction.

Treatment
Remove the dressing and don't use that type again (it is usually the adhesive). Try and remove any residual adhesive. Depending on the severity of the inflammatory dermatitis reaction this may be possible with solvent

TABLE 12.4 Risk of local recurrence of BCC depending on clearance as measured histologically

BCC type	<0.38 mm	0.38–0.75 mm	>0.75 mm
Solid	40%	10%	4%
Multifocal sclerosing infiltrative	80%	45%	20%

Note: the significance of a close margin varies depending on the subtype of BCC.
Adapted from Dixon AY et al. J Cutan Pathol 1993;20:137–42.

TABLE 12.5 Factors influencing recurrence and metastasis of SCC

	Local recurrence %	Metastasis %
Size		
<2 cm	7.4	9.1
>2 cm	15.2	30.3
Depth		
<4 mm/Clark Lv 1 to ii	5.3	6.7
>4 mm/Clark Lv iv–v	17.2	45.7
Differentiation		
Well differentiated	13.6	9.2
Poorly differentiated	28.6	32.8
Site		
Sun-exposed	7.9	5.2
Ear	18.7	11.0
Lip	10.5	13.7
Scar SCC (non-sun-exposed)	N/A	37.9
Previous treatment	23.3	30.3
Perineural involvement	47.2	47.3
Immunosuppression	N/A	12.9

Adapted from Rowe DE, Carroll RJ, Day CL Jr. J Am Acad Dermatol 1992;26:976.

TABLE 12.6 Complications associated with flaps

Cause	Complication
Preoperative	
Surgeon	Poor flap design, especially kinking or tension Haematomas (evacuate urgently) Inadequate flap size Design of the flap in traumatised tissue
Patient	Smoking Hypertension Hypotension Poor overall health (diabetes, malnutrition, renal failure) Steroids Age
Intraoperative	
Technical errors	Injuring the blood supply Creating too much tension Twisting or kinking the flap pedicle
Postoperative	
Early	Infection Dehiscence Flap necrosis Haematoma/seroma

ether, which is the most efficient solvent for this. Otherwise, use sterile water/normal saline. Pat dry and apply a steroid ointment tds – not a cream as these hurt more.

Monitor for infection. Try and leave uncovered.

Life-threatening complications

Life-threatening complications are extremely rare with cutaneous surgery. Careful selection of patients who are only suitable for operations in hospitals with a full resuscitation unit must be made. Such patients are those with severe cardiovascular disease, uncontrolled endocrine illness (especially diabetes) and past history of coaguloapathies/DVT and where the operation will be long and difficult. Smoking has also been associated with poor outcomes.

The most common potential life-threatening complication is a DVT. Preventive measures should be mandatory in all patients: never compress calves and early ambulation.

Other possible emergencies are:

- vaso-vagal reactions
- myocardial infarction/arrhythmias
- anaphylaxis.

Immediate-type hypersensitivity manifests as urticaria, angio-oedema or anaphylaxis and represents a potentially fatal complication. This type of allergy to amide local anaesthetics (e.g. lignocaine, mepivacaine,

articaine) is rare, but cases have been reported [73]. Allergy to ester-type local anaesthetics (e.g. procaine, benzocaine, amethocaine (tetracaine)) is more common because of their metabolism to *p*-aminobenzoic acid (PABA), a potential allergen. Anaphylaxis caused by chlorhexidine has been reported in rare cases [74].

Is CPR a waste of time?

Shockable, survivable rhythms such as ventricular fibrillation decay – sometimes quickly – into unshockable more lethal rhythms, including asystole. Prompt defibrillation works. The CPR that precedes it may not. Rescue breathing is already being questioned and it is time to apply the same critical thinking to chest compressions [75].

Complications of flaps

These are essentially the same as complications in general but are summarised here for convenience (Table 12.6).

- Haematoma/seroma: good haemostasis is essential to prevent haematomas and seromas. Pressure/conforming bandages are helpful. Elevate leg wounds above the heart and moderate exercise for 48 hours. Drain or aspirate haematomas whenever possible to prevent induration and irregularity of the operative field. Seromas often resolve without treatment but should be aspirated as needed.

- Infection is uncommon in clean surgery. Most infections come from the patient's own skin. Clean technique and site preparation are important. Waterproof dressings secured and left on are best. Perioperative antibiotics are used for diabetics and others at risk. Swab culture and sensitivity should be done and systemic and topical antibiotics commenced immediately. Abscessed wounds require incision and drainage.

- Wound dehiscences can occur as the result of poor surgical technique, poor patient compliance or poor patient healing ability (old and fragile or 'steroid' skin). Patients with renal failure, undergoing chemotherapy, the malnourished or those who have been irradiated heal poorly. A judicious method of dealing with minor dehiscence is to allow the patient to heal then attempt repair at 6 months after the scar has matured and normal healthy tissue surrounds the original defect.

- Flap necrosis is more serious and is usually due to a design flaw or an error in execution of the reconstruction. These errors include the use of too small a flap for a given defect, damage to the flap's blood supply, extending the flap beyond its blood supply or closing the defect in such a way that it is subject to too much tension. Flap necrosis usually can be avoided by more precise flap design and avoidance of undue tension upon closure of the wound. Treatment of distal necrosis is conservative and may include allowing certain areas to heal by secondary intention and/or subsequent surgical revision of the area. However, in areas where the flap was placed to prevent a deforming scar contracture, such as the eyelid, a new reconstruction should be performed as soon as the wound condition permits.

Late complications

- Unfavourable scarring: occurs when scars are placed outside of the direction of the skin tension lines. Scars that lie in the wrong direction can be revised with a Z-plasty or a W-plasty.

- Pin-cushioning (trapdoor deformity): arises from a curvilinear scar. Correction of the pin-cushion deformity should not be performed until the scar matures. Options for correction include excision of the old scar, defatting of the flap and closure with Z-plasties or a W-plasty.

- Hypertrophic scars: are uncommon on the face.

- Keloids: can be problematic. Warn any patient with a personal or family history of keloids or a personal history of hypertrophic scars about the risk of developing a keloid or a hypertrophic scar. Once a keloid forms, many treatment options are available, most of which are only partially effective in minimising the scar. Pressure, topical silicone, steroid injections and massage are the standard treatments as detailed above.

These complications are avoided for the most part by experience and careful planning of the flap reconstruction.

REFERENCES

[1] Eaglstein WH. Experiences with biosynthetic dressings. J Am Acad Dermatol 1985;12:434–40.

[2] Eaglstein WH. Occlusive dressings. J Dermatol Surg Oncol 1993;19:716–20.

[3] Klode J, Schöttler L, Stoffels I, et al. Investigation of adhesion of modern wound dressings: a comparative analysis of 56 different wound dressings. J Eur Acad Dermatol Venereol 2011;25:933–9.

[4] Goetze S, Ziemer M, Kaatz M, et al. Treatment of superficial surgical wounds after removal of seborrheic keratosis: a single-blinded randomized-controlled clinical study. Derm Surg 2006;5:661–8.

[5] Castelli ML, Di Lisi D, Marcato P, et al. Is pressure dressing necessary after ear surgery? Ann Otol Rhinol Laryngol 2001;110:254–6.

[6] Wasserman DI, Tucker D, Zeltser R, et al. "Trapdoor" ear dressing for auricular surgery. Dermatol Surg 2008;34(4):567–70.

[7] Telfer NR, Moy RL. Wound care after office procedures. J Dermatol Surg Oncol 1993; 19:722.

[8] Abercrombie M, James DW. Long-term changes in the size and collagen content of scars in the skin of rats. J Embryol Exp Morph 1956;4:167–75.

[9] Baumann LS, Spencer J. The effects of topical vitamin E on the cosmetic appearance of scars. Dermatol Surg 1999;25(4):311–15.

[10] Lai Y, Di Nardo A, Nakatsuji T, et al. Commensal bacteria regulate Toll-like receptor 3-dependent inflammation after skin injury. Nat Med 2009;15:1377–82.

[11] Heal CF, Buettner PG, Cruickshank R, et al. Does single application of topical chloramphenicol to high risk sutured wounds reduce incidence of wound infection after minor surgery? Prospective randomised placebo controlled double blind trial. BMJ 2009;338:a2812.

[12] Draelos ZD, Rizer RL, Trookman NS. A comparison of postprocedural wound care treatments: do antibiotic-based ointments improve outcomes? J Am Acad Dermatol 2011;64(3, Suppl. 1):S23–9.

[13] Taylor SC, Averyhart AN, Heath CR. Postprocedural wound-healing efficacy following removal of dermatosis papulosa nigra lesions in an African American population: A comparison of a skin protectant ointment and a topical antibiotic. J Am Acad Dermatol 2011;64(3, Suppl. 1):S30–5.

[14] Trookman NS, Rizer RL, Weber T. Treatment of minor wounds from dermatologic procedures: a comparison of

three topical wound care ointments using a laser wound model. J Am Acad Dermatol 2011;64:S8.

[15] Bode LG, Kluytmans JA, Wertheim HF, et al. Preventing surgical-site infections in nasal carriers of Staphylococcus aureus. N Engl J Med 2010;362:9–17.

[16] Lawrence WT, Murphy RC, Robson MC, et al. The detrimental effect of cigarette smoking on flap survival: an experimental study in the rat. Br J Plast Surg 1984;37(2):216–19.

[17] Aker JS, Mancoll J, Lewis B, et al. The effect of pentoxifylline on random-pattern skin-flap necrosis induced by nicotine treatment in the rat. Plast Reconstr Surg 1997;100(1):66–71.

[18] Karacaoğlan N, Akbaş H. Effect of parenteral pentoxifylline and topical nitroglycerin on skin flap survival. Otolaryngol Head Neck Surg 1999;120(2):272–4.

[19] Weatherhead SC, Lawrence CM. Antibiotics for skin surgery. Preoperative integrity of skin surface predicts infection risk. BMJ 2009;338:b516.

[20] Duff AJ. Incorporating psychological approaches into routine paediatric venepuncture. Arch Dis Child 2003;88:931–7.

[21] Nir Y, Paz A, Sabo E, et al. Fear of injections in young adults: prevalence and associations. Am J Trop Med Hyg 2003;68:341–4.

[22] Hamilton JG. Needle phobia: a neglected diagnosis. J Fam Pract 1995;2:169–75.

[23] American Psychiatric Association (APA). Diagnostic and statistical manual of mental disorders DSM-IV-TR. Washington, DC: APA; 2000.

[24] Lin J, Ziegler D, Lai CW, et al. Convulsive syncope in blood donors. Ann Neurol 1982;59:122–4.

[25] Poles F, Boycott M. Syncope in blood donors. Lancet 1942;2:531–5.

[26] National Alliance on Mental Illness. Cognitive-behavioral therapy. Available: <http://www.nami.org/Template.cfm?Section=About_Treatments_and_Supports&template=/ContentManagement/ContentDisplay.cfm&ContentID=7952>; 2003 [accessed 7 March 2007].

[27] Horan TC, Gaynes RP, Martone WJ, et al. CDC definitions of nosocomial surgical site infections, 1992: a modification of CDC definitions of surgical wound infections. Am J Infect Control 1992;20:271–4.

[28] Dixon AJ, Dixon MP, Dixon JB. Prospective study of skin surgery in patients with and without known diabetes. Dermatol Surg 2009a;35:1035–40.

[29] Futoryan T, Grande D. Postoperative wound infection rates in dermatologic surgery. Dermatol Surg 1995;21:509–14.

[30] Maragh SL, Otley CC, Roenigk RK, et al. Antibiotic prophylaxis in dermatologic surgery: updated guidelines. Dermatol Surg 2006;32(6):819–27.

[31] Heal C, Buettner P, Browning S. Risk factors for wound infection after minor surgery in general practice. Med J Aust 2006;185(5):255–8.

[32] Darouiche RO, Wall MJ Jr, Itani KM, et al. Chlorhexidine–alcohol versus povidone–iodine for surgical-site antisepsis. N Engl J Med 2010;362:18–26.

[33] Rappaport WD, Hunter GC, Allen R, et al. Effect of electrocautery on wound healing in midline laparotomy incisions. Am J Surg 1990;160(6):618–20.

[34] Dixon AJ, Dixon MP, Askew DA, et al. Prospective study of wound infections in dermatologic surgery in the absence of prophylactic antibiotics. Dermatol Surg 2006;32(6):819–26, discussion 826–27.

[35] Dixon AJ, Dixon MP, Dixon JB, et al. Prospective study of skin surgery in smokers vs. nonsmokers. Br J Dermatol 2009b;16(2):365–7.

[36] West SW, Otley CC, Nguyen TH, et al. Cutaneous surgeons cannot predict blood-thinner status by intraoperative visual inspection. Plast Reconstr Surg 2002;110(1):98–103.

[37] Shimizu I, Jellinek NJ, Dufresne RG, et al. Multiple antithrombotic agents increase the risk of postoperative hemorrhage in dermatologic surgery. J Am Acad Dermatol 2008;58(5):810–16.

[38] Schanbacher CF, Bennett RG. Postoperative stroke after stopping warfarin for cutaneous surgery. Dermatol Surg 2000;26(8):785–9.

[39] Kovich O, Otley CC. Thrombotic complications related to discontinuation of warfarin and aspirin therapy perioperatively for cutaneous operation. J Am Acad Dermatol 2003;48(2):233–7.

[40] Lewis KG, Dufresne RG Jr. A meta-analysis of complications attributed to anticoagulation among patients following cutaneous surgery. Dermatol Surg 2008;34(2):160–5.

[41] Cook-Norris RH, Michaels JD, Weaver AL, et al. Complications of cutaneous surgery in patients taking clopidogrel-containing anticoagulation. J Am Acad Dermatol 2011;65(3):584–91.

[42] Aronberg J, Kluser F. Surgical pearl: securing surgical dressing with acetone. J Am Acad Dermatol 2003;48:611–12.

[43] Zeitani J, Bertoldo F, Bassano C, et al. Superficial wound dehiscence after median sternotomy: surgical treatment versus secondary wound healing. Ann Thorac Surg 2004;77:672–5.

[44] Byrne P. Randomised clinical trial of suture compared with adhesive strip for skin closure after HRT implant. Br J Obstet Gynaecol 2002;109:1178–80.

[45] Conolly WB, Hunt TK, Zederfeldt B, et al. Clinical comparison of surgical wounds closed by suture and adhesive tapes. Am J Surg 1969;117:318–22.

[46] Pepicello J, Yavorek H. Five year experience with tape closure of abdominal wounds. Surg Gynecol Obstet 1989;169:310–14.

[47] Chao TC, Tsaez FY. Paper tape in the closure of abdominal wounds. Am J Gynecol Obstet 1990;171:65–7.

[48] Katz S, Izhar M, Mirelman D. Bacterial adherence to surgical sutures. A possible factor in suture induced infection. Ann Surg 1981;194(1):35–41.

[49] Roenigk R, Roenigk H, editors. Dermatologic surgery: principles and practice. New York: Marcel Dekker; 1989.

[50] Eichler MJ, Carlson MA. Modeling dermal granulation tissue with the linear fibroblast-populated collagen matrix: a comparison with the round matrix model. J Dermatol Sci 2006;41(2):97–108.

[51] Romo R III. Skin wound healing. Emedicine. Available: <http://emedicine.medscape.com/article/884594-overview>; 2005 [accessed 4 January 2013].

[52] James WD. Military dermatology (Textbook of military medicine – Part 3, Disease and the environment, vol 1). Department of the Army, USA; 1994.

[53] Stadelmann WK, Digenis AG, Tobin GR. Physiology and healing dynamics of chronic cutaneous wounds. Am J Surg 1998;176(2):26S–38S.

[54] DiPietro LA, Burns AL, editors. Wound healing: methods and protocols. Totowa, NJ: Humana Press; 2003.

[55] Lorenz HP, Longaker MT. Wounds: biology, pathology, and management. Stanford University Medical Center; 2003.

[56] Chi SG, Kim JY, Lee WJ, et al. Ear keloids as a primary candidate for the application of mitomycin C after shave excision: in vivo and in vitro study. Dermatol Surg 2011;37(2):168–75.

[57] Martin-García RF, Busquets AC. Postsurgical use of imiquimod 5% cream in the prevention of earlobe keloid recurrences: results of an open-label, pilot study. Dermatol Surg 2005;31(11):1394–8.

[58] Berman B, Kaufman J. Pilot study of the effect of postoperative imiquimod 5% cream on the recurrence rate of excised keloids. J Am Acad Dermatol 2002;47:S209–11.

[59] Jimenez SA, Freudlich B, Rosenbloom J. Selective inhibition of diploid fibroblast collagen synthesis by Interferons. J Clin Invest 1984;74:1112–16.

[60] Berman B, Villa A. Imiquimod 5% cream for keloid management. Dermatol Surg 2003;29:1050–1.

[61] Berman B, Duncan MR. Short-term keloid treatment in vivo with human interferon alpha-2b results in a selective and persistant normalization of keloidal fibroblast collagen, glycosaminoglycan, and collagenase production in vitro. J Am Acad Dermatol 1989;21:694–706.

[62] Patel PJ, Skinner RB Jr. Experience with keloids after excision and application of 5% imiquimod cream. Dermatol Surg 2006;32(3):462.

[63] Fikrle T, Pizinger K. Cryosurgery in the treatment of earlobe keloids: report of seven cases. Dermatol Surg 2005;31:1728–31.

[64] Music EN, Engel G. Earlobe keloids: a novel and elegant surgical approach. Dermatol Surg 2010;36:395–400.

[65] Malvehy J, Puig S, Braun RP. Handbook of dermoscopy. London: Taylor & Francis; 2006. p. 54.

[66] Seretis K, Thomaidis V, Karpouzis A, et al. Epidemiology of surgical treatment of nonmelanoma skin cancer of the head and neck in Greece. Dermatol Surg 2010;36(1):15–22.

[67] Bisson MA, Dunkin CS, Suvarna SK, et al. Do plastic surgeons resect basal cell carcinomas too widely? A prospective study comparing surgical and histological margins. Br J Plast Surg 2002;55:293–7.

[68] Gooding CA, White G, Yatsuhashi M. Significance of marginal extension in excised basal-cell carcinoma. N Engl J Med 1965;273:923–4.

[69] De Silva SP, Dellon AL. Recurrence rate of positive margin basal cell carcinoma: results of a five-year prospective study. J Surg Oncol 1985;28:72–4.

[70] Richmond JD, Davie RM. The significance of incomplete excision in patients with basal cell carcinoma. Br J Plast Surg 1987;40:63–7.

[71] Robinson JK, Fisher SG. Recurrent basal cell carcinoma after incomplete resection. Arch Dermatol 2000;136:1318–24.

[72] Wolf DJ, Zitelli JA. Surgical margins for basal cell carcinoma. Arch Dermatol 1987;123(3):340–4.

[73] Klein CE, Gall H. Type IV allergy to amide-type local anesthetics. Contact Dermatitis 1991;25(1):45–8.

[74] Schechter JF, Wilkinson RD, Del Carpio J. Anaphylaxis following the use of bacitracin ointment. Report of a case and review of the literature. Arch Dermatol 1984;120(7):909–11.

[75] Bardy GH. A critic's assessment of our approach to cardiac arrest. N Engl J Med 2011;364:374–5.

What operation where

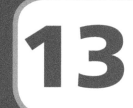

13

If there are six surgeons in a room there will be six different operations proposed for the same lesion.

Anonymous

It is essential for any practitioner who wishes to embark on minor or skin surgery to get training. This training, as in the whole of medicine, benefits from exposure to a variety of teachers. Surgeons each have their favourites, based on very good reasons, but primarily a favourite is an operation that achieves the best results with the least complications for that surgeon. However, there are always other ways and frequently better ways. Try to train with as many different surgeons as possible. This book provides the fundamentals and, where evidenced, recommendations. It is therefore most interesting and helpful to see how our colleagues operate.

There are, however, some glaring and reprehensible practices best avoided, seemingly around the world. For example, 'Grafts are done too often … Given the superior aesthetic results of flaps, grafts should be done at the last resort, after all possible flaps have been considered and rejected' [1]. It would seem some of our colleagues still practice grafting noses when a flap would have given a far better result. Moreover, unfortunately excising a lesion to heal by secondary intention attracts no Medicare rebate in Australia, and so the inner canthi of erstwhile pretty young women now sport mismatched, pin-cushioned grafts, which otherwise may have been invisible if allowed to heal by secondary intention. Similarly, the dreadful scars that are the result of sewing up a lesion under tension, with no respect for the natural wrinkles or skin lines and with what must have been rope, are also anathema.

Not every operation can be perfect but at least we can strive for it to be so. It is essential to learn subcuticular suturing, optimise incision lines, undermine and use deep sutures where necessary to reduce tension.

Scar spread on the back is a problem. Deep sutures with prolonged absorption or even permanent ones reduce this spread. PDS II and its equivalents (Assut, Monoslow) with a life of 180 days are the only absorbable sutures to use to try and prevent scar spread (shorter absorption sutures can be used to close the dead space or minimise tension of the skin edges of the wound). Nylon eventually absorbs after some 14 years, and some surgeons are using it too. The technique, of course, is to ensure the knots are inverted and deep so as to prevent irritation. But despite all best prophylaxis, back scars can still spread.

Always consider a side-by-side diamond excision to preserve as much normal skin as possible.

MARGINS

The most important factor is to cut the cancer with evidenced correct margins and/or Mohs pathology to best assess complete clearance and thus save the patient's life. These margins may be compromised by the site (noses especially), the practitioner's training and speciality.

Important points to note:

- Minor variations exist between countries as to the recommended margins.
- Until the 1980s wide margins of 4–5 cm were performed for melanomas based on anecdotal evidence from 1907 [2]. These were disfiguring and subsequently found not to be necessary:
  - Prospective studies by the World Health Organization in the USA and Europe found that, for melanomas less than 2 mm thick, a 1 cm margin was safe [3].
  - Further prospective studies in the USA and UK found 2-cm and 3-cm margins were safe for lesions greater than 2 mm and 4 mm thick, respectively [4, 5].
- Wide local excision reduces local recurrence rates but has no statistically significant effect on survival [5, 6].

- Narrow margins risk local recurrence. Margins less than 1 cm result in increased loco-regional recurrence. Beyond 1 cm the figures are less clear [7].

Margins and quality control

WIDE EXCISION PERFORMANCES

Plastic surgeons	=	26% with a further 26% in combination with others
Dermatologists	=	24% with a further 16% in combination with others
General surgeons	=	8%
General practitioners	=	6%
Adequate margins	=	31%
Margins too narrow	=	37%
Margins too large	=	32%

MARGIN ADEQUACY BY SPECIALITY

Dermatologists	=	45%
Plastic surgeons	=	38%
General Practitioners	=	31%
General surgeons	=	19%

LOCATION AND MARGIN ADEQUACY

Face	=	78% too narrow
Trunk	=	57% too large
With no prior biopsy	=	58% too narrow

IN SITU MELANOMA MARGINS

36% were less than 3 mm. This is considered inexcusable. Melanoma in situ excision should be curative with 5-mm margins. Narrow margins can result in residual tumour, high recurrence rates, metastasis and death.

Adapted from Kelly et al. The management of primary cutaneous melanoma in Victoria in 1996 and 2000. Med J Aust 2007;187(9):511–14.

SCAR SHAPE

Although getting the cancer out with the correct margins is the essential aim, bear in mind how the final scar will look. There may be a way to still get the correct margin with a smaller scar. The final scar shape is also to be kept in mind. Conversely, never compromise the correct margins.

The **one hammer rule** is: 'If you only have a hammer you will use it to do all jobs'. If the practitioner's knowledge is limited to the basics, he too will use the one flap when there is a better one. Knowing in one's mind's eye how the scars of different flaps finally look is of primary importance for flap selection. As an example, the rhomboid flap results in an ugly scar and should be avoided on the face if at all possible in this author's opinion. Yet, it comes highly recommended by others. A small rhomboid flap on the nose may be acceptable but a large one on a woman's cheek looks more like a brand or a mutilation. The resulting operation scars are drawn in Chapter 8, 'Flaps'. Be aware of and refer to these before planning the operation. The best flap is the one that allows the correct margin to be taken and the defect to be repaired with the fewest complications and minimal scarring. Knowing the harvest areas where there is loose available tissue to mobilise and how tissues move is also of primary importance.

Aids to better scars and what operation where

- A curved line is usually more discrete that a straight one.
- A longer curve is often more discrete than a short, straight one.
- Place incisions in cosmetic unit borders if possible.
- Elsewhere, place incisions in wrinkle lines.
- Ask the patient to posture and grimace to see where these lines are.
- Ensure no tension.
- Do not cauterise flap edges.
- Use the finest sutures possible.
- An A-T can usually do what a bilateral advancement flap can do, only better.
- An A-T can usually do what most flaps can do – only better.
- Remove sutures ASAP.
- Secure-strip the wound and cover with paper tape.
- Simple ellipse (diamonds) A-T, O-S(Z) and bilobed flaps will cover at least 90% of clinic operations.

Possible operations for a primary skin cancer

As to the actual excision, it is essential to consider all options and possibilities and not be restricted. Expertise will increase with experience – but this is the same for all and grafts can then be minimised.

1 Side-by-side – rhomboid/diamond
2 Secondary intention
3 Advancement flap
4 Rotation flap
5 Transposition flap

6 Island flap
7 Graft
8 Interpolation flap
9 Free flap
10 Tissue expansion

Although some sites and lesions suggest a preference, the above list must always be considered.

- A simple ellipse heals best.
- An A-T can usually be buried in wrinkle lines/cosmetic borders and has no potential for tip necrosis or pin-cushioning.
- An O-S (Z) is preferred over joints as it has an inbuilt extension design.

TISSUE WASTAGE

A diamond excision (as noted previously) wastes the least amount of normal tissue. This is easily visualised and understood. What is less well understood is that if, for example, 20-mm margins are taken in a circle surrounding a 10-mm melanoma, four times as much tissue is excised as for 10-mm margins.

The correct margins must be taken, but wider margins are not necessary and are more tissue wasteful than may be thought.

CLOSURES AND TECHNIQUES

A survey conducted in the USA on the 'Frequency of use of suturing and repair techniques preferred by dermatologic surgeons' noted that: 'There are many closure techniques and suture types available to cutaneous surgeons. Evidence-based data are not available regarding the frequency of use of these techniques by experienced practitioners'. The survey set out 'to quantify, by anatomic site, the frequency of use of common closure techniques and suture types by cutaneous surgeons'. This was done by 'a prospective survey of the members of the Association of Academic Dermatologic Surgeons that used length-calibrated visual-analogue scales to elicit the frequency of use of specific suture techniques' [8].

This survey revealed that cutaneous surgeons trained through dermatology tend to repair similar-sized wounds with similar closure techniques. The relative uniformity of suture techniques included similarity in the major method chosen (e.g. primary closure, local flap, etc), preparation of the wound for repair (e.g. undermining, electrocoagulation), suture material composition and the number of suture layers and suturing style (e.g. simple interrupted, simple running, vertical mattress, subcuticular, etc). Additionally, there was consistency across surgeons in how these parameters were varied for defects at different anatomic sites. Their conclusions as to operation type are given in Table 13.1.

TABLE 13.1 Primary strategies used for repair

Repair method	Percentile value (%)		
	25th	**50th**	**75th**
Primary closure	45	54	65
Local flap	12	20	25
Skin graft	5	10	10
Secondary intent	5	10	10
Referred for repair	1	5	10

Note: Displayed values include the median, or 50th percentile, as well as the highest values of the bottom quarter of respondents, or the 25th percentile, and the lowest values of the top quarter, or 75th percentile.
Adapted from Adams B, Levy R, Rademaker AE et al. Frequency of use of suturing and repair techniques preferred by dermatologic surgeons. Dermatol Surg 2006;32(5):682–9.

TABLE 13.2 Westmead Mohs surgery unit cases from 2007

Repair method	Percentage
Side-to-side	25.8%
Flaps	47.5%
Grafts	14.1%
Oculoplastics	11.8%
Secondary intention	0.8%

Source: Westmead Mohs surgery unit.

FLAPS AND THEIR USES

Rotation flaps
Rotation flaps are most commonly used for:

- Large defects
  - Midface – malar-maxilla
  - Large medial cheek lesions [9]
- Small to mid-size lesions
  - Nose
  - Canthus
  - Eyelids
  - Lateral face
  - Scalp
  - Temple
  Do not use on forehead or glabella.

Transposition flaps
The straight line of transposition flaps can be oriented parallel to skin creases.
  Uses:

- Forehead
- Glabella

TABLE 13.3 Suggested closure options

Location	Area	Options
Head and neck	Scalp	Ellipse, rotation flap, O-S (Z), pinwheel flap, ellipse with central 2° intention, 2° intention
	Lateral forehead	Ellipse, A-T flap, rotation flap
	Mid forehead	Ellipse – vertical, A-T flap, rotation flap
	High brow	Ellipse – horizontal, ellipse – vertical, A-T flap
	Eyebrow	Ellipse – vertical, A-T flap, bilateral advancement flap
	Temple	Ellipse – horizontal, A-T flap, bilobed flap, Mercedes flap, rotation flap, rhomboid flap
	Cheek – preauricular	Ellipse – vertical, Burow's exchange flap
	Cheek – central	Ellipse in RSTL, lazy S, rhomboid transposition, A-T flap
	Cheek – nasofacial	Ellipse – vertical (use N/L groove), Burow's exchange advancement from below, rotation flap
	Cheek – mandibular margin	Ellipse – horizontal, A-T flap, rhomboid, banner flap, second intention
	Nose – inner canthus	Ellipse, A-T flap
	Nasal root	Ellipse – vertical or horizontal, bilobed flap, rotation flap
	Nasal dorsum	Ellipse – vertical or horizontal, A-T flap, rotation flap
	Nasal tip	Side-to-side – vertical or horizontal, trilobed flap, A-T flap, asymmetrical ellipse
	Nasal ala	Bilobed flap, 2° intention ± purse-strings, nasolabial flap
	Nasal sidewall	Ellipse, A-T flap, Burow's advancement flap, bilobed flap
	Upper lip (periala)	Ellipse – vertical, ellipse – vertical (nasolabial fold), A-T flap, wedge, rotation flap
	Upper lip (lateral)	Ellipse – vertical, A-T flap, wedge, Burow's exchange advancement, rotation flap, transposition
	Upper lip (medial)	Ellipse, wedge, A-T flap, bilateral advancement
	Lower lip	Ellipse, wedge, bilateral advancement flap
	Chin	Ellipse, advancement T-plasty, rotation single or double flap, transposition (for lateral chin)
	Ear, postauricular sulcus	Ellipse
	Postauricular ear surface	Ellipse, A-T flap, bilobed flap, rotation flap, advancement flap
	Ear lobe	Simple ellipse, wedge
	Helical rim – anterior $\frac{1}{3}$	Hatchet/7/L-plasty flap
	Helical rim – upper $\frac{1}{3}$	Ellipse, wedge, transposition flap
	Helical rim – middle $\frac{1}{3}$	Ellipse, helical rim advancement flap, helical rim rotation flap, wedge
	Anterior ear	Ellipse
	Conchal bowl	2° intention
	Anterior neck	Ellipse, A-T flap, transposition flap, advancement flap
	Posterior neck	Ellipse, A-T flap
Trunk and limbs		Ellipse, lazy S flap, O-S (Z) flap (esp over joints), transposition flap, rotation flap, Mercedes flap – shoulder tip
	Hand – dorsal surface	Ellipse (don't cross wrist joint), A-T flap, rhomboid – radial harvest
Grafts*	Helix, anterior ear, concha, forehead, temple, inner canthus, nose, upper lip, neck	Full thickness (FTSG)
	Scalp, temple, concha, lower limb	Split thickness (STSG)

*Every attempt should be made to avoid grafts, but they may be needed on these areas.
Notes:
• Ellipse = simple ellipse (fusiform), primary closure or side-to-side.
• Island pedicle and myocutaneous flaps have not been considered.

Bilobed flaps

- Cheek, especially near the nose
- Upper nose
- Trunk
- Limb

O-S (Z) flaps

- Use where the skin is very tight.
- Use across joints.

SOME SUGGESTED OPERATIONS

Head

On the forehead eyebrow elevation has to be guarded against and, as in Figure 13.1, an A-T flap prevents this. However, further up the forehead a simple ellipse (side-to-side) is often possible. In the midline a vertical incision is often made as there is sufficient lax skin either side, but this can leave an obvious scar. A horizontal excision using the frown creases, however, often allows scar minimisation.

Bilobed and trilobed flaps

These are the most used flaps for the lower third of the nose, replacing most other repairs, and can cover defects of the nasal ala, distal nose and nasal tip where skin is less mobile and provide reconstruction of the primary defect with matching skin. The base of the flap is placed laterally on the sidewall of the nose for nasal tip defects,

whereas the base is medial on the dorsum of the nose for repairing alar defects. Defects less than 1.5 cm in diameter are most suitable as larger defects can pose a problem because of the limited lax donor skin from the upper nose. The nasolabial flap also provides a good match, but it has limitations in reaching the nasal tip area and it can distort the alar contour.

Bilobed flaps are frequently used for repairing defects of the temporal forehead. Primary closure and other local flaps can distort the eyebrow, scalp hairline and lateral canthus of the eye. Use of the bilobed flap corresponds to the 'Robin Hood principle' (i.e. borrowing from the rich laxity of the cheek and transposing it to the relatively poor inelastic temporal forehead without distortion).

Bilobed flaps in skin cancer of the face

The bilobed Zitelli flap for covering defects in the area of the face shows very few complications and good aesthetic results. When used to treat 285 consecutive patients, 51.9% involved the nose, 17.9% the cheeks, 12.6% the preauricular region, 9.5% the perilabial region and chin and 8.1% the periorbital region. The size of the defect following tumour removal was between 1 and 4 cm. Completely acceptable aesthetic and functional deficits were obtained in 96.4% patients. 3.6% patients suffered postoperative complications. Two cases of local infection, one case of complete flap necrosis and seven cases of partial revision due to flap necrosis occurred. The level of satisfaction with the surgical long-term result reported by the patients was high [10].

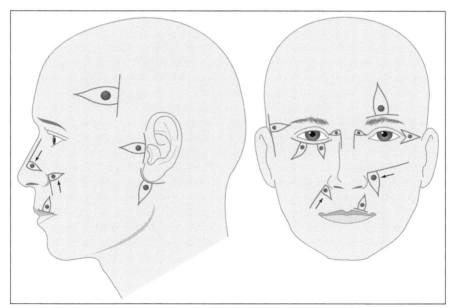

Figure 13.1 Suggested operations on the head
Here the versatility of the A-T flap and its lack of resultant distortion (eyebrow lift, ectropion) are evident. Further, the horizontal arm can invariably be hidden and there is no threatened necrosis. M-plasty would seem the only option at the external canthus and lateral lip. Burow's advancement flaps are also shown here and in Figure 13.2, where they use skin folds such as the nasolabial groove and the ala crease to advantage.

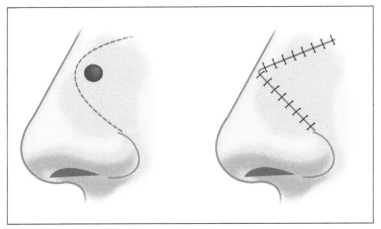

Figure 13.2 Burow's advancement flaps

Limbs
Please refer Figure 13.3.

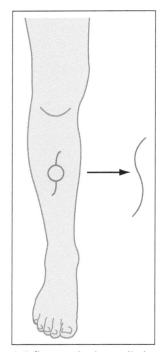

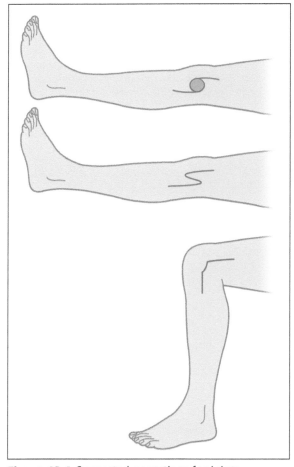

Figure 13.3 O-S flap on the lower limb

The lower limb is a great problem area due to poor blood supply and tight skin. The obese and diabetics can make it a nightmare when only an STSG will do. Otherwise an O-S flap is most usual. Here, it provides a more vertical central scar, which does not cut as horizontally as an O-Z and thus may not compromise the blood supply as much.

Figure 13.4 Suggested operations for joints

Joints

Please insert Figure 13.4.

An O-Z flap provides a central 'spring' or an inbuilt scar elongation when the joint is flexed whereas a straight scar contracts and would impede later movement. The bottom flap incision should arguably be sited on the limb that flexes most (e.g. the lower leg with the upper incision on the thigh to maximise movement).

In the same way do not extend an ellipse across the wrist even if the size of the lesion dictates and it is possible. Instead, an A-T flap works very well.

Hands

To plan dorsal hand excisions, make a fist and flex. The skin will stretch but use a cock-up splint. Don't cross the wrist joint with a linear scar/ellipse as scars contract by up to 30% and may limit future flexion.

REFERENCES

[1] Buchen D. Skin flaps in facial surgery. New York: McGraw Hill; 2006. p. 81.

[2] Handley WS. The pathology of melanocytic growths in relation to their operative treatment. Lancet 1907;1:927–33.

[3] Veronesi U, Cascinelli N. Narrow excision (1-cm margin). A safe procedure for thin cutaneous melanoma. Arch Surg 1991;126:438–41.

[4] Balch CM, Soong SJ, Smith T, et al. Long-term results of a prospective surgical trial comparing 2 cm vs. 4 cm excision margins for 740 patients with 1–4 mm melanomas. Ann Surg Oncol 2001;8:101–8.

[5] Thomas JM, Newton-Bishop J, A'Hern R, et al. Excision margins in high-risk malignant melanoma. N Engl J Med 2004;350:757–66.

[6] Lens MB, Nathan P, Bataille V. Excision margins for primary cutaneous melanoma: updated pooled analysis of randomized controlled trials. Arch Surg 2007;142:885–91, 891–3.

[7] McKinnon JG, Starritt EC, Scolyer RA, et al. Histopathologic excision margin affects local recurrence rate. Ann Surg 2005;241(2):326–33.

[8] Adams B, Levy R, Rademaker AE, et al. Frequency of use of suturing and repair techniques preferred by dermatologic surgeons. Dermatol Surg 2006;32(5):682–9.

[9] McGregor IA. Local skin flaps in facial reconstruction. Otolaryngol Clin North Amer 1982;15:77–98.

[10] Salgarelli AC, Cangiano A, Sartorelli F, et al. The bilobed flap in skin cancer of the face: Our experience on 285 cases. J Craniomaxillofac Surg 2010;38:460–4.

Hints, tips, tricks and reminders

14

Use every trick, ancillary aid and piece of equipment that makes your job easier.

Many of the following are covered in detail in their respective chapters. They are listed here as quick reminders. More details and figures are given for new hints.

AK TO SCC

Rapid growth, erosion and pain often indicate transition to an SCC. Squeeze.

LOCAL ANAESTHETIC

- Pain reduction: sodium bicarbonate, 'bicarb', and warm
- Dental vials for biopsies
- Snapping anaesthetic ampoules
- Painless injections

ANATOMY

Know the four danger zones of the face.

Always draw in the danger zones and try to palpate the facial and superficial temporal artery.

BELL RINGERS

- BCC – micronodular, infiltrative, morphoeic, scirrhous, basosquamous, H-zone face
- SCC – undifferentiated, ear, lip, fast growing, >20 mm
- Melanoma – Clark level 2 signifies infiltration through the basement membrane

BIOPSY

If the biopsy site can't be identified, infiltrate the suspected site with local anaesthetic in the dermis. The previous biopsy site may form a blister due to the separation of the epidermis from the dermis.

Better still, photograph the sites.

Stretch the skin in the opposite direction to RSTL for a punch biopsy so it forms an oval along the RSTL when released.

Punch biopsies up to 6 mm can be hyfrecated; thereafter, patients prefer sutures.

BLEEDING

Do not stop anticoagulants. The doctor who prescribed it is the only person to do so, even though many people are on aspirin when they have no cardiovascular risks. Also see 'Clopidogrel' below.

BLUEY FACE DOWN PRE-CUT

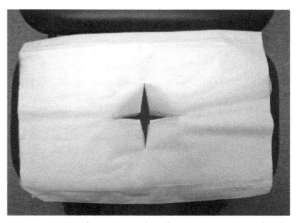

Figure 14.1 'Blueys' are absorbent paper on a plastic waterproof back used under procedures, but they also provide a clean pillow cover that patients should expect

For procedures on backs if the operating table has a face hole, a pre-cut cross in the Bluey reassures the patient that he is provided with a clean tissue on which to place his face.

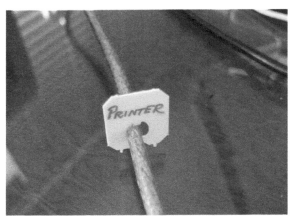

Figure 14.2 Bread tags for identifying cables

Hyfrecator – insulated tip

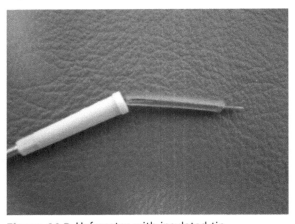

Figure 14.3 Hyfrecator with insulated tip
If the spot to be hyfrecated/cauterised involves the risk of peripheral damage, leave the plastic electrode sheath on but cut it so just the tip is exposed. The insulated shaft prevents collateral damage to adjoining tissue.

CABLE IDENTIFICATION
Use bread tags (Figure 14.2).

CATCHERS
To prevent blood running down the patient, place some gauze swabs below the proposed incision and secure with paper tape. These can be pre-made. Ensure they do not intrude into the fenestrated hole in the drape/sterile area.

CAUTERY
Bipolar cautery is recommended as the current only passes between the forceps heads causing far less char and giving better haemostasis. Further, the instrument is sterile as the cables and forceps are autoclaved. Finally, it is safe for use with pacemakers/defibrillators.

Monopolar hyfrecation goes right through the patient and can give the unwary operator a shock if touching any metal on the table. It causes more damage/char to the tissues, and the tips and the handle are not sterile. Although the handle may be put in a sterile glove, penrose tube or special sheath, the latter and the tips are invariably not sterile and the operator is deluded that the heat is sterilising the tip. The handle and cable are autoclavable in modern models and reusable autoclavable electrode tips are also now available.

CLOPIDOGREL
Clopidogrel causes more bleeding than other anticoagulants, which increases with each combination (aspirin, warfarin).

CHLORAMPHENICOL FOR NARES
The nostrils are the most germ contaminated area of the body. It is circumspect, and arguably good practice, to instil chloramphenicol (shown to be superior to other topical antibiotics) around their margins for any operations in the area.

COMPLAINTS
BLAST:

- **B**elieve
- **L**isten
- **A**pologise
- **S**olve
- **T**hank

CRYOSURGERY PAIN
Post-cryosurgery pain: dabbing with an alcohol swab helps some.

CURETTES

If no curette is available, a 6–8 mm punch biopsy will do.

DERMABRASION

This is normally performed using a hand-held drill/wire brush, which can 'get away' and do too much and is expensive.

Silicon–carbide sandpaper from 80 grade (medium used to gently remove varnish) to 220 grade (very fine sanding of bare wood) can be used with one's fingers or wrapped around a 3-cc or 5-cc syringe. Cut into 5 × 5 cm squares (or whatever best suits) and autoclave. The aim is to sand the skin flat, as with pin-cushioning, or to bevel the edges of a depression to make it less noticeable.

Hyfrecation is used for this purpose by some, but the 'blending' setting on a Surgitron® is arguably better.

DESIGN AND EQUIPMENT

Don't let technicians, managers or anyone other than yourself decide where equipment is to go. Technicians will always install equipment to best suit themselves (viz. the computer server under your desk, the printer on your desk and the mouse cord too short).

Avoid floor lamps – they invariably get in the way.

LED light is better than halogen.

Theatre lights should be fully enclosed for hygiene/cleaning and there should be multiple sources to obviate shadows.

DRAPES AND HAIR

Put gauze on hair to stop sticky drapes ripping out hair. The recommended sterile drapes are ultra-sticky and, at the end of a long operation on the face, the surgeon may forget and remove it along with the patient's eyebrows and such. It is a good idea to place gauze swabs over the eyebrows and hair or trim any other hairy areas if sticky drapes are being used.

DRESSINGS

Adherence:

- Acetone to clean skin
- Tinct Benz Co

- Skin-Prep

Removal of sticky residue:

- Solvent ether best
- 'Remove' or 'Zoff' can be used

DROPPED NEEDLES

To retrieve lost fine suture needles in OT:

1 magnet – auto supply shops sell with a long lead
2 75–100-mm adhesive paper tape, sticky side down on a pad (gauze) moving out in increasing circles
3 put a stocking over the vacuum cleaner nozzle.

DYSPLASTIC NAEVI

- Mild – observe.
- Moderate – excise with 2-mm margins.
- Severe – excise with 5-mm margins.

EARS

For operations always plug the external auditory meatus with a pledget of cotton wool.

EXAMINATIONS

Start with the inner canthi. Look at the eyelids.

Pull toes well apart.

Ask patients to mark lesions of concern.

GRAFTS

Flaps, if possible, give a better result.

The ear conchae give the best match for nose grafts (and heal by secondary intention).

HAEMOSTASIS

Gauze: push up at dissection edge of excision to provide a bloodless field.

Chalazion clamps: can provide a bloodless field on the distal nose. They come in three sizes but, unfortunately, only the smallest seems to be available in Australia, which often doesn't provide for adequate margins. The largest size is recommended. The eyes of scissors can also be used.

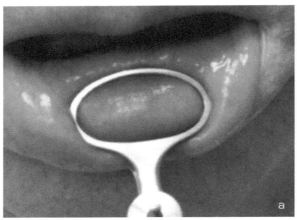
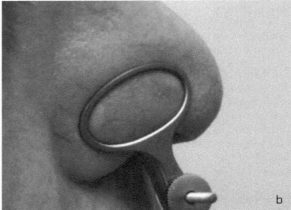

Figure 14.4 A large chalazion clamp provides both a bloodless field and controlled haemostasis
a Lip. **b** Nose.

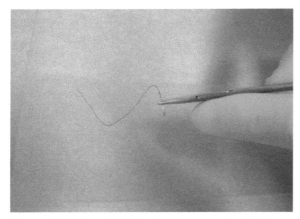

Figure 14.5 Hand stabilisation even works with the stabilising hand free and not resting on anything, as here, or by placing the stabilising hand/finger on the patient

HAIR

To pick up hair from a clean-shaved site, use paper adhesive tape.

Mesh gauze on the scalp provides a hair-free site.

Ensure total hair restraint: minimal removal is favoured but long hair intruding into the surgical site is more than annoying. Use ibis clips, paper tape, mesh gauze or all three, but ensuring the site is free of hair that can escape to intrude will avoid bother, frustration and delays.

Use blue sutures.

HAND STABILISATION

Two hands are better than one. Dentists are taught to stabilise their working hand with the other. This is good technique (Figure 14.5).

HEALING

Wounds heal best under waterproof dressings.

KERATOACANTHOMA

All KAs should be excised to exclude SCC or to avoid scarring.

LEG ULCERS

Biopsy leg ulcers that do not improve with treatment. In one study, 10.4% of such cases were malignant: 9 SCCs, 5 BCCs, 1 melanoma and 1 leiomyosarcoma [1].

LIGHTS

Autoclaved aluminium foil can provide a no-cost sterile wrap for adjusting lights if operating alone.

If the sterile glove packet is still sterile, it too can be used.

MEASURING LESIONS

Any and all lesions over 10 mm should be photographed with a measure as proof for Medicare claims.

Most pathology labs provide transparent rulers. Some doctors even use vernier calipers.

Identification of the patient can be made with a sticky-label if a digital camera is used or directly into their files if a computerised digital dermatoscope is used.

NEEDLE STICKS

Do not recap needles using both hands. Jam the cap into the hilt of some forceps, place on a bench and reinsert keeping the other hand away from the cap and forceps.

NOSE

The use of instilled antibiotic ointment in the nostrils has been shown to reduce *S. aureus* infections. Chloramphenicol is the most effective topical ointment.

OPENING SEALED PACKS – SUTURES AND SYRINGES

Refer to Figure 14.6.

PHOTODAMAGE

Perhaps 95% of the visible and histological cutaneous epidermal/dermal damage or photoageing is directly proportional to the quantity of UVR received over the course of a whole lifetime, with older men at most risk.

Only some 25% of UVR damage occurs before age 18 years. Patients should be educated that sun protection is equally important in older and younger patients.

UVA (the 'ageing rays') penetrates glass and is the cause of solar lentigo.

SKIN MARKERS

'Sharpie' or similar alcohol-based commercially available markers have been found to be best for marking skin for excisions.

SKIN PREP

2% chlorhexidine with 70% alcohol is the best skin prep.

SPITZ NAEVI

All Spitz/Reed naevi should be excised.

STATISTICS

Sensitivity = probability of a positive test or result.

The sensitivity of a test refers, for example, to how many cases of melanoma a particular test/algorithm can find. A very sensitive test is likely to give a fair number of false-positive results, but almost no true positives will be missed.

Tests with a high sensitivity are often used to *screen* for disease. Screening tests tend to cast a wide net in order to pick up all cases of a disease, in this case a melanoma on dermoscopy, and not miss one, but they often include some accidental positive results (people who don't actually have a melanoma).

Specificity = probability of a negative test or result.

The specificity of a test refers to how accurately it diagnoses a melanoma, for example, without giving false-positive results.

Tests with a high specificity are used to *confirm* the results of sensitive, but less specific, screening tests. People who came up positive on a very sensitive screening test may come up negative on a specific confirmatory test.

Statistics example

Of 10 pigmented lesions, 5 are tentatively diagnosed as melanomas (1–5) and 5 as benign pigmented naevi (6–10). The test results determine that lesions 1, 2, 3, 4, 7 and 9 are melanomas.

The test sensitivity would be: 4/5 = 80% (because it correctly identified 4 of the 5 melanomas).

The test specificity would be: 3/5 = 60% (because it correctly identified 3 of the 5 benign pigmented lesions as 'not melanoma').

Ideally, it is desirable that a test be both very sensitive, in that it picks up almost all true positives, and very

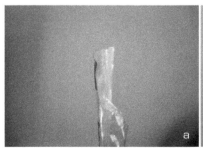 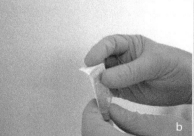 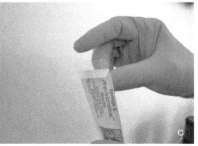

Figure 14.6 Opening sealed packs

a When the plastic front is almost welded to the paper back, as in sutures, syringes and other sterile packs, this can be eminently frustrating. **b** Fold the plastic front over towards the backing paper. **c** The paper remains folded down while the plastic front springs back; the two are now separated and opening is easy. This simple trick saves much time and annoyance.

specific, in that it has almost no false-negatives. Neither sensitivity nor specificity is less important than the other. A test with low sensitivity does a relatively poor job at detecting occurrences of a condition when the condition exists and a test with low specificity does a relatively poor job at detecting non-occurrences of a condition when the condition doesn't exist.

A useful aide mémoire

- Se**N**sitivity of a test: related to the rate of false **N**egatives
- S**P**ecificity of a test: related to the rate of false **P**ositives

Alternatively written:

- Se**N**sitive: **N**o **N**on-**N**egatives
- S**P**ecific: **P**uny **P**seudo-**P**ositives

Confidence interval: gives a range of values within which there is a high probability (95%) that the true population value can be found. There is nothing special about 95%. It is used most commonly and is convention. If it is assumed that the sample is randomly selected from some population, it means there is 95% surety that the confidence interval includes the population mean. How good is the estimate? It depends on how large the sample is. It can never be known for sure whether or not the confidence interval contains the true mean.

Probability value (P): is a probability with a value ranging from zero to one. It is the answer to the question: 'If the populations really have the same mean overall, what is the probability that random sampling would lead to a difference between sample means as large (or larger) than observed?' It is the statistical significance of the overall result or the test for overall effect. The information required to derive P is the magnitude of change(s), sample size and standard deviation.

A result is regarded as significant if $p < 0.05$. $P < 0.05$ means there is less than 5% chance that the difference between sample means could have occurred by chance. The P value assesses only the play of chance and gives no information about bias or confounding.

STERILISATION

Make sure your autoclave is validated and what it is validated (maximum challenge load) for. Check your validator's credentials. Use Emulating indicators (ISO class 6) to monitor all critical parameters until you have discussed this with the validation engineer.

A vacuum autoclave is better than one without a vacuum.

SUNSCREENS

There have been no deleterious side effects, other than occasional allergy, to sunscreens since their commercial introduction in 1928. They do, however, protect against SCC and melanoma if used every day.

SUNGLASSES

Small amounts of sun over the years speed up cataracts, pterygia and lid cancers. Twice as many cataract operations are performed in Australia as in Europe. 48% of Australians leave their sunglasses behind for quick lunch-time breaks.

SURGERY

Cut it out early and cut it out widely. The first operation is the best chance.

Know the correct margins.

Mohs

Do Mohs pathology on all melanomas, SCCs and difficult BCCs on the face and on undifferentiated SCCs elsewhere.

Lentigo maligna melanoma

Have always spread beyond the visible margins until proven otherwise.

MIS

Recommended margins are now 9 mm.

Incision markers

Wounds fall apart when lesions are excised. This occurs with simple ellipses due to tension vectors and retraction as well as with flaps. Drawing aligning marks across the excision to make sure the sutures line up is simple, easy and a fail-safe protocol. Let these dry as long as possible before skin prep as prepping often dissolves those not completely dry.

Orientate

Nick the lesion to be excised before it is excised. Mark saucerised lesions with typewriter fluid.

12 o'clock is the usual place to mark and what labs take as the default marker site unless advised otherwise.

Alar groove

Do not incise against the ala: Leave a 1-mm(+) strip of tissue to provide a lip or edge to suture to.

Face

Remember to avoid eyebrow lift and ectropions with horizontal excisions.

Umbilical lesions

Place deep sutures at either end of the lesion, then use traction to evert and display the lesion and provide more stability.

Incise outwards

Excising outwards (i.e. angling the blade slightly out and away from the vertical centre) gives a wider clearance of the lesion and facilitates better eversion.

Dog-ear minimisation

Short wide excisions lead to dog-ears. If unavoidable, have an assistant stretch the wound lengthways until there are no dog-ears, then sew up.

Skin stretches

Even after 20 minutes, wound edges can be approximated without previous tension. Dog-ears and deformities often settle. Leave and review.

Compress wide wound edges

Have an assistant push the wound edges together. This is especially helpful with subcuticular sutures.

SUTURES

Withdrawing sutures to needle holder

Read the manufacturer's instructions. Different manufacturers have different methods to open their sutures to best present the needle. In addition, some provide in-built measures. Don't just rip them open. One brand (Assut) which provides 75 cm 6/0 has a small 'U' notch in the cardboard envelope that prevents knots and tangles if the suture is pulled out through this U.

Use 75 cm

At least one manufacturer charges the same for 75 cm as for 45 cm and, although 75 cm may be more unwieldy, you are not compromised. Even so, cut free ends short. 'All wounds need one more stitch'.

Sutures on the same side

Ensuring the first throw is across the incision makes the sutures drape laterally and not along the wound.

Suture length to cut

1 cm would seem a good suggestion. If not, cross the sutures where you want the assistant to cut.

Deep sutures

Ensure the wound first throw (usually free) is aligned along the suture and not cinched. If right-handed this is best achieved by having the end of the suture to the left. Then, when the needle holder is wound around the needle end of the suture to make the first throw and the distal/free end on the left is grabbed, the needle holder is passed under the left wrist, hands changed and the throws will align along the suture. If the free end is to the right and the needle holder is again passed to the left, a cinch will result.

Cutting deep sutures

Carefully run the scissors down the thread until the knot halts progress, then angle the scissors 15–30° and cut.

Suture memory erasure

Nylon and many other monofilament sutures have a memory in that they return to their coiled packaged state, which can be extremely irritating and counterproductive. Grab the thread below the needle (never the needle as it is designed to break off) between the index fingers and thumbs of both hands and stretch it or run it through under tension to straighten it out.

Four throws for 6/0 slippery

Some slippery sutures, especially 6/0, fail to lock with the usual three throws. If a suture is that slippery, use four or more throws to secure. There is no limit to the throws as long as it pulls together and doesn't pull apart.

Tightening arrested knots

The more throws, the more difficult to close. Try not pulling both ends but rather fix one and pull the other or seesaw/pull-relax-pull the other end.

Knots

First knot can be loose so as not to cut in or be too tight. Then the third knot can be tightened against the second throw to lock and provide security.

Mixed sutures

Use any mix of gauge and type of suture you want as long as they will survive the required time (e.g. the wound may be closed with deep absorbable sutures but these are just as good as nylon to close superficially if they last as long as wanted). 4/0 may be needed to initially approximate wound edges under tension, but the skin will relax and the rest of the wound can be done with 5/0 or 6/0 for better cosmesis.

In the same way, a pulley stitch may be needed to close the wound centrally but, by the time the operation is finished, the skin has stretched and this can be replaced by a more discrete and lesser gauge suture.

Short end and one more suture needed

Perhaps the fifth law of surgery is that 'the number of sutures needed always requires one more, which requires opening a new pack'. Always make the free end as short as possible. If there is only a short length left and only one more suture is needed, use non-toothed forceps to

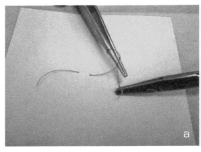 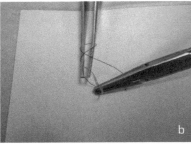 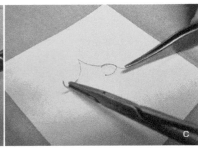

Figure 14.7 Short suture ends

a When there is only a short length of suture left and winding it around the jaws of the needle holder makes it too short to grasp, use forceps. The needle holder still holds the needle and pulling the minimum amount of suture through that will allow it to be wound around the closed forceps jaws. **b** Use the forceps to grasp the short suture end. Here, toothed forceps are used but this requires the jaws to be opened wider than non-toothed and only makes it more difficult as opening the forceps jaws pulls the short end through more and often makes it too short to grasp. Use Adson's plain fine forceps, which will fully close and grasp 6/0 securely. **c** Once the first throw has been secured, it is easy to do the second.

wind the needle end around and to grab the free end (Figure 14.7). Needle holder jaws are too large in these instances, taking too much thread to wind around them and more as they are opened. Finally, check all the forceps you use and ensure they will actually grab 6/0 sutures and only use these.

Blue sutures for hair
Refer to Figure 14.8.

Mouth sutures
Leave mucosal sutures long (Figure 14.9). This is less irritating than short ends that stick and prick.

TAPE STRIPS
Tape strips can be made to adhere better if the skin is cleaned/degreased with acetone (usually in nail polish remover) or Tinct Benz Co or Smith & Nephew's Skin Prep to make skin tacky. They are not recommended to

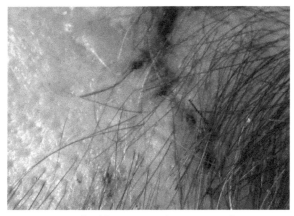

Figure 14.8 The blue sutures here are easily seen facilitating ROS

At 6 o'clock the black suture is not so easily seen and may be missed. Further, these were 5/0 sutures. 6/0 is more the gauge of hair and even more difficult to see.

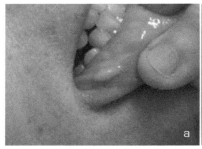 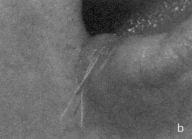 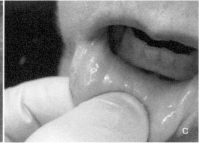

Figure 14.9 Leaving sutures long

a Lesion for excision. **b** Excised and sutured with rapidly absorbing sutures. These are left long so that stubs don't stick in and irritate. Although the aesthetic urge may be to cut them shorter, don't make them too short. Patients don't notice the length, just the short end that sticks in. **c** 7 days later. The mucosa heals rapidly and well.

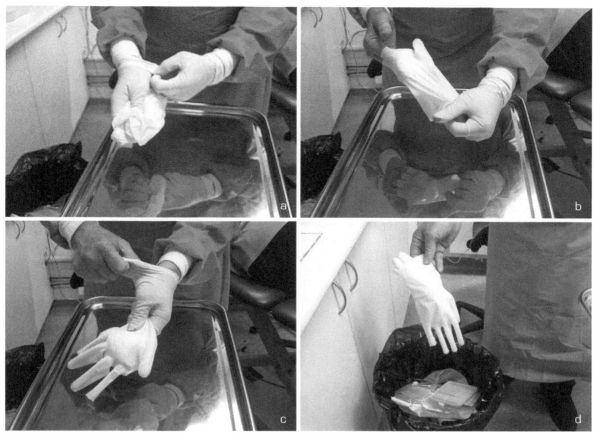

Figure 14.10 Tidying up gloves
a Surgical gloves can be folded over to enclose soft, small postoperative debris. Collect and grasp these with one hand. **b** Fold that glove over the debris. **c** Fold the other glove completely over the first debris-containing glove. **d** The doubly enclosed and now secured debris can be discarded.

secure wound closure and only recommended to secure wounds after ROS.

All face wounds should be taped after ROS.

Give the patient an extra pack of tapes in case they peel off.

Fixomull cut strips are much cheaper, provide excellent adhesion and can be stretched to provide 'dumbbell' increased traction. A healed and sealed wound does not need sterile strips.

TIDYING UP – GLOVES
Refer to Figure 14.10.

TOES
Refer to Figure 14.11.

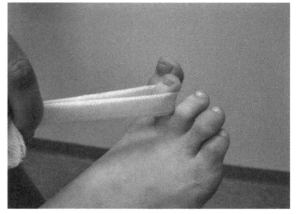

Figure 14.11 Digits can be isolated and better presented by unfolding a gauze square, which makes a perfect sling to either present the slung digit or get one out of the way

TOWEL CLAMP

The towel clamp (Figure 14.12) is a locking clamp with two sharp points separated by 60° [2]. It can serve many other uses in skin surgery, including the following:

1 Approximation of wide wounds (particularly on the scalp or back) [2]: the clamp is positioned across the widest part of the excision and closed as much as is adjudged possible without tearing. It is left in position for as long as the surgeon has time. Skin stretches and, after 15–30 minutes, the width can be significantly reduced to allow closure.

2 Epidermoid cysts: the clamp is locked into the tissue a little away from the distal (to the surgeon) incision end. The clamp serves as a secure/non-slip retractor, allowing this end to be moved in any direction to provide excellent retraction either unassisted (non-dominant hand) or assisted.

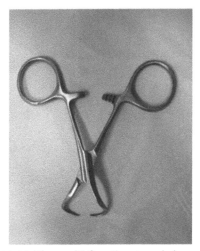

Figure 14.12 The multi-function towel clamp

It is particularly useful for the unassisted surgeon [3, 4].

TOURNIQUETS

Surgical gloves can be used as finger tourniquets [5–7]. Generally, the glove and the antiseptic develop a non-slip environment, and exsanguination cannot be properly performed. Moreover, during the procedure, a second haemostat is necessary to fix the ring glove at the base of the finger to prevent slippage of the tourniquet during surgery. Not infrequently, in patients with hair on the fingers, the procedure is traumatic and may lead to hair pulling.

Use a spray dressing (Opsite, Smith & Nephew) just before the application of the finger of the surgical glove. It is a transparent, quick-drying film. It contains an acrylic polymer dissolved in ethyl acetamide and acetone and adheres to skin. The outside surface is not adherent. Opsite spray dressing facilitates the rolling of latex upon itself and thereby augments the exsanguination process and helps fix the ring glove at the base of the finger. In this way, slippage of the tourniquet is prevented.

WARTS

In a recent study, the average rate of cure was 23% for the placebo, 52% for salicylic acid, 49% for cryotherapy, 54% for aggressive cryotherapy and 58% for the combination of salicylic acid and cryotherapy. These two treatments must therefore be considered as priority [8].

FINGER WEB DRESSINGS

Fold a non-stick dressing (Telfa/Cutilin/Melolin) in half or where holes are wanted (Figure 14.13). Cut semicircles, which open to full holes. Bend back and tape.

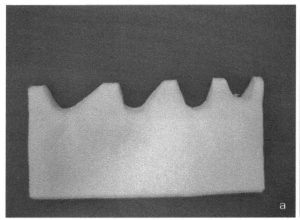
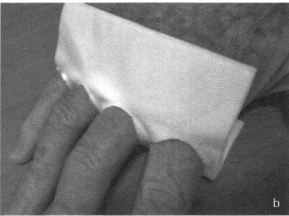

Figure 14.13 Finger web dressings
a Fold a large non-stick dressing in half. Cut four semicircles out along the folded spine. **b** Open and insert the fingers through these holes with the non-stick dressing bedding into the web space. The folded-back and taped-down remainder of the dressing provides further protection to the entire area.

REFERENCES

[1] Senet P, Combemale P, Debure C, et al; for the Angio-Dermatology Group of the French Society of Dermatology. Malignancy and chronic leg ulcers. The value of systematic wound biopsies: a prospective, multicenter, cross-sectional study. Arch Dermatol 2012;148:704–8.

[2] Liu CM, McKenna J, Griess A. Surgical pearl: the use of towel clamps to reapproximate wound edges under tension. J Am Acad Dermatol 2004;50:273–4.

[3] Chen HH, Chen JS, Changchien CR, et al. Hemorrhoidectomy with self-retaining retraction. Dis Colon Rectum 1996;39:1058–9.

[4] Link MJ. A new technique for single-person fascia lata harvest. Neurosurgery 2008;63(4 Suppl. 2):359–61, discussion 361.

[5] Smith IM, Austin OM, Knight SL. A simple and fail safe method for digital tourniquet. J Hand Surg 2002;27:363–4.

[6] Harrington AC, Cheyney JM, Kinsley-Scott T, et al. A novel digital tourniquet using a sterile glove and hemostat. Dermatol Surg 2004;30:1065–7.

[7] Goyal N, Colver G. British-style digital tourniquet. Dermatol Surg 2005;31:729.

[8] Kwok CS, Holland R, Gibbs S. Efficacy of topical treatments for cutaneous warts: a meta-analysis and pooled analysis of randomized controlled trials. Br J Dermatol 2011;165:233–46.

Index

Page numbers followed by 'f' indicate figures, 't' indicate tables, and 'b' indicate boxes.

Lightning Source UK Ltd.
Milton Keynes UK
UKHW052048160522
403082UK00003B/71

9 780729 539326